Hormone Action: Metabolism

Hormone Action: Metabolism

Edited by **Estelle Jones**

FOSTER
ACADEMICS

New Jersey

Published by Foster Academics,
61 Van Reypen Street,
Jersey City, NJ 07306, USA
www.fosteracademics.com

Hormone Action: Metabolism
Edited by Estelle Jones

International Standard Book Number: 978-1-63242-233-0 (Hardback)

Printed in the United States of America.

Contents

Preface

The aim of this book is to emphasize on current aspects of the complex regulation of hormonal action, specifically metabolism. Novel approaches to the pathology and physiology of endocrine glands are established on molecular and cellular research of peptide, protein cascade, hormones, and genes at distinct levels. All these aspects are described throughout the book so that the reader can be provided with the state-of-the-art endocrine knowledge.

This book is a comprehensive compilation of works of different researchers from varied parts of the world. It includes valuable experiences of the researchers with the sole objective of providing the readers (learners) with a proper knowledge of the concerned field. This book will be beneficial in evoking inspiration and enhancing the knowledge of the interested readers.

In the end, I would like to extend my heartiest thanks to the authors who worked with great determination on their chapters. I also appreciate the publisher's support in the course of the book. I would also like to deeply acknowledge my family who stood by me as a source of inspiration during the project.

Editor

Metabolism

The Gut Peptide Hormone Family, Motilin and Ghrelin

Ichiro Sakata and Takafumi Sakai
Saitama University
Japan

1. Introduction

Endocrine hormones are a system of glands, each of which secretes a type of hormone into the bloodstream to regulate multiple physiology of the body. In the past several decades, many hormones from the gastrointestinal tract has been identified and cloned, and their physiological functions have been studied. Although the pituitary gland was considered to be the main endocrine organ of the body in early studies, there are other organs that produce endocrine hormones such as adipose tissue, reproductive organ, adrenal gland, and gastrointestinal tract. Among those, the gastrointestinal tract is the largest endocrine organ of the body in volume, and hormones produced in the gastrointestinal tract are physiologically important for their roles in development, growth, cardiovascular, gastric motility, behavior and maintenance of energy homeostasis. Many hormones have been identified in each different parts of the gastrointestinal tract. For instance, in the stomach, gastrin, histamine (Dornonville de la Cour, et al. 2001), somatostatin (Bolkent, et al. 2001), neuropeptide Y (Wang, et al. 1987), ghrelin (Sakata, et al. 2002) and leptin (Bado, et al. 1998) are produced in the mucosal layer and/or myentric plexus, and cholecystokinin (CCK) (Miyamoto and Miyamoto 2004), glucagon-like peptide-1 (Theodorakis, et al. 2006), motilin (Sakai, et al. 1994a) (Satoh, et al. 1995), serotonin (Ku, et al. 2004) and PYY$_{3-36}$ (Rozengurt, et al. 2006) are produced in the upper and lower intestine. Motilin and ghrelin are considered to comprise a peptide family based on similarity of their structures and also their similarity in each specific G protein coupled receptor, growth hormone secretagogue receptor (GHS-R) and motilin receptor (MTL-R, also known as GPR38). In this chapter, we review recent research and knowledge of the peptides, motilin and ghrelin regarding their structures, distribution of motilin- and ghrelin-producing cells, distribution of their receptors, plasma profies and secretion of motilin and ghrelin, and the role of motilin and ghrelin in gastric motility. However, there is a lack of basic information for motilin study such as information on the detailed distribution of motilin and motilin receptor in the body and changes in motilin release under some physiological states. One of the reasons for the difficulty in motilin study is that rodents such as rats and mice cannot be used for motilin study because the motilin gene is inactivated in the common ancestor of mice and rats (He, et al. 2010). For this reason, motilin has been studied using relatively large- sized animals, such as dogs and rabbits, which has made it difficult to investigate in detail the mechanisms underlying the actions of motilin. Recently, we characterized the *house musk shrew* (Suncus murinus, order: Insectivora, suncus named as laboratory strain) as a motilin- and ghrelin-producing small animal model for studies on gastric motility, and we therefore also provide some information on suncus motilin and ghrelin.

2. Structures of motilin and ghrelin

Motilin was initially isolated from a side fraction produced during the purification of secretin by Brown et al. in 1971 (Brown, et al. 1971), and the complete amino acid sequence of motilin was determined in 1973 (Brown, et al. 1973). Mature motilin is a 22-amino-acid polypeptide with a molecular weight of 2698, and motilin has been isolated from humans (Strausberg, et al. 2002), pigs (Khan, et al. 1990) (Bond, et al. 1988), dogs (Ohshiro, et al. 2008), cats (Xu, et al. 2003), guinea pigs (Xu, et al. 2001), rabbits (Banfield, et al. 1992), and chickens (De Clercq, et al. 1996). We recently identified and cloned suncus motilin as a useful small animal model, and the mature region of suncus motilin is highly conserved between these species (Tsutsui, et al. 2009). The precursor of motilin consists of 133 amino acids and includes a 25-amino-acid signal peptide followed by a 22-amino-acid motilin sequence and a motilin-associated peptide (MAP) (Banfield et al. 1992). The amino acid sequence of MAP is also conserved between species, but the functional and physiological roles of MAP have not been elucidated.

Ghrelin was identified from rat and human stomach extracts by Kojima et al. in 1999 using a "reverse pharmacology" strategy (Kojima, et al. 1999). In mice, rats and humans, ghrelin is a 28-amino-acids polypeptide and, interestingly, ghrelin has an acyl modification at the third serine by n-octanoate, one of the medium chain fatty acids (Kojima et al. 1999). Ghrelin exists as two different molecular forms, acyl ghrelin (modified form) and des-acyl ghrelin (unmodified form), in both gastric ghrelin-producing cells and circulation (Ariyasu, et al. 2001; Fujimiya, et al.). Ghrelin has been identified in many species, including mammlas, avians (Kaiya, et al. 2002; Wada, et al. 2003), amphibians (Kaiya, et al. 2001; Kaiya, et al. 2006), reptilian (Kaiya, et al. 2004), and fish (Kaiya, et al. 2009; Kaiya, et al. 2003; Miura, et al. 2009), and the sequence of first seven amino acids of the N-terminal region of ghrelin are highly conserved between species (Kojima, et al. 2008). In addition, it has been reported that the first four or five amino acids are sufficient for calcium mobilization *in vitro* (Bednarek, et al. 2000).

3. Distributions of motilin- and ghrelin-producing cells

The distribution of motilin-producing cells in the gastrointestinal tract has been studied by using immunohistochemistry and *in situ* hybridization techniques. Since motilin is genetically knockdown in rats and mice, the distribution and morphology of motilin-producing cells were investigated using rabbits (Satoh et al. 1995), monkeys, and humans (Helmstaedter, et al. 1979). In rabbits, motilin-immunopositive cells were found in the epithelia of the crypts and villi throughout the gastrointestinal tract from the gastric antrum to the distal colon, but no immunostaining was observed in the gastric body (Satoh et al. 1995), and motilin-producing cells were localized abundantly in the upper small intestine. Cell densities (cells/mm^2, mean ± SE) were 0.41 ± 0.16 in the gastric antrum, 8.2 ± 0.8 in the duodenum, 1.9 ±0.5 in the jejunum, 0.62 ± 0.14 in the ileum, 0.19 ± 0.05 in the cecum, 0.13 ± 0.03 in the proximal colon, and 0.39 ± 0.18 in the distal colon (Satoh et al. 1995). Immunoelectron microscopic observations revealed that the motilin-producing cell is characterized by relatively small (180 nm in man; 200 nm in the dog) solid granules with a homogeneous core and closely applied membrane, round in man and round to irregularly-shaped in the dog. Recently, we succeeded in identification of suncus motilin cDNA and amino acid sequence (Tsutsui et al. 2009), and immunohistochemical analysis was performed in all regions of the gastrointestinal tract and also *in situ* hybridization analysis was performed to detect motilin mRNA-expressing cells. Motilin-immunopositive and expressing cells in suncus were observed in the mucosal layer but not in the myenteric plexus and were abundantly distributed in the upper intestine. However, the density of motilin mRNA-expressing cells was slightly higher than that of motilin-immunopositive cells, suggesting low accumulation of motilin in the cytoplasm. In addition, motilin-producing cells in suncus were closed- and opened-type cells as previously reported in other mammals.

Gastric ghrelin cells had been classified as X/A-like cells by their round, compact, electron-dense secretory granules that distinguish them electron-microscopically from other previously characterized gastric endocrine cell types before the discovery of ghrelin (Dornonville de la Cour et al. 2001) (Date, et al. 2000). The distribution of ghrelin-producing cells in the gastrointestinal tract has been studied in many species. Ghrelin-producing cells were most dense in the gastric body and were found in the mucosal layer but not in the myenteric plexus in all of the examined regions of rats (Sakata et al. 2002). In the stomach, most of the ghrelin cells were observed in the glandular base to body of the fundic gland, and a few ghrelin cells were observed in the glandular neck. In rodents, in addition to the stomach, ghrelin-producing cells were observed in all regions of the gastrointestinal tract, including the duodenum, ileum, cecum and colon (Sakata et al. 2002). In the duodenum, ileum, cecum and colon, ghrelin cells were scattered in the epithelia of crypts and villi, and the densities of ghrelin cells were dramatically decreased toward the lower gastrointestinal tract. In the stomach, ghrelin-producing cells were observed as small and round-shaped cells (called closed-type cells). On the other hand, in the duodenum, ileum, cecum and colon, ghrelin cells were found as two different types of endocrine cells, closed-type cells with triangular or elongated shapes and opened-type cells with their apical cytoplasmic process in contact with the lumen. In suncus, ghrelin-producing cells were abundant in the stomach and most of the ghrelin cells were closed-type cells with relatively rich cytoplasm and scattered in the glandular body and base of the gastric mucosa (Ishida, et al. 2009). Using electron microscopic observation, immunogold labeling for ghrelin has been shown to be localized on round and electron-dense granules in gastric mucosal cells. The diameters of granules containing ghrelin in mice (277.7 ± 11.1 nm) and rats (268.8 ± 13.0 nm) were similar; however, those in hamsters (200.8 ± 8.8 nm) were significantly smaller than those in mice or rats. Rindi et al. demonstrated that mouse and canine ghrelin-immunoreactive cells closely resembled those of the human stomach, though it has been shown that dog ghrelin cells have obviously larger granules (273 ± 49 nm) than those of rats (183 ± 37 nm) and humans (147 ± 30 nm).

Co-localization of motilin and ghrelin was examined in the human biopsy and tissues from pig by immunohistochemistry and *in situ* hybridization in a study by Wierup et al. (Wierup, et al. 2007). They showed that ghrelin and motilin are coproduced in the same cells in the duodenum and jejunum of humans and pigs and that ghrelin and motilin are stored in all secretory granules of such cells in humans, suggesting that motilin and ghrelin are co-secreted by the same stimulus (Wierup et al. 2007). As mentioned above, suncus is a small laboratory animal that produces both motilin and ghrelin, and further studies are therefore needed to examine the co-localization of motilin and ghrelin in the duodenum and lower intestine of suncus.

4. Distributions of motilin and ghrelin receptors

The receptor for motilin was identified from the human gastrointestinal tract by Feighner et al. in 1999 (Feighner, et al. 1999) and it is now called GPR38 or motilin receptor. Growth hormone secretagogue receptor (GHS-R) was initially identified from the pituitary gland and brain in 1996 (Howard, et al. 1996), and GHS-R had been known as the orphan receptor until ghrelin was discovered. In the process of exploring the natural ligand for the GHS-R using reverse pharmacology, ghrelin was discovered as an endogenous ligand for GHS-R. Both motilin and ghrelin receptors belong to the seven transmembrane G protein-coupled receptor family (McKee, et al. 1997), and these receptors showed high sequence homology of 52 % to each other in humans (Takeshita, et al. 2006). The tissue distribution of motilin and ghrelin receptors has been mainly examined using binding assays or mRNA analysis with RT-PCR. Motilin binding sites were found on smooth muscle layers of the gastric antrum, duodenum and colon, but no positive binding reaction was detected in the smooth muscle layer of the cecum (Sakai, et al. 1994b). Specific binding sites were particularly abundant in the circular muscle layers, with low concentrations in longitudinal muscle layers of the gastric antrum, duodenum and colon, and no motilin binding sites were found in the mucosa of the gastrointestinal tract and pancreas (Sakai et al. 1994b). mRNA analysis showed that motilin receptor was expressed in the gastrointestinal tract in humans (Takeshita et al. 2006; Ter Beek, et al. 2008), dogs (Ohshiro et al. 2008), guinea pigs (Xu, et al. 2005) and chickens (Yamamoto, et al. 2008). It has also been shown that motilin receptor immunoreactivity was present in muscle cells and the myenteric plexus, but not in mucosal or submucosal cells in humans (Takeshita et al. 2006). In dogs, motilin receptor immunoreactivity was observed among muscle fibers on both the longitudinal and circular muscle layers (Ohshiro et al. 2008). In the guinea pig stomach, motilin receptor immunoreactivity was also found in the myenteric plexus, consistent with findings in humans and dogs (Xu et al. 2005). In addition to gastrointestinal tract, Depoortere et al. reported that specific binding sites for the motilin receptor were observed in the hippocampus, thalamus, hypothalamus and amygdaloid body in the central nervous system (Depoortere, et al. 1997).

On the other hand, distribution of the ghrelin receptor (GHS-R) has been studied in detail in several species, and it has been shown that the ghrelin receptor is expressed widely in the body from the central nervous system to peripheral organs. In rodents, expression of ghrelin receptor mRNA was observed in the various of regions of the brain, with high expression levels in Arcuate nucleus (Arc), Ventromedial nucleus, Ventral tegmental area (VTA), hippocampus and the nucleus of solitary tract (NTS) (Zigman, et al. 2006) (Mondal, et al. 2005) (Guan, et al. 1997). In addition, high expression levels of GHS-R were found in the pituitary gland (Kamegai, et al. 2001) (Gnanapavan, et al. 2002) and pancreas (Kageyama, et al. 2005) (Volante, et al. 2002). In the gastrointestinal tract, ghrelin receptor mRNA expression was also found throughout the stomach and intestines, and expression of the ghrelin receptor was detected in the muscle layer but not in the mucosal layer in the stomach (Date et al. 2000). Moreover, it has been reported that ghrelin receptor immunoreactivity was found within neuronal cell bodies and fibers in rats (Dass, et al. 2003) and that ghrelin receptor mRNA transcripts were found in longitudinal muscle/myenteric plexus preparations and in cultured myenteric neurons of the guinea pig (Xu et al. 2005)

5. Roles of motilin and ghrelin in gastric motility

According to the origin of its name, the main function of motilin is to stimulate gastric motility. Migrating motor complex (MMC) is characterized by the appearance of gastrointestinal motility in the interdigestive state. It has been reported that these coordinated contractions consist of three phases, phase I (period of motor quiescence), phase II (period of preceding irregular contractions) and phase III (period of clustered potent contractions). It has been shown that plasma concentration of motilin changed in a cyclic fashion and that it has rhythmus occurring every 90-100 min. In fact, administration of motilin has been shown to induce phase III-like contraction via the cholinergic pathway, and endogenous motilin is thought to be physiologically important for phase III contraction (Vantrappen, et al. 1979) (Itoh, et al. 1978).

Since the ghrelin receptor is expressed in the gastrointestinal tract, the effect of ghrelin on gastric motility has also been examined. In rats, ghrelin exerts stimulatory effects on motility of the antrum and duodenum in both fed and fasted states (Fujimiya, et al. 2008), and Taniguchi et al. reported that ghrelin infusion significantly increased motility index of phase III-like contractions at the antrum and jejunum in a dose dependent manner (Taniguchi, et al. 2008). As well as the rat stomach, phase III-like contractions in mice were observed in the interdigestive state, and no spontaneous phase III-like contractions were found in vagotomized mice, suggesting that ghrelin-induced gastric phase III-like contractions are mediated via vagal cholinergic pathways in mice (Zheng, et al. 2009). In humans, administration of ghrelin induced a premature gastric phase III of the MMC, which was not mediated through release of motilin (Tack, et al. 2006).

As a new model to study gastric motility, we established an *in vitro* and *in vivo* functional assay system using suncus. Administration of suncus motilin showed almost the same contractile effect as that of human motilin *in vitro* (Tsutsui et al. 2009). During the fasted state, the suncus stomach and duodenum showed clear migrating phase III contractions (intervals of 80-150 min) as found in humans and dogs, and motilin injection also increased the gastric motility index in a dose-dependent manner (Sakahara, et al. 2010). Moreover, pretreatment with atropine completely abolished the motilin-induced gastric phase III contractions (Sakahara et al. 2010). Since suncus has almost the same GI motility and motilin response as those found in humans and dogs, suncus would be a suitable model to analyze the interaction of motilin and ghrelin in gastric motility.

6. Plasma profiles and secretion of motilin and ghrelin in the gastrointestinal tract

Motilin is mainly produced in the duodenum and secreted into the blood stream. During the interdigestive state, it was found that plasma motilin concentration increased in complete accordance with the cyclical interdigestive contractions of the stomach in dogs (Itoh et al. 1978). Furthermore, plasma motilin concentration was lowered by ingestion of food, and it remained low as long as the gastric motor activity was in the digestive pattern (Itoh et al. 1978). It has been demonstrated that plasma motilin is released at about 100-min intervals in the interdigestive state in humans (Vantrappen et al. 1979) and dogs (Itoh et al. 1978). Zietlow et al. also reported that the peak of plasma motilin levels was always observed in the period of gastric phase III contractions (Zietlow, et al. 2010).

Inverse correlations were found between plasma motilin concentration and glucose and between motilin concentration and insulin, suggesting that glucose and/or insulin are important in suppressing motilin secretion during feeding (Funakoshi, et al. 1985). Dopamine infusion caused a significant decline of plasma motilin levels, and dopamine antagonism with domperidone caused a significant elevation of motilin (Funakoshi, et al.

1983). Atropine suppressed the basal levels of motilin but did not alter the increment of motilin levels after domperidone administration, suggesting that dopaminergic mechanisms exert a tonic inhibitory effect on motilin secretion in normal subjects (Funakoshi et al. 1983). Using an enzymatic method, dispersed cells from the canine duodenojejunal mucosa were separated by centrifugal counterflow elutriation to enrich motilin content, and carbachol dose-dependently stimulated the release of motilin from its enriched cells (Poitras, et al. 1993). Moreover, bombesin, morphine, and erythromycin stimulated motilin release *in vivo*, but did not influence the secretion of motilin *in vitro* (Poitras et al. 1993). Serotonin, GIP, CCK, pentagastrin, cisapride, neosynephrine, isoproterenol, and muscimol also had no effect on motilin release in an *in vitro* model (Poitras et al. 1993). The response to carbachol was abolished by atropine but was not affected by somatostatin, serotonin, secretin, CCK, or GIP (Poitras et al. 1993). These results suggest that muscarinic receptors are present on the motilin cell membrane and that acetylcholine is a major regulator of motilin release.

It is well known that the stomach is a major source of circulation plasma ghrelin, and the levels were elevated in a fasting state and returned to basal levels after re-feeding (Cummings, et al. 2001; Cummings, et al. 2002). In contrast, peptide content of ghrelin in the stomach decreased after fasting, indicating that cytoplasmic ghrelin released from gastric ghrelin cells caused an increase in plasma ghrelin levels (Toshinai, et al. 2001). The effects of nutrients on ghrelin release have been studied in detail. Oral and intravenous glucose administration sharply reduced plasma ghrelin concentration in rodents, and this effect of glucose on ghrelin inhibition was similar to that found in humans (Broglio, et al. 2004; Soriano-Guillen, et al. 2004). In addition to glucose, it has been reported that duodenal and jejunal infusions of lipids reduced ghrelin levels in rats and that infusion of amino acids also induced ghrelin suppression in rats (Overduin, et al. 2005). Although further studies are needed to elucidate the molecular mechanisms of ghrelin secretion from the stomach by nutrients, nutrients may be directly involved in the rapid decline of plasma ghrelin concentration after feeding.

Ghrelin secretion is regulated by peptide and steroid hormones. For example, ghrelin cells are located close to somatostatin-producing D cells, and somatostatin inhibits ghrelin secretion in rats and humans (Broglio, et al. 2002; Shimada, et al. 2003). Ghrelin secretion from the perfused stomach was also stimulated by glucagon treatment in a dose-dependent manner (Kamegai, et al. 2004), and this effect was shown to be mediated by glucagon receptors on ghrelin cells (Katayama, et al. 2007). de la Cour et al. found that epinephrine, norepinephrine, endothelin and secretin stimulated ghrelin release (de la Cour, et al. 2007). In addition, steroid hormone is involved in ghrelin regulation. In humans, estrogen regulates plasma ghrelin concentration (Paulo, et al. 2008) (Kellokoski, et al. 2005). In female rats, the levels of gastric ghrelin mRNA and plasma ghrelin and the number of ghrelin cells were found to be transiently increased by ovariectomy (Matsubara, et al. 2004), and treatment of gastric mucosal cells with estrogen showed that estrogen stimulated ghrelin expression and ghrelin secretion (Sakata, et al. 2006) (Zhao, et al. 2008). Recently, ghrelin-producing cell lines have been generated by different two groups. Iwakura et al. generated ghrelin cell lines from the stomach and showed that insulin decreased ghrelin secretion into culture medium (Iwakura, et al. 2010). Zhao et al. also established different ghrelin cell lines from the stomach and pancreas, and they showed that adrenaline and noradrenaline stimulated ghrelin secretion and that ghrelin-secreting cells express high levels of mRNA encoding beta(1)-adrenergic receptors (Zhao, et al. 2010). Moreover, they reported that fasting-induced increase in plasma ghrelin was blocked by treatment with reserpine to deplete adrenergic neurotransmitters from sympathetic neurons and that inhibition was also seen following administration of atenolol, a selective beta1-adrenergic antagonist, suggesting that sympathetic neurons are involved in ghrelin secretion by directly acting on beta1 receptors (Zhao et al. 2010).

7. Conclusion and future perspectives

Although ghrelin was discovered more than twenty years after motilin was identified, the biological and physiological functions of ghrelin have been studied in more detail than those of motilin. The major reason for this is due to the lack of a motilin gene in experimental rodents like mice and rats, which are used for biological and physiological analysis. So far, dogs and/or rabbits have been used for motilin studies, but these animals are too large to perform detailed analysis. Research has also been limited by the ban on use of genetically engineered mice. To resolve this problem and expand studies on motilin and its relationship with ghrelin, we established suncus as a novel motilin- and ghrelin-producing laboratory animal for motilin study. It has been shown that suncus motilin exerted phase III contraction in MMC using *in vivo* and *in vitro* experiments. This new suncus model will enable the detailed molecular and physiological analysis that were difficult using dogs and rabbits, and suncus will therefore be a powerful tool to understand the detailed mechanisms of motilin- and/or ghrelin-induced gastrointestinal motility.

8. References

Ariyasu H, Takaya K, Tagami T, Ogawa Y, Hosoda K, Akamizu T, Suda M, Koh T, Natsui K, Toyooka S, et al. 2001 Stomach is a major source of circulating ghrelin, and feeding state determines plasma ghrelin-like immunoreactivity levels in humans. *J Clin Endocrinol Metab* 86 4753-4758.

Bado A, Levasseur S, Attoub S, Kermorgant S, Laigneau JP, Bortoluzzi MN, Moizo L, Lehy T, Guerre-Millo M, Le Marchand-Brustel Y, et al. 1998 The stomach is a source of leptin. *Nature* 394 790-793.

Banfield DK, MacGillivray RT, Brown JC & McIntosh CH 1992 The isolation and characterization of rabbit motilin precursor cDNA. *Biochim Biophys Acta* 1131 341-344.

Bednarek MA, Feighner SD, Pong SS, McKee KK, Hreniuk DL, Silva MV, Warren VA, Howard AD, Van Der Ploeg LH & Heck JV 2000 Structure-function studies on the new growth hormone-releasing peptide, ghrelin: minimal sequence of ghrelin necessary for activation of growth hormone secretagogue receptor 1a. *J Med Chem* 43 4370-4376.

Bolkent S, Yilmazer S, Kaya F & Ozturk M 2001 Effects of acid inhibition on somatostatin-producing cells in the rat gastric fundus. *Acta Histochem* 103 413-422.

Bond CT, Nilaver G, Godfrey B, Zimmerman EA & Adelman JP 1988 Characterization of complementary deoxyribonucleic acid for precursor of porcine motilin. *Mol Endocrinol* 2 175-180.

Broglio F, Gottero C, Prodam F, Destefanis S, Gauna C, Me E, Riganti F, Vivenza D, Rapa A, Martina V, et al. 2004 Ghrelin secretion is inhibited by glucose load and insulin-induced hypoglycaemia but unaffected by glucagon and arginine in humans. *Clin Endocrinol (Oxf)* 61 503-509.

Broglio F, Koetsveld Pv P, Benso A, Gottero C, Prodam F, Papotti M, Muccioli G, Gauna C, Hofland L, Deghenghi R, et al. 2002 Ghrelin secretion is inhibited by either somatostatin or cortistatin in humans. *J Clin Endocrinol Metab* 87 4829-4832.

Brown JC, Cook MA & Dryburgh JR 1973 Motilin, a gastric motor activity stimulating polypeptide: the complete amino acid sequence. *Can J Biochem* 51 533-537.

Brown JC, Mutt V & Dryburgh JR 1971 The further purification of motilin, a gastric motor activity stimulating polypeptide from the mucosa of the small intestine of hogs. *Can J Physiol Pharmacol* 49 399-405.

Cummings DE, Purnell JQ, Frayo RS, Schmidova K, Wisse BE & Weigle DS 2001 A preprandial rise in plasma ghrelin levels suggests a role in meal initiation in humans. *Diabetes* 50 1714-1719.

Cummings DE, Weigle DS, Frayo RS, Breen PA, Ma MK, Dellinger EP & Purnell JQ 2002 Plasma ghrelin levels after diet-induced weight loss or gastric bypass surgery. *N Engl J Med* 346 1623-1630.

Dass NB, Munonyara M, Bassil AK, Hervieu GJ, Osbourne S, Corcoran S, Morgan M & Sanger GJ 2003 Growth hormone secretagogue receptors in rat and human gastrointestinal tract and the effects of ghrelin. *Neuroscience* 120 443-453.

Date Y, Kojima M, Hosoda H, Sawaguchi A, Mondal MS, Suganuma T, Matsukura S, Kangawa K & Nakazato M 2000 Ghrelin, a novel growth hormone-releasing acylated peptide, is synthesized in a distinct endocrine cell type in the gastrointestinal tracts of rats and humans. *Endocrinology* 141 4255-4261.

De Clercq P, Depoortere I, Macielag M, Vandermeers A, Vandermeers-Piret MC & Peeters TL 1996 Isolation, sequence, and bioactivity of chicken motilin. *Peptides* 17 203-208.

de la Cour CD, Norlen P & Hakanson R 2007 Secretion of ghrelin from rat stomach ghrelin cells in response to local microinfusion of candidate messenger compounds: a microdialysis study. *Regul Pept* 143 118-126.

Depoortere I, Van Assche G & Peeters TL 1997 Distribution and subcellular localization of motilin binding sites in the rabbit brain. *Brain Res* 777 103-109.

Dornonville de la Cour C, Bjorkqvist M, Sandvik AK, Bakke I, Zhao CM, Chen D & Hakanson R 2001 A-like cells in the rat stomach contain ghrelin and do not operate under gastrin control. *Regul Pept* 99 141-150.

Feighner SD, Tan CP, McKee KK, Palyha OC, Hreniuk DL, Pong SS, Austin CP, Figueroa D, MacNeil D, Cascieri MA, et al. 1999 Receptor for motilin identified in the human gastrointestinal system. *Science* 284 2184-2188.

Fujimiya M, Asakawa A, Ataka K, Chen CY, Kato I & Inui A Ghrelin, des-acyl ghrelin, and obestatin: regulatory roles on the gastrointestinal motility. *Int J Pept* 2010.

Fujimiya M, Asakawa A, Ataka K, Kato I & Inui A 2008 Different effects of ghrelin, des-acyl ghrelin and obestatin on gastroduodenal motility in conscious rats. *World J Gastroenterol* 14 6318-6326.

Funakoshi A, Ho LL, Jen KL, Knopf R & Vinik AI 1985 Diurnal profile of plasma motilin concentrations during fasting and feeding in man. *Gastroenterol Jpn* 20 446-456.

Funakoshi A, Matsumoto M, Sekiya K, Nakano I, Shinozaki H & Ibayashi H 1983 Cholinergic independent dopaminergic regulation of motilin release in man. *Gastroenterol Jpn* 18 525-529.

Gnanapavan S, Kola B, Bustin SA, Morris DG, McGee P, Fairclough P, Bhattacharya S, Carpenter R, Grossman AB & Korbonits M 2002 The tissue distribution of the mRNA of ghrelin and subtypes of its receptor, GHS-R, in humans. *J Clin Endocrinol Metab* 87 2988.

Guan XM, Yu H, Palyha OC, McKee KK, Feighner SD, Sirinathsinghji DJ, Smith RG, Van der Ploeg LH & Howard AD 1997 Distribution of mRNA encoding the growth hormone secretagogue receptor in brain and peripheral tissues. *Brain Res Mol Brain Res* 48 23-29.

He J, Irwin DM, Chen R & Zhang YP 2010 Stepwise loss of motilin and its specific receptor genes in rodents. *J Mol Endocrinol* 44 37-44.

Helmstaedter V, Kreppein W, Domschke W, Mitznegg P, Yanaihara N, Wunsch E & Forssmann WG 1979 Immunohistochemical localization of motilin in endocrine non-enterochromaffin cells of the small intestine of humans and monkey. *Gastroenterology* 76 897-902.

Howard AD, Feighner SD, Cully DF, Arena JP, Liberator PA, Rosenblum CI, Hamelin M, Hreniuk DL, Palyha OC, Anderson J, et al. 1996 A receptor in pituitary and hypothalamus that functions in growth hormone release. *Science* 273 974-977.

Ishida Y, Sakahara S, Tsutsui C, Kaiya H, Sakata I, Oda S & Sakai T 2009 Identification of ghrelin in the house musk shrew (Suncus murinus): cDNA cloning, peptide purification and tissue distribution. *Peptides* 30 982-990.

Itoh Z, Takeuchi S, Aizawa I, Mori K, Taminato T, Seino Y, Imura H & Yanaihara N 1978 Changes in plasma motilin concentration and gastrointestinal contractile activity in conscious dogs. *Am J Dig Dis* 23 929-935.

Iwakura H, Li Y, Ariyasu H, Hosoda H, Kanamoto N, Bando M, Yamada G, Hosoda K, Nakao K, Kangawa K, et al. 2010 Establishment of a novel ghrelin-producing cell line. *Endocrinology* 151 2940-2945.

Kageyama H, Funahashi H, Hirayama M, Takenoya F, Kita T, Kato S, Sakurai J, Lee EY, Inoue S, Date Y, et al. 2005 Morphological analysis of ghrelin and its receptor distribution in the rat pancreas. *Regul Pept* 126 67-71.

Kaiya H, Kodama S, Ishiguro K, Matsuda K, Uchiyama M, Miyazato M & Kangawa K 2009 Ghrelin-like peptide with fatty acid modification and O-glycosylation in the red stingray, Dasyatis akajei. *BMC Biochem* 10 30.

Kaiya H, Kojima M, Hosoda H, Koda A, Yamamoto K, Kitajima Y, Matsumoto M, Minamitake Y, Kikuyama S & Kangawa K 2001 Bullfrog ghrelin is modified by n-octanoic acid at its third threonine residue. *J Biol Chem* 276 40441-40448.

Kaiya H, Kojima M, Hosoda H, Moriyama S, Takahashi A, Kawauchi H & Kangawa K 2003 Peptide purification, complementary deoxyribonucleic acid (DNA) and genomic DNA cloning, and functional characterization of ghrelin in rainbow trout. *Endocrinology* 144 5215-5226.

Kaiya H, Sakata I, Kojima M, Hosoda H, Sakai T & Kangawa K 2004 Structural determination and histochemical localization of ghrelin in the red-eared slider turtle, Trachemys scripta elegans. *Gen Comp Endocrinol* 138 50-57.

Kaiya H, Sakata I, Yamamoto K, Koda A, Sakai T, Kangawa K & Kikuyama S 2006 Identification of immunoreactive plasma and stomach ghrelin, and expression of stomach ghrelin mRNA in the bullfrog, Rana catesbeiana. *Gen Comp Endocrinol* 148 236-244.

Kaiya H, Van Der Geyten S, Kojima M, Hosoda H, Kitajima Y, Matsumoto M, Geelissen S, Darras VM & Kangawa K 2002 Chicken ghrelin: purification, cDNA cloning, and biological activity. *Endocrinology* 143 3454-3463.

Kamegai J, Tamura H, Shimizu T, Ishii S, Sugihara H & Oikawa S 2001 Regulation of the ghrelin gene: growth hormone-releasing hormone upregulates ghrelin mRNA in the pituitary. *Endocrinology* 142 4154-4157.

Kamegai J, Tamura H, Shimizu T, Ishii S, Sugihara H & Oikawa S 2004 Effects of insulin, leptin, and glucagon on ghrelin secretion from isolated perfused rat stomach. *Regul Pept* 119 77-81.

Katayama T, Shimamoto S, Oda H, Nakahara K, Kangawa K & Murakami N 2007 Glucagon receptor expression and glucagon stimulation of ghrelin secretion in rat stomach. *Biochem Biophys Res Commun* 357 865-870.

Kellokoski E, Poykko SM, Karjalainen AH, Ukkola O, Heikkinen J, Kesaniemi YA & Horkko S 2005 Estrogen replacement therapy increases plasma ghrelin levels. *J Clin Endocrinol Metab* 90 2954-2963.

Khan N, Graslund A, Ehrenberg A & Shriver J 1990 Sequence-specific 1H NMR assignments and secondary structure of porcine motilin. *Biochemistry* 29 5743-5751.

Kojima M, Hosoda H, Date Y, Nakazato M, Matsuo H & Kangawa K 1999 Ghrelin is a growth-hormone-releasing acylated peptide from stomach. *Nature* 402 656-660.

Kojima M, Ida T & Sato T 2008 Structure of mammalian and nonmammalian ghrelins. *Vitam Horm* 77 31-46.

Ku SK, Lee HS & Lee JH 2004 An immunohistochemical study of gastrointestinal endocrine cells in the BALB/c mouse. *Anat Histol Embryol* 33 42-48.

Matsubara M, Sakata I, Wada R, Yamazaki M, Inoue K & Sakai T 2004 Estrogen modulates ghrelin expression in the female rat stomach. *Peptides* 25 289-297.

McKee KK, Tan CP, Palyha OC, Liu J, Feighner SD, Hreniuk DL, Smith RG, Howard AD & Van der Ploeg LH 1997 Cloning and characterization of two human G protein-coupled receptor genes (GPR38 and GPR39) related to the growth hormone secretagogue and neurotensin receptors. *Genomics* 46 426-434.

Miura T, Maruyama K, Kaiya H, Miyazato M, Kangawa K, Uchiyama M, Shioda S & Matsuda K 2009 Purification and properties of ghrelin from the intestine of the goldfish, Carassius auratus. *Peptides* 30 758-765.

Miyamoto Y & Miyamoto M 2004 Immunohistochemical localizations of secretin, cholecystokinin, and somatostatin in the rat small intestine after acute cisplatin treatment. *Exp Mol Pathol* 77 238-245.

Mondal MS, Date Y, Yamaguchi H, Toshinai K, Tsuruta T, Kangawa K & Nakazato M 2005 Identification of ghrelin and its receptor in neurons of the rat arcuate nucleus. *Regul Pept* 126 55-59.

Ohshiro H, Nonaka M & Ichikawa K 2008 Molecular identification and characterization of the dog motilin receptor. *Regul Pept* 146 80-87.

Overduin J, Frayo RS, Grill HJ, Kaplan JM & Cummings DE 2005 Role of the duodenum and macronutrient type in ghrelin regulation. *Endocrinology* 146 845-850.

Paulo RC, Brundage R, Cosma M, Mielke KL, Bowers CY & Veldhuis JD 2008 Estrogen elevates the peak overnight production rate of acylated ghrelin. *J Clin Endocrinol Metab* 93 4440-4447.

Poitras P, Dumont A, Cuber JC & Trudel L 1993 Cholinergic regulation of motilin release from isolated canine intestinal cells. *Peptides* 14 207-213.

Rozengurt N, Wu SV, Chen MC, Huang C, Sternini C & Rozengurt E 2006 Colocalization of the alpha-subunit of gustducin with PYY and GLP-1 in L cells of human colon. *Am J Physiol Gastrointest Liver Physiol* 291 G792-802.

Sakahara S, Xie Z, Koike K, Hoshino S, Sakata I, Oda S, Takahashi T & Sakai T 2010 Physiological characteristics of gastric contractions and circadian gastric motility in the free-moving conscious house musk shrew (Suncus murinus). *Am J Physiol Regul Integr Comp Physiol* 299 R1106-1113.

Sakai T, Satoh M, Koyama H, Iesaki K, Umahara M, Fujikura K & Itoh Z 1994a Localization of motilin-immunopositive cells in the rat intestine by light microscopic immunocytochemistry. *Peptides* 15 987-991.

Sakai T, Satoh M, Sonobe K, Nakajima M, Shiba Y & Itoh Z 1994b Autoradiographic study of motilin binding sites in the rabbit gastrointestinal tract. *Regul Pept* 53 249-257.

Sakata I, Nakamura K, Yamazaki M, Matsubara M, Hayashi Y, Kangawa K & Sakai T 2002 Ghrelin-producing cells exist as two types of cells, closed- and opened-type cells, in the rat gastrointestinal tract. *Peptides* 23 531-536.

Sakata I, Tanaka T, Yamazaki M, Tanizaki T, Zheng Z & Sakai T 2006 Gastric estrogen directly induces ghrelin expression and production in the rat stomach. *J Endocrinol* 190 749-757.

Satoh M, Sakai T, Koyama H, Shiba Y & Itoh Z 1995 Immunocytochemical localization of motilin-containing cells in the rabbit gastrointestinal tract. *Peptides* 16 883-887.

Shimada M, Date Y, Mondal MS, Toshinai K, Shimbara T, Fukunaga K, Murakami N, Miyazato M, Kangawa K, Yoshimatsu H, et al. 2003 Somatostatin suppresses ghrelin secretion from the rat stomach. *Biochem Biophys Res Commun* 302 520-525.

Soriano-Guillen L, Barrios V, Martos G, Chowen JA, Campos-Barros A & Argente J 2004 Effect of oral glucose administration on ghrelin levels in obese children. *Eur J Endocrinol* 151 119-121.

Strausberg RL, Feingold EA, Grouse LH, Derge JG, Klausner RD, Collins FS, Wagner L, Shenmen CM, Schuler GD, Altschul SF, et al. 2002 Generation and initial analysis of more than 15,000 full-length human and mouse cDNA sequences. *Proc Natl Acad Sci U S A* 99 16899-16903.

Tack J, Depoortere I, Bisschops R, Delporte C, Coulie B, Meulemans A, Janssens J & Peeters T 2006 Influence of ghrelin on interdigestive gastrointestinal motility in humans. *Gut* 55 327-333.

Takeshita E, Matsuura B, Dong M, Miller LJ, Matsui H & Onji M 2006 Molecular characterization and distribution of motilin family receptors in the human gastrointestinal tract. *J Gastroenterol* 41 223-230.

Taniguchi H, Ariga H, Zheng J, Ludwig K & Takahashi T 2008 Effects of ghrelin on interdigestive contractions of the rat gastrointestinal tract. *World J Gastroenterol* 14 6299-6302.

Ter Beek WP, Muller ES, van den Berg M, Meijer MJ, Biemond I & Lamers CB 2008 Motilin receptor expression in smooth muscle, myenteric plexus, and mucosa of human inflamed and noninflamed intestine. *Inflamm Bowel Dis* 14 612-619.

Theodorakis MJ, Carlson O, Michopoulos S, Doyle ME, Juhaszova M, Petraki K & Egan JM 2006 Human duodenal enteroendocrine cells: source of both incretin peptides, GLP-1 and GIP. *Am J Physiol Endocrinol Metab* 290 E550-559.

Toshinai K, Mondal MS, Nakazato M, Date Y, Murakami N, Kojima M, Kangawa K & Matsukura S 2001 Upregulation of Ghrelin expression in the stomach upon fasting, insulin-induced hypoglycemia, and leptin administration. *Biochem Biophys Res Commun* 281 1220-1225.

Tsutsui C, Kajihara K, Yanaka T, Sakata I, Itoh Z, Oda S & Sakai T 2009 House musk shrew (Suncus murinus, order: Insectivora) as a new model animal for motilin study. *Peptides* 30 318-329.

Vantrappen G, Janssens J, Peeters TL, Bloom SR, Christofides ND & Hellemans J 1979 Motilin and the interdigestive migrating motor complex in man. *Dig Dis Sci* 24 497-500.

Volante M, Allia E, Gugliotta P, Funaro A, Broglio F, Deghenghi R, Muccioli G, Ghigo E & Papotti M 2002 Expression of ghrelin and of the GH secretagogue receptor by pancreatic islet cells and related endocrine tumors. *J Clin Endocrinol Metab* 87 1300-1308.

Wada R, Sakata I, Kaiya H, Nakamura K, Hayashi Y, Kangawa K & Sakai T 2003 Existence of ghrelin-immunopositive and -expressing cells in the proventriculus of the hatching and adult chicken. *Regul Pept* 111 123-128.

Wang YN, McDonald JK & Wyatt RJ 1987 Immunocytochemical localization of neuropeptide Y-like immunoreactivity in adrenergic and non-adrenergic neurons of the rat gastrointestinal tract. *Peptides* 8 145-151.

Wierup N, Bjorkqvist M, Westrom B, Pierzynowski S, Sundler F & Sjolund K 2007 Ghrelin and motilin are cosecreted from a prominent endocrine cell population in the small intestine. *J Clin Endocrinol Metab* 92 3573-3581.

Xu L, Depoortere I, Tang M & Peeters TL 2001 Identification and expression of the motilin precursor in the guinea pig. *FEBS Lett* 490 7-10.

Xu L, Depoortere I, Thielemans L, Huang Z, Tang M & Peeters TL 2003 Sequence, distribution and quantification of the motilin precursor in the cat. *Peptides* 24 1387-1395.

Xu L, Depoortere I, Tomasetto C, Zandecki M, Tang M, Timmermans JP & Peeters TL 2005 Evidence for the presence of motilin, ghrelin, and the motilin and ghrelin receptor in neurons of the myenteric plexus. *Regul Pept* 124 119-125.

Yamamoto I, Kaiya H, Tsutsui C, Sakai T, Tsukada A, Miyazato M & Tanaka M 2008 Primary structure, tissue distribution, and biological activity of chicken motilin receptor. *Gen Comp Endocrinol* 156 509-514.

Zhao TJ, Sakata I, Li RL, Liang G, Richardson JA, Brown MS, Goldstein JL & Zigman JM 2010 Ghrelin secretion stimulated by {beta}1-adrenergic receptors in cultured ghrelinoma cells and in fasted mice. *Proc Natl Acad Sci U S A* 107 15868-15873.

Zhao Z, Sakata I, Okubo Y, Koike K, Kangawa K & Sakai T 2008 Gastric leptin, but not estrogen and somatostatin, contributes to the elevation of ghrelin mRNA expression level in fasted rats. *J Endocrinol* 196 529-538.

Zheng J, Ariga H, Taniguchi H, Ludwig K & Takahashi T 2009 Ghrelin regulates gastric phase III-like contractions in freely moving conscious mice. *Neurogastroenterol Motil* 21 78-84.

Zietlow A, Nakajima H, Taniguchi H, Ludwig K & Takahashi T 2010 Association between plasma ghrelin and motilin levels during MMC cycle in conscious dogs. *Regul Pept* 164 78-82.

Zigman JM, Jones JE, Lee CE, Saper CB & Elmquist JK 2006 Expression of ghrelin receptor mRNA in the rat and the mouse brain. *J Comp Neurol* 494 528-548.

Functions of Adipose Tissue and Adipokines in Health and Disease

Francisca Lago[1], Rodolfo Gómez[2], Javier Conde[2],
Morena Scotece[2], Carlos Dieguez[3] and Oreste Gualillo[2]
[1]SERGAS Santiago University Clinical Hospital, Research Laboratory 7
(Molecular and Cellular Cardiology), Santiago de Compostela,
[2]SERGAS Santiago University Clinical Hospital, Research Laboratory 9
(NEIRID LAB, Laboratory of Neuro Endocrine Interactions in Rheumatology
and Inflammatory Diseases), Santiago de Compostela,
[3]University of Santiago de Compostela, Department of Physiology,
Santiago de Compostela,
Spain

1. Introduction

The notion of white adipose tissue (WAT) as an active contributor to whole-body homeostasis, rather than as a mere fat depot, began to take identity with the discovery of leptin in 1994 [1]. This 16 kDa protein secreted by adipocytes was found to be the product of the gene obese (ob), which is mutated in a murine form of hereditary obesity. From this point on, WAT has been found to produce more than 50 cytokines and other molecules. These "adipokines" participate, through endocrine, paracrine, autocrine or juxtacrine mechanisms of action, in a wide variety of physiological or physiopathological processes, including food intake, insulin sensitivity, vascular sclerotic processes, immunity and inflammation [2,3,4]. They are currently considered to play a crucial role in crosstalk among the adrenal, immune and central and peripheral nervous systems, among others.

Obesity, the condition originally motivating the spate of research on WAT, is now regarded as a pro-inflammatory state, several markers of inflammation having been found to be elevated in obese subjects [5]. It is thought that excess WAT can contribute to the maintenance of this state in three ways: through inflammation-inducing lipotoxicity; by secreting factors that stimulate the synthesis of inflammatory agents in other organs; and by secreting inflammatory agents itself. Adipokines include a variety of pro-inflammatory peptides (including TNFα, secretion of which by adipocytes was observed even before the discovery of leptin [6]). These pro-inflammatory adipokines appear to contribute significantly to the "low-grade inflammatory state" of obese subjects with metabolic syndrome [7], a cluster of metabolic abnormalities including insulin resistance, dyslipidaemia and alteration of coagulation that is associated with increased risk of cancer, type II diabetes, cardiovascular complications and autoimmune inflammatory diseases.

WAT also produces, possibly as an adaptive response, anti-inflammatory factors such as IL1 receptor antagonist (which binds competitively to the interleukin 1 receptor without triggering activity within the cell) and IL10 (circulating levels of which are also elevated in obese individuals).

2. Cellular and molecular alterations of white adipose tissue in obesity

One of the consequences of the production and local release of cytokines and adipokines by adipocytes is the recruitment of large numbers of immune cells, including monocytes and T-lymphocytes, into adipose tissue. In particular, pro-inflammatory cytokine levels and macrophage density in visceral fat depots are much higher than in subcutaneous adipose tissue. While the mechanisms underlying the recruitment and activation of macrophages in adipose tissue remain poorly understood, there is emerging evidence that adipose tissue-secreted chemokines are largely responsible for the recruitment, retention and activation of macrophage precursors (monocytes) in fat. Monocyte chemoattractant protein-1 (MCP-1) has been implicated as one of the major mediators of the monocyte recruitment that occurs in adipose tissue, while macrophage colony stimulating factor (M-CSF) is believed to mediate the conversion of monocytes to macrophages in adipose tissue. Other candidate adipocyte-derived molecules that have also been implicated in macrophage recruitment/activation in adipose tissue include free fatty acids and lipoprotein lipase.

The primary function of resident macrophages of adipose tissue remains still unclear. It has been proposed that macrophages clear dead (apoptotic and necrotic) cells. Actually, adipocytes undergoing necrosis secondary to hypertrophy may lead to macrophage activation (with the accompanying release of inflammatory mediators) and their subsequent elimination from adipose tissue Another potentially important role of adipose tissue macrophages is modulation of adipocyte function. Cross-talk between adipocytes and macrophages is evidenced by the ability of each cell type to enhance the production of protein mediators by the other. For instance, adipocyte conditioned media can elicit large increases in the production/release of TNFa, IL-6 and NO by macrophages, while TNF-a released from macrophages inhibits the production of adiponectin by adipocytes. Likely consequences of this cross-talk between macrophages and adipocytes include amplification and perpetuation of the inflammatory phenotype that is induced by the expanding mass of body fat.

In humans, macrophage infiltration is correlated with both adipocyte size and BMI and is reduced after surgery-induced weight loss in morbidly obese subjects. There is also a preferential infiltration of macrophages into omental *vs.* subcutaneous fat, a phenomenon exaggerated by central. The majority of macrophages in obese adipose tissue aggregates in "crown-like structures" completely surrounding dead (necrotic-like) adipocytes and scavenging adipocyte debris.

3. Leptin

Leptin is a 16 kDa non-glycosylated peptide hormone encoded by the gene obese (ob), the murine homologue of the human gene LEP [1]. Structurally, it belongs to the class I cytokine superfamily, consisting of a bundle of four α-helices. It is mainly produced by adipocytes, and circulating leptin levels are directly correlated with WAT mass. It decreases food intake and increases energy consumption by acting on hypothalamic cell populations [8,9], inducing anorexigenic factors (CART, POMC) and inhibiting orexigenic neuropeptides

(NPY, AGRP and orexin), and leptin levels are negatively correlated with glucocorticoids [10] and positively with insulin [11]. Its own synthesis is mainly regulated by food intake and eating-related hormones, but also depends on energy status, sex hormones (being inhibited by testosterone and increased by ovarian sex steroids) and a wide range of inflammation mediators [12, 13] (being increased or suppressed by pro-inflammatory cytokines depending on whether their action is acute or chronic). Through the mediation of these latter agents, leptin synthesis is increased by acute infection and sepsis. As a result of the effects of sex hormones, leptin levels are higher in women than in men even when adjusted for BMI, which may be relevant to the influence of sex on the development or frequency of certain diseases [14], such as osteoarthritis [56]. Thus leptin appears to act not only as an adipostatin, the function in relation to which it was discovered, but also as a general signal of energy reserves [2] that is involved in a wide variety of other functions, including glucose metabolism, the synthesis of glucocorticoids, the proliferation of CD4+ T lymphocytes, cytokine secretion, phagocytosis, regulation of the hypothalamic-pituitary-adrenal axis, reproduction, and angiogenesis [15]. It can accordingly be described as a cytokine-like hormone with pleiotropic actions.

Leptin exerts its biological actions by binding to its receptors. These are encoded by the gene diabetes (db) and belong to the class I cytokine receptor superfamily, which includes receptors for IL6, LIF, CNTF, OSM, G-CSF and gp130. Alternative splicings of db give rise to six receptor isoforms: the soluble form Ob-Re, which lacks a cytoplasmic domain; four forms with short cytoplasmic domains (Ob-Ra, Ob-Rc, Ob-Rd and Ob-Rf); and the long form Ob-Rb, which is found in almost all tissues and appears to be the only form capable of transducing the leptin signal.

As in the case of other class I cytokine receptors, the main routes by which Ob-Rb appears to transmit the extracellular signal it receives are JAK-STAT pathways [16], which involve JAK2 phosphorylating tyrosines in the cytoplasmic domain of the receptor. In particular, mutation of the intracellular tyrosine Y1138 of murine Ob-Rb prevents STAT3 activation and results in hyperphagia, obesity and impaired thermoregulation, and replacing Y1138 with a serine residue likewise causes pronounced obesity in knock-in mice. However, since Y1138S knock-in mice do not exhibit other defects of db/db mice, such as infertility, the role of leptin in the processes that are disrupted in these latter conditions must be independent of STAT3 [17]. Indeed, the other two cytoplasmic tyrosines of murine Ob-Rb, Y985 and Y1077, have been shown to bind other intracellular signalling molecules [16, 18]. The early studies of leptin focused on its anorexigenic action. Both in humans and rodents, leptin levels are closely correlated with body mass index, and defects of the genes encoding for leptin and its receptors give rise to severe obesity and diabetes. Treating leptin-deficient mice with leptin induces a reduction in food intake accompanied by an increase in metabolic rate and weight loss. Mutations of these genes in humans appear to be rare, but the cases that are known have occurred in families with a high prevalence of morbid obesity; again, leptin administration has ameliorated all the problems associated with leptin deficiency. As noted in previous sections, leptin participates in the control of food intake by acting on an intricate neuronal circuit involving hypothalamic and brainstem nuclei [19], where it integrates a variety of different orexigenic and anorexigenic signals.

Leptin therapy is not an effective treatment for morbid obesity that is not due to congenital deficiency of leptin or leptin receptors. In these noncongenital types of obesity, leptin concentrations are already high as a consequence of increased fat mass. The persistence of obesity in spite of high leptin levels suggests that high leptin levels can induce leptin resistance. This may occur due to a leptin-induced increase of SOCS3, which blocks intracellular transmission of the leptin signal [20], but our understanding of leptin resistance is still limited.

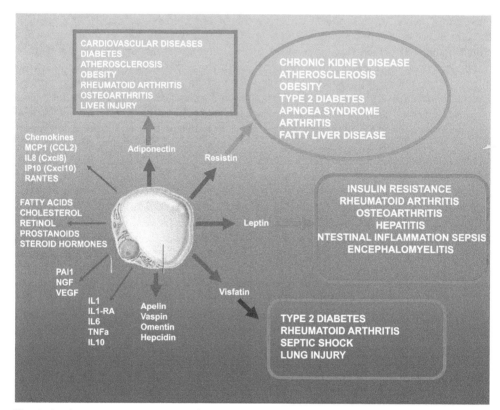

Fig. 1. A schematic representation of white adipose tissue (wat) functions. Besides to be the main energy store of the body and the site of synthesis of steroids and prostanoids, wat is also a source of a plethora of novel factors that modulate the immune/inflammatory response and promote atherosclerosis, vascular dysfunction and insulin resistance.

Db/db mice, which lack leptin receptors, suffer from thymus atrophy [21], and ob/ob mice, which lack leptin, are immunodeficient. Leptin must therefore play a role in immunity. This presumably explains why the murine immune system is depressed by acute starvation and reduced caloric intake, both of which result in low leptin levels [33], and why this depression is reverted by administration of exogenous leptin.

It promotes phagocyte function [24] and induces the synthesis of eicosanoids [25], nitric oxide [26] and several pro-inflammatory cytokines [26] in macrophages and monocytes. It increases IFNγ-induced production of nitric oxide synthase in murine macrophages [26]. It induces chemotaxis and the release of reactive oxygen species by neutrophils [27, 28]. It influences the proliferation, differentiation, activation and cytotoxicity of natural killer (NK) cells [29].

It may protect dendritic cells from apoptosis and promote their lipopolysaccharide-induced maturation and a cytokine production profile featuring low levels of IL10 and high levels of IL12, TNFα and costimulatory molecules, which favours the proliferation of allogeneic CD4+ T cells (whereas leptin receptor deficiency and sequestration of leptin have the opposite effects and result in depressed proliferation of allogeneic CD4+ T cells) [30]. Finally, it modifies T-cell balance, induces T-cell activation, and alters the pattern of T-cell cytokine production by directing T-cell differentiation towards a T_{H1} response [31, 32].

Leptin also prevents glucocorticoid-induced thymocyte apoptosis, and increases thymic cell counts [33]. The low circulating CD4+ T-cell counts, impaired T-cell proliferation and impaired release of T-cell cytokines exhibited by young human patients with morbid obesity due to congenital leptin deficiency are all ameliorated by administration of recombinant human leptin. The fact that several T-cell antigens are expressed aberrantly in both ob/ob and db/db mice suggests that leptin may influence the growth, differentiation and activation of T cells by interacting with T-cell co-stimulatory antigens such as CTLA4 and dipeptidyl peptidase IV [34]. It is possible, however, that in the thymus T cells are affected by leptin only indirectly, via other signalling molecules: fetal db/db thymi develop normally when transplanted into wild-type hosts; neither the thymus weight and cellularity nor the cellular and humoral immune responses of wild-type mice are affected by transplantation of bone marrow cells from db/db mice more than by transplantation from db/+ mice; and thymus weight and cellularity are decreased when bone marrow cells are transplanted from wild-type mice to db/db mice [47].

A salient aspect of the effects of leptin in the immune system is its action as a pro-inflammatory cytokine: it is produced by inflammatory cells [35], and leptin mRNA expression and circulating leptin levels are increased by a number of inflammatory stimuli, including IL1, IL6 and lipopolysaccharide (LPS) [36]. Leptin-deficient mice are less prone than non-leptin-deficient mice to develop inflammatory diseases, regardless of whether these involve innate or adaptive immunity; reported conditions include experimentally induced colitis, experimental autoimmune encephalomyelitis, type I diabetes and experimentally induced hepatitis [2]. In the innate case, a reported imbalance between pro- and anti-inflammatory cytokines [37] suggests that leptin is able to modify the cytokine secretion pattern of monocytes and macrophages through a STAT3-mediated mechanism [38]. In the adaptive case, resistance may be due to the above-noted influence of leptin deficiency on T_{H1}/T_{H2} balance [39]. When transferred to T-cell-deficient mice, murine CD4+ CD45RBhigh T cells from db/db mice do not induce colitis as rapidly as do CD4+ CD45RBhigh T cells from non-db/db mice, which feature leptin receptors [40]. Also, in rats with chemically induced intestinal inflammation, circulating leptin levels are elevated, and correlate with the degree of inflammation and the development of anorexia, during the first day following the induction of inflammation [41]. Serum leptin levels are likewise high in human patients with acute ulcerative colitis, in whom inflamed colonic epithelial cells secrete leptin into the intestinal lumen, where it is able to activate NFkB [42]. Thus leptin appears to play a significant role in intestinal inflammation as well as in the development of associated anorexia.

Mice in which experimental autoimmune encephalomyelitis (EAE) has been induced by inoculation of appropriate self-antigens constitute an animal model of human multiple sclerosis, a disease in which leptin levels in serum and cerebrospinal fluid are high and are negatively correlated with CD4+ CD25+ regulatory T cells [43]. Ob/ob mice do not develop EAE in response to EAE-inducing antigens, but this resistance is abolished by administration of leptin, and the abolition of resistance is accompanied by a switch from a T_{H2} to a T_{H1} pattern of cytokine release [44]. Also, the onset of EAE in wild-type mice is preceded by an increase in circulating leptin and is delayed by acute starvation [35]. Of particular interest is the finding that during the active phase of EAE leptin is secreted by both macrophages and T cells that have infiltrated the central nervous system (CNS), and that secretion by activated T cells appears to constitute an autocrine loop sustaining their proliferation [35]. By contrast, however, leptin secretion by T cells seems to have at most a marginal role in experimentally induced colitis and hepatitis, in which conditions no differences have been found between ob/ob and wild-type T cells regarding their ability to induce inflammation [45].

Serum leptin levels increase preceding not only the onset of EAE [35], but also the onset of diabetes in female non-obese diabetic (NOD) mice, in which leptin administration augments inflammatory infiltrates, increases interferon γ production by peripheral T cells, and speeds up the destruction of pancreatic β cells [46]. These latter findings suggest that leptin may promote the development of type 1 diabetes through a T_{H1} response.

Finally, leptin administration increases both inflammatory and platelet responses in humans during caloric deprivation [48], and in WAT-less mice increases T-cell–mediated hepatic inflammation [49]. Together with a number of other neuroendocrine messengers, leptin appears to play a major role in autoimmune diseases such as rheumatoid arthritis. In patients with rheumatoid arthritis, circulating leptin levels are high [51, 52], and leptin production is much higher in osteoarthritic cartilage than in normal cartilage [55].

Of all the connective tissues that compose a skeletal joint, articular cartilage is the most damaged by rheumatic disease. Under pathological conditions, control of the balance between synthesis and degradation of extracellular matrix by chondrocytes is lost, and the production of a host of inflammation mediators by these cells eventually leads to complete loss of cartilage structure [53, 54]. The finding that administration of exogenous leptin increases IGF1 and TGFβ1 production by rat knee joint cartilage has suggested that high circulating leptin levels in obese individuals may protect cartilage from osteoarthritic degeneration [55]. However, most of the evidence points the other way: in rheumatoid arthritis patients a fasting-induced fall in circulating leptin is associated with CD4+ lymphocyte hyporeactivity and increased IL4 secretion [50]; experimental antigen-induced arthritis is less severe in leptin-deficient ob/ob mice than in wild-type mice [39]; and in cultured chondrocytes type 2 nitric oxide synthase (NOS2) is activated by the combination leptin plus IFNγ (though by either without the other) [57], and NOS2 activation by IL1 is increased by leptin [58] (nitric oxide has well-documented pro-inflammatory effects on joint cartilage, triggering the loss of chondrocyte phenotype, chondrocyte apoptosis, and the activation of metalloproteases). Intracellularly, the joint action of IL1 and leptin involves JAK2, PI3K, MEK1 and p38.

A pro-inflammatory effect of leptin on cartilage would be in keeping with the fact that, in comparison with men, women have both higher circulating leptin levels and a greater propensity to develop osteoarthritis [56]. It would also explain association between obesity and inflammatory conditions, especially those related with alterations of cartilage homeostasis.

4. Adiponectin

Adiponectin, also called gelatin binding protein 28 (GBP28), adipose most abundant gene transcript 1(apM1), and 30 kDa adipocyte complement-related protein (Acrp30, AdipoQ), is a 244-residue protein that, as far as is known, is produced prevalently by WAT. It increases fatty acid oxidation and reduces the synthesis of glucose in the liver [61]. Ablation of the adiponectin gene has no dramatic effect on knock-out mice on a normal diet, but when placed on a high-fat, high-sucrose diet they develop severe insulin resistance and exhibit lipid accumulation in muscles [62]. Circulating adiponectin levels tend to be low in morbidly obese patients and increase with weight loss and with the use of thiazolidinediones, which enhance sensitivity to insulin [67].

Adiponectin acts mainly via two receptors, one (AdipoR1) found mainly in skeletal muscle and the other (AdipoR2) in liver (for a third route, see the next section). Transduction of the adiponectin signal by AdipoR1 and AdipoR2 involves the activation of AMPK, PPAR (α and γ) and presumably other signalling molecules also. Adiponectin exhibits structural homology with collagen VIII and X and complement factor C1q, and circulates in the blood in relatively large amounts in oligomeric forms (mainly trimers and hexamers, but also a 12-18-mer form [59]), constituting about 0.01% of total plasma protein. Whether the various oligomers have different activities, which would make the effect of adiponectin controlable through its oligomerization state, is somewhat controversial and may depend on target cell type: although authors working with myocytes reported that trimers activated AMP-activated protein kinase (AMPK) whereas higher oligomers activated NFκb, it has also been reported that 12-18-mers promote AMPK in hepatocytes [60].

Although adiponectin was discovered nearly at the same time as leptin, its role in protection against obesity and obesity-related disorders only began to be recognized some years later. It is now beginning to be recognized that, in addition, it has a wide range of effects in pathologies with inflammatory components, such as cardiovascular disease, type 2 diabetes, metabolic syndrome and rheumatoid arthritis. One indication of a relationship between adiponectin and inflammation is provided by the finding that its secretion by cultured adipocytes is inhibited by pro-inflammatory cytokines such as IL6 [65] and TNFα [66]. More recently, an explanation of how hypoadiponectinaemia might contribute to the development of inflammation-related diseases has been suggested by the finding that adiponectin promotes the phagocytosis of apoptotic cells (by interacting with calreticulin on the phagocyte surface), since the accumulation of apoptotic débris is known to be able to cause inflammation and immune system dysfunction [67]. In the remainder of this section we look at the relationship of adiponectin to inflammatory processes in several types of pathology.

Adiponectin has been described as a potent anti-atherogenic factor that protects vascular endothelium against atherogenic inflammation through multiple effects on the endothelium itself and other vascular structures [63]. It inhibits the adhesion of monocytes to endothelial cells, reduces the synthesis of adhesion molecules and tumor necrosis factor, and reduces NFκB levels [64]. Subnormal levels of adiponectin have been linked to inflammatory atherosclerosis in humans [69], and in animal models they are associated with increased vascular smooth cell proliferation in response to injury, increased free fatty acid levels, and insulin resistance [70]. The conjunction of pro-diabetic and pro-atherogenic effects of reduced adiponectin levels, as seen in metabolic syndrome, make adiponectin a link between obesity and inflammation.

In contrast to its protective role against obesity and vascular diseases, it appears that in skeletal joints adiponectin is pro-inflammatory and involved in matrix degradation. Plasma adiponectin levels in rheumatoid arthritis patients are higher than in healthy controls [51] (and adiponectin levels in synovial fluid are higher in rheumatoid arthritis patients than in patients with osteoarthritis [72]). In human synovial fibroblasts adiponectin selectively induces, via the p38 MAPK pathway, two of the main mediators of rheumatoid arthritis, IL6 and matrix metalloproteinase 1 [71]. Chondrocytes also present functional adiponectin receptors, activation of which leads to the induction of type 2 NOS via a signalling pathway that involves PI3 kinase; and adiponectin-treated chondrocytes similarly increase IL6, TNFα and MCP1 synthesis (but not release of prostaglandin E_2 or leukotriene B_4). Taken together, these results suggest that it may be worth considering adiponectin as a potential target of treatment for degenerative joint diseases. On the other hand, the high adiponectin levels of patients with rheumatoid arthritis can also be interpreted as an attempt to overcome the well-known pro-inflammatory effect of leptin, for example by counteracting the pro-inflammatory effects of TNFα and reducing the production of IL6 and CRP in rheumatoid arthritis [73].

In experimental models of liver injury, adiponectin has been reported to have anti-inflammatory effects: in rodents, adiponectin administration improves liver function in both alcoholic and non-alcoholic fatty liver disease as the result of TNF suppression, and in mice it reduces liver enzyme levels, hepatomegaly and steatosis [74], attenuates liver fibrosis [75], and protects against LPS-induced liver injury [76].

Finally, there is also evidence that adiponectin may influence the development of certain neoplasias and the course of wound healing [77, 78].

5. Resistin

Resistin is a dimeric protein that received its name from its apparent induction of insulin resistance in mice. It belongs to the FIZZ (found in inflammatory zones) family (now also known as RELMs, i.e. resistin-like molecules). The first member this family to be discovered, FIZZ1 (also known as RELMα), is a protein that is found in above-normal levels in the bronchoalveolar fluid of mice with experimentally induced asthma [79]. FIZZ2 (RELMβ) was discovered in the proliferating epithelium of intestinal crypt [80]. Resistin (FIZZ3) has been found in adipocytes, macrophages and other cell types. In rodents, a fourth FIZZ protein, RELMγ, has been identified in WAT and haematopoietic tissues [81].

As noted above, it has been postulated that resistin mediates insulin resistance, but this role may be limited to rodents. Initial enthusiasm for this theory, which provides a direct link between adiposity and insulin resistance [83], was quickly quenched by contradictory findings in both mice and humans. It nonetheless appears safe to assert that resistin levels depend upon both nutritional state and hormonal environment; that they are low during fasting and restored by refeeding; and that growth hormone, catecholamines and endothelin 1 are all able to increase resistin secretion [82].

5.1 Resistin and inflammation
That resistin is involved in inflammatory conditions in humans is suggested by its secretion in appreciable quantities by mononuclear cells. Also, resistin levels are correlated with those

of cell adhesion molecules such as ICAM1 in patients with obstructive sleep apnoea [87], and in atherosclerotic patients are positively associated with other markers of inflammation, such as soluble TNF-R type II and lipoprotein-associated phospholipase A2 [88]. Furthermore, LPS has been reported to induce resistin gene expression in primary human and murine macrophages via a cascade involving the secretion of pro-inflammatory cytokines [86]; and in human peripheral blood mononuclear cells resistin appears both to induce [85] and be induced by [84] IL6 and TNFa (induction of these cytokines by resistin occurring via the NFκB pathway [85]). However, both TNFα and IL6 downregulate resistin or have no effect in adipocytes [84].

A pro-inflammatory role of resistin in atherosclerosis is suggested by reports that in vascular endothelial cells it induces the inflammation marker long pentraxin 3 [90] and promotes the release of endothelin 1 and production of VCAM1, ICAM1 and monocyte chemotactic protein 1 (MCP1) [89]. In murine models of atherosclerosis, resistin is present in sclerotic lesions at levels that are proportional to the severity of the lesion [92]. In humans resistin is associated with coronary artery calcification, a quantitative marker of atherosclerosis [91].

There are indications that resistin may also be involved in the pathogenesis of rheumatoid arthritis: resistin has been found in the plasma and the synovial fluid of rheumatoid arthritis patients [92], and injection of resistin into mice joints induces an arthritis-like condition, with leukocyte infiltration of synovial tissues, hypertrophy of the synovial layer and pannus formation [85]. However, plasma resistin levels in rheumatoid arthritis patients appear to be no different from those found in healthy controls [51,85]; and although in some studies of rheumatoid arthritis patients resistin levels were higher in synovial fluid than in serum (which shows that circulating levels of adipokines do not necessarily reflect the situation in the joint), the discrepancy may be due simply to the increased permeability of inflamed synovial membrane [93].

6. Other adipokines

6.1 Visfatin

Visfatin is an insulin-mimetic adipokine that was originally discovered in liver, skeletal muscle and bone marrow as a growth factor for B lymphocyte precursors (whence its alternative name, pre-B-colony enhancing factor, or PBEF). It is up-modulated in models of acute lung injury and sepsis. It was re-discovered by Fukuhara et al. [94] using a differential display technique to identify genes that are relatively specifically expressed in abdominal fat. Circulating visfatin levels are closely correlated with WAT accumulation, visfatin mRNA levels increase in the course of adipocyte differentiation, and visfatin synthesis is regulated by several factors, including glucocorticoids, TNFα, IL6 and growth hormone. In an experimental model of obesity-associated insulin resistance, circulating visfatin levels increased during the development of obesity, apparently due solely to secretion by abdominal WAT (since visfatin mRNA increased only in this tissue, not in subcutaneous WAT or liver). However, visfatin is not only produced by WAT, but also by endotoxin-challenged neutrophils, in which it prevents apoptosis through a mechanism mediated by caspases 3 and 8 [95]. Also, patients with inflammatory bowel diseases have increased circulating visfatin levels and increased levels of visfatin mRNA in their intestinal epithelium; and visfatin has been shown to induce chemotaxis and the production of IL1β, TNFα, IL6 and costimulatory molecules by CD14+ monocytes, and to increase their ability to induce alloproliferative responses in lymphocytes, effects which are mediated intracellularly by p38 and MEK1 [96]. Visfatin is therefore certainly pro-inflammatory in some circumstances. In addition, circulating visfatin is higher in patients with rheumatoid arthritis than in healthy controls [51]. Even though it is currently unclear what is visfatin physiological role or relevance in the context of rheumatoid arthritis, it may reflect modulation of the inflammatory or immune response by visfatin; or it may forms part of a compensatory mechanism that facilitates the accumulation of intra-abdominal fat so as to prevent rheumatoid cachexia; or it may simply be an epiphenomenon.

6.2 Apelin

Apelin is a bioactive peptide that was originally identified in bovine stomach extracts as the endogenous ligand of the orphan G protein-coupled receptor APJ [97]. It is derived from a 77-amino-acid prepropeptide that is cleaved into a 55-amino-acid fragment and then into shorter forms. The physiologically active form is thought to be apelin 36, although the pyroglutamylated form of apelin 13, which is also produced endogenously, is more potent. Boucher et al. [98] recently found that apelin is produced and secreted by mature human and murine adipocytes, and that the apelin mRNA levels found in these cells are similar to those found in the stroma-vascular fraction (which contains other cell types present in adipose tissue) and in organs such as kidney and heart [98]. In obese humans plasma apelin levels are significantly higher than in lean controls [98,100], and that this may be due to production by WAT is suggested by the finding that in several murine models of obesity above-normal plasma apelin levels are accompanied by above-normal apelin mRNA levels in adipocytes [98]. TNFα increases both apelin production in adipose tissue and blood plasma apelin levels when administered to mice by intraperitoneal injection [99]. Intriguingly, in mice with diet-induced obesity, macrophage counts and the levels of pro-inflammatory agents such as TNFα seem to rise progressively in adipose tissue before a rise in circulating insulin levels indicates the onset of insulin resistance [101]. So, it could be conceivable that in adipocytes there is a substantial regulation of apelin synthesis exerted by TNFα, leading to sustained apelin secretion in obesity.

Thus, one may envisage that over-production of apelin in the obese may be an adaptive response that attempts to forestall the onset of obesity-related disorders such as mild chronic inflammation, hypertension and cardiovascular dysfunctions. Accordingly, further elucidation of the role of apelin is of major interest.

6.3 Vaspin

Vaspin (visceral-adipose-tissue-derived serpin) was discovered by Hida et al. [102] as a serpin (serine protease inhibitor) that was produced in the visceral adipose tissue of Otsuka Long–Evans Tokushima Fatty rats at the age when obesity and plasma insulin concentrations reach a peak; thereafter, vaspin production decreased as diabetes worsened and body weight fell in untreated mice, but serum vaspin levels were maintained by treatment with insulin or pioglitazone. Administration of vaspin to obese mice improved glucose tolerance and insulin sensitivity, and reversed altered expression of genes that may promote insulin resistance.

Kloting et al. [103] reported that human vaspin mRNA is not detectable in the adipose tissue of normal, lean, glucose-tolerant individuals, but can be induced by increased fat mass, decreased insulin sensitivity, and impaired glucose tolerance. The regulation of vaspin gene expression seems to be fat depot-specific. The induction of vaspin by adipose tissue may constitute a compensatory mechanism in response to obesity, severe insulin resistance and type 2 diabetes.

7. Conclusions

It is now clear that adipokines play multiple important roles in the body, and the increasing research effort in this area is gradually revealing the intricate adipokine-mediated interplay among white adipose tissue, metabolic diseases and inflammatory (auto)immune illnesses. Although many issues remain foggy, in this section we outline several possible avenues for therapeutic action that this work has already opened.

There is now a huge amount of data on the promotion of inflammation by high circulating leptin levels. It might perhaps be possible to control the amount of bioavailable circulating leptin, and hence to prevent leptin-induced inflammation, by means of a soluble, high-affinity leptin-binding molecule analogous to the soluble TNFα receptors used to treat rheumatoid arthritis. Alternatively, it might be possible to block the leptin receptor with monoclonal humanized antibodies or mutant leptins that are able to bind to the receptor without activating it. An obvious proviso here is that receptors mediating the influence of leptin on food intake should not be blocked, lest the patient develop hyperphagia and obesity; but the fact that this influence is exerted in the brain, on the other side of the blood-brain barrier, would seem to make such discrimination possible. At present, little is known in this area because current anti-leptin agents were developed to control the adipostatic effects of leptin, and hence to cross the blood brain barrier.

The anti-atherosclerotic and vasoprotective effects of adiponectin are another source of inspiration for possible pharmacological approaches to inflammatory diseases. In particular, one strategy against diabetes and relevant cardiovascular and metabolic diseases might be to tackle the hypoadiponectinaemia associated with these conditions. Given the high levels of adiponectin in the blood, exogenous administration of the adipokine itself would probably have little effect; but drugs that specifically enhance endogenous adiponectin production, such as thiazolidinediones, might well prove to be effective. It should not be forgotten, of course, that the primary causes of obesity are generally nutritional and lifestyle factors such as overeating and physical inactivity, and that front line treatment of obesity-related hypoadiponectinemia and obesity-related hyperproduction of detrimental adipokines therefore essentially involves the correction of these factors.

8. Acknowledgements

Part of the research described in this chapter was supported by the Spanish Ministry of Health through the Fondo de Investigación Sanitaria, Instituto de Salud Carlos III and by the Xunta de Galicia. The work of Oreste Gualillo and Francisca Lago is funded by the Instituto de Salud Carlos III and the Xunta de Galicia (SERGAS) through a research staff stabilization contract.
We apologize to the authors of the many relevant papers, mention of which in this chapter has been prevented by shortage of space.

9. References

[1] Zhang Y, Proenca R, Maffei M, Barone M, Leopold L, Friedman JM. Positional cloning of the mouse obese gene and its human homologue. Nature. 1994; 372(6505):425-32.

[2] Otero M, Lago R, Lago F, Casanueva FF, Dieguez C, Gomez-Reino JJ, Gualillo O. Leptin, from fat to inflammation: old questions and new insights. FEBS Lett. 2005; 579(2):295-301.

[3] Trayhurn P, Wood IS. Adipokines: inflammation and the pleiotropic role of white adipose tissue. Br J Nutr. 2004; 92(3):347-55.

[4] Trayhurn P, Wood IS. Signalling role of adipose tissue: adipokines and inflammation in obesity. Biochem Soc Trans. 2005; 33(Pt 5):1078-81.

[5] Lau DC, Dhillon B, Yan H, Szmitko PE, Verma S. Adipokines: molecular links between obesity and atherosclerosis. Am J Physiol Heart Circ Physiol. 2005; 288(5):H2031-41.

[6] Hotamisligil GS, Shargill NS, Spiegelman BM. Adipose expression of tumor necrosis factor-alpha: direct role in obesity-linked insulin resistance. Science. 1993; 259(5091):87-91.

[7] Trayhurn P, Bing C, Wood IS. Adipose tissue and adipokines--energy regulation from the human perspective. J Nutr. 2006; 136(7):1935S-9S.

[8] Ahima RS, Prabakaran D, Mantzoros C, et al. Role of leptin in the neuroendocrine response to fasting. Nature 1996; 382: 250-252

[9] Chan JL, Heist K, DePaoli AM, Veldhuis JD, Mantzoros CS. The role of falling leptin levels in the neuroendocrine and metabolic adaptation to short-term starvation in healthy men. J Clin Invest. 2003; 111: 1409-21.

[10] Zakrzewska KE, Cusin I, Sainsbury A, Rohner-Jeanrenaud F, Jeanrenaud B. Glucocorticoids as counterregulatory hormones of leptin: toward an understanding of leptin resistance. Diabetes 1997; 46: 717-9.

[11] Boden G, Chen X, Kolaczynski JW, Polansky M. Effects of prolonged hyperinsulinemia on serum leptin in normal human subjects. J. Clin. Inv 1997; 100: 1107-13

[12] Sarraf P, Frederich RC, Turner EM, et al. Multiple cytokines and acute inflammation raise mouse leptin levels: potential role in inflammatory anorexia. J. Exp. Med. 1997; 185: 171-5.

[13] Gualillo O, Eiras S, Lago F, Dieguez C, Casanueva FF. Elevated serum leptin concentrations induced by experimental acute inflammation. Life Sci. 2000; 67: 2433-41.

[14] Blum WF, Englaro P, Hatsch S, et al. Plasma leptin levels in healthy children and adolescents: dependence on body mass index, body fat mass, gender, pubertal stage, and testosterone. Clin. Endocrinol. Metab. 1997; 82: 2904-10.

[15] Otero M, Lago R, Gomez R, Dieguez C, Lago F, Gomez-Reino J, Gualillo O. Towards a pro-inflammatory and immunomodulatory emerging role of leptin. Rheumatology (Oxford). 2006; 45(8):944-50

[16] Fruhbeck G. Intracellular signalling pathways activated by leptin. Biochem J. 2006; 393: 7-20

[17] Bates, S.H., Stearns, W.H., Dundon, T.A., Schubert, M., Tso, A.W., Wang, Y., Banks, A.S., Lavery, H.J., Haq, A.K., Maratos-Flier, E., Neel, B.G., Schwartz, M.W. and Myers Jr., M.G. STAT3 signalling is required for leptin regulation of energy balance but not reproduction. Nature 2003 , 421 (6925), 856–859.

[18] Gualillo O, Eiras S, White DW, Dieguez C, Casanueva FF. Leptin promotes the tyrosine phosphorylation of SHC proteins and SHC association with GRB2. Mol Cell Endocrinol. 2002; 190: 83-9.

[19] Prodi F, Obici S. The brain as a molecular target for diabetic therapy. Endocrinology 2006; 147(6): 2664-9.

[20] Bjorbaek C, Elmquist JK, Frantz JD, Flier JS. The role of SOCS3 in leptin signalling and leptin resistance. J Biol Chem 1999; 274: 30059-65.

[21] Kimura M, Tanaka S, Isoda F, Sekigawa K, Yamakawa T, Sekihara H. T lymphopenia in obese diabetic (db/db) mice is non-selective and thymus independent. Life Sci. 1998; 62: 1243-50

[22] Tilg H, Moschen AR. Adipocytokines: mediators linking adipose tissue, inflammation and immunity. Nature Reviews Immunology 2006; 6:772-783.

[23] Matarese G, Moschos S, Mantzoros CS. Leptin in immunology. J Immunol. 2005; 174: 3137-42.

[24] Zarkesh-Esfahani H, Pockley G, Metcalfe RA, et al. High-dose leptin activates human leukocytes via receptor expression on monocytes. J Immunol. 2001; 167: 4593-9

[25] Mancuso P, Canetti C, Gottschalk A, Tithof PK, Peters-Golden M. Leptin augments alveolar macrophage leukotriene synthesis by increasing phospholipase activity and enhancing group IVC iPLA2 (cPLA2gamma) protein expression. Am J Physiol Lung Cell Mol Physiol. 2004; 287: 497-502.

[26] Raso GM, Pacilio M, Esposito E, Coppola A, Di Carlo R, Meli R. Leptin potentiates IFN-gamma-induced expression of nitric oxide synthase and cyclo-oxygenase-2 in murine macrophage J774A.1. Br J Pharmacol. 2002; 137: 799-804

[27] Caldefie-Chezet F, Poulin A, Tridon A, Sion B, Vasson MP. Leptin: a potential regulator of polymorphonuclear neutrophil bactericidal action? J Leukoc Biol. 2001; 69: 414-8.

[28] Caldefie-Chezet F, Poulin A, Vasson MP. Leptin regulates functional capacities of polymorphonuclear neutrophils. Free Radic Res. 2003; 37: 809-14.

[29] Tian Z, Sun R, Wei H, Gao B. Impaired natural killer (NK) cell activity in leptin receptor deficient mice: leptin as a critical regulator in NK cell development and activation. Biochem Biophys Res Commun. 2002; 298: 297-302.

[30] Lam, Q. L. K., Liu, S., Cao, X. and Lu, L., Involvement of leptin signaling in the survival and maturation of bone marrow-derived dendritic cells. Eur. J. Immunol. 2006. 36(12): 3118-3130.

[31] Farooqi IS, Matarese G, Lord GM, et al. Beneficial effects of leptin on obesity, T cell hyporesponsiveness, and neuroendocrine/metabolic dysfunction of human congenital leptin deficiency. J Clin Invest. 2002;110: 1093-103.

[32] Lord GM, Matarese G, Howard JK, Baker RJ, Bloom SR, Lechler RI. Leptin modulates the T-cell immune response and reverses starvation-induced immunosuppression. Nature. 1998; 394: 897-901.

[33] Howard JK, Lord GM, Matarese G, et al. Leptin protects mice from starvation-induced lymphoid atrophy and increases thymic cellularity in ob/ob mice. J Clin Invest. 1999; 104: 1051-9.

[34] Ruter J, Hoffmann T, Demuth HU, Moschansky P, Klapp BF, Hildebrandt M. Evidence for an interaction between leptin, T cell costimulatory antigens CD28, CTLA-4 and CD26 (dipeptidyl peptidase IV) in BCG-induced immune responses of leptin- and leptin receptor-deficient mice. Biol Chem. 2004; 385:537-41.

[35] Sanna V, Di Giacomo A, La Cava A, et al. Leptin surge precedes onset of autoimmune encephalomyelitis and correlates with development of pathogenic T cell responses. J Clin Invest. 2003; 111: 241-50

[36] Faggioni R, Feingold KR, Grunfeld C. Leptin regulation of the immune response and the immunodeficiency of malnutrition. FASEB J. 2001; 14: 2565-71.

[37] Faggioni R, Fantuzzi G, Gabay C, et al. Leptin deficiency enhances sensitivity to endotoxin-induced lethality. Am J Physiol. 1999; 276: 136-42

[38] Williams L, Bradley L, Smith A, Foxwell B. Signal transducer and activator of transcription 3 is the dominant mediator of the anti-inflammatory effects of IL-10 in human macrophages. J Immunol. 2004; 172: 567-76.

[39] Busso N, So A, Chobaz-Peclat V, et al. Leptin signaling deficiency impairs humoral and cellular immune responses and attenuates experimental arthritis. J Immunol. 2002; 168: 875-82

[40] Siegmund B, Sennello JA, Jones-Carson J, et al. Leptin receptor expression on T lymphocytes modulates chronic intestinal inflammation in mice. Gut. 2004; 53: 965-72.

[41] Barbier M, Cherbut C, Aube AC, Blottiere HM, Galmiche JP. Elevated plasma leptin concentrations in early stages of experimental intestinal inflammation in rats. Gut 1998; 43: 783-790

[42] Tuzun A, Uygun A, Yesilova Z, et al. Leptin levels in the acute stage of ulcerative colitis. J Gastroenterol Hepatol. 2004; 19:429-32

[43] Matarese G, Carrieri PB, La Cava A, et al. Leptin increase in multiple sclerosis associates with reduced number of CD4(+)CD25+ regulatory T cells. Proc Natl Acad Sci. 2005; 102: 5150-5

[44] Matarese G, Di Giacomo A, Sanna V, et al. Requirement for leptin in the induction and progression of autoimmune encephalomyelitis. J Immunol. 2001; 166: 5909-16

[45] Fantuzzi G, Sennello JA, Batra A, et al. Defining the role of T cell-derived leptin in the modulation of hepatic or intestinal inflammation in mice. Clin Exp Immunol. 2005; 142: 31-8

[46] Matarese G, Sanna V, Lechler RI, et al. Leptin accelerates autoimmune diabetes in female NOD mice. Diabetes. 2002; 51: 1356-61

[47] Palmer G, Aurrand-Lions M, Contassot E, Talabot-Ayer D, Ducrest-Gay D, Vesin C, Chobaz-Peclat V, Busso N, Gabay C. Indirect effects of leptin receptor deficiency on lymphocyte populations and immune response in db/db mice. J Immunol. 2006 Sep 1;177(5):2899-907.

[48] Canavan B, Salem RO, Schurgin S, et al. Effects of physiological leptin administration on markers of inflammation, platelet activation, and platelet aggregation during caloric deprivation. J Clin Endocrinol Metab. 2005; 90: 5779-85.

[49] Sennello J.A,, Fayad R., Morris A.M., et al. Regulation of T cell-mediated hepatic inflammation by adiponectin and leptin. Endocrinology. 2005; 146: 2157-64

[50] Fraser DA, Thoen J, Reseland JE, Forre O, Kjeldsen-Kragh J. Decreased CD4+ lymphocyte activation and increased interleukin-4 production in peripheral blood of rheumatoid arthritis patients after acute starvation. Clin Rheumatol 1999; 18: 394-401.

[51] Otero M, Lago R, Gomez R, Lago F, Dieguez C, Gomez-Reino JJ, Gualillo O. Changes in fat-derived hormones plasma concentrations: adiponectin, leptin, resistin and visfatin in rheumatoid arthritis subjects. Ann Rheum Dis. 65(9):1198-201

[52] Bokarewa M, Bokarew D, Hultgren O, Tarkowski A. Leptin consumption in the inflamed joints of patients with rheumatoid arthritis. Ann Rheum Dis 2003; 62: 952-6

[53] Goldring MB. The role of the chondrocyte in osteoarthritis. Arthritis Rheum. 2000; 43: 1916-26.

[54] Goldring MB, Berenbaum F. The regulation of chondrocyte function by proinflammatory mediators: prostaglandins and nitric oxide. Clin Orthop Relat Res. 2004; 427: 37-46

[55] Dumond H, Presle N, Terlain, B, et al. Evidence for a key role of leptin in osteoarthritis. Arthritis Rheum. 2003; 48: 3118-29.

[56] Teichtahl AJ, Wluka AE, Proietto J, Cicuttini FM. Obesity and the female sex, risk factors for knee osteoarthritis that may be attributable to systemic or local leptin biosynthesis and its cellular effects. Med Hypotheses. 2005; 65: 312-5.

[57] Otero M, Gomez Reino JJ, Gualillo O. Synergistic induction of nitric oxide synthase type II: in vitro effect of leptin and interferon-gamma in human chondrocytes and ATDC5 chondrogenic cells. Arthritis Rheum. 2003; 48: 404-9.

[58] Otero M, Lago R, Lago F, Reino JJ, Gualillo O. Signalling pathway involved in nitric oxide synthase type II activation in chondrocytes: synergistic effect of leptin with interleukin-1. Arthritis Res Ther. 2005; 7: 581-591.

[59] Kadowaki T, Yamauchi T, Kubota N, Hara K, Ueki K, Tobe K. Adiponectin and adiponectin receptors in insulin resistance, diabetes, and the metabolic syndrome.J Clin Invest. 2006; 116(7):1784-1792.

[60] Ronti T, Lupattelli G, Mannarino E, The endocrine role of adipose tissue: an update. Clin Endocrinol 2006; 64:355-365.

[61] Berg AH, Scherer PE. Adipose tissue, inflammation, and cardiovascular disease.Circ Res. 2005; 96(9):939-49.

[62] Whitehead JP, Richards AA, Hickman IJ, MacDonald GA, Prins JB. Adiponectin, a key adipokine in the metabolic syndrome. Diabetes, Obesity and Metabolism 2006; 8:264-280.

[63] Kadowaki T, Yamauchi T. Adiponectin and adiponectin receptors. Endocrine Rev 2005 26: 439-451.

[64] Tan KC, Xu C, Chow WS, Lam MC, Ai VH, Tam SC, Lam KS. Hypoadiponectinemia is associated with impaired endothelium-dependent vasodilation. J Clin Endocrinol Metab 2004; 89: 765-760.

[65] Fasshuer M, Kralish S, Klier M, Lossner U, Bluher M, Klein J,Paschke R. Adiponectin gene expression and secretion is inhibited by IL-6 in 3T3-L1 adipocytes. Biochem Biophys Res Comm 2003; 301:1045-1050.

[66] Bruun JM, Lihn AS, Verdich C, Pedersen SB, Toubro S, Astrup A, Richelsen B. Regulation of adiponectin by adipose tissue derived cytokines: in vivo and in vitro investigations in humans. Am J Physiol Endocrinol Metab, 2003; 285: E527-E533.

[67] Takemura Y, Ouchi N, Shibata R, Aprahamian T, Kirber MT, Summer RS, Kihara S, and Walsh K. Adiponectin modulates inflammatory reactions via calreticulin

receptor–dependent clearance of early apoptotic bodies. J Clin Invest .Published January 25, 2007. 10.1172/JCI29709

[68] Maeda N, Takahashi M, Funahashi T, Kihara S, Nishizawa H, Kishida K,Nagaretani H, Matsuda M, Komuro R, Ouchi N, Kuriyama H, Hotta K, Nakamura T,Shimomura I, Matsuzawa Y.   PPARgamma ligands increase expression and plasma concentrations of adiponectin, an adipose-derived protein.Diabetes. 2001; 50(9):2094-9.

[69] Funahashi T, Nakamura T, Shimomura I, Maeda K, Kuriyama H, Takahashi M, Arita Y, Kihara S, Matsuzawa Y.   Role of adipocytokines on the pathogenesis of atherosclerosis in visceral obesity. Intern Med. 1999; 38(2):202-6.

[70] Pischon T, Girman CJ, Hotamisligil GS, Rifai N, Hu FB, Rimm EB. Plasma adiponectin levels and risk of myocardial infarction in men. JAMA. 2004; 291(14):1730-7.

[71] Ehling A, Schaffler A, Herfarth H, Tarner IH, Anders S, Distler O, Paul G, Distler J, Gay S, Scholmerich J, Neumann E, Muller-Ladner U. The potential of adiponectin in driving arthritis. J Immunol. 2006;176(7):4468-78.S

[72] Schaffler A, Ehling A, Neumann E, Herfarth H, Paul G, Tarner I, et al. Adipocytokines in synovial fluid. JAMA 2003; 290:1709–10.

[73] Fantuzzi G. Adipose tissue, adipokines, and inflammation. J Allergy Clin Immunol, 2005; 115 (5): 911-919.

[74] Xu A, Wang Y, Keshaw H, Xu LY, Lam KS, Cooper GJ.   The fat-derived hormone adiponectin alleviates alcoholic and nonalcoholic fatty liver diseases in mice.J Clin Invest. 2003; 112(1):91-100.

[75] Kamada Y, Tamura S, Kiso S, Matsumoto H, Saji Y, Yoshida Y, Fukui K, Maeda N, Nishizawa H, Nagaretani H, Okamoto Y, Kihara S, Miyagawa J, Shinomura Y,Funahashi T, Matsuzawa Y. Enhanced carbon tetrachloride-induced liver fibrosis in mice lacking adiponectin. Gastroenterology. 2003; 125(6):1796-807

[76] Masaki T, Chiba S, Tatsukawa H, Yasuda T, Noguchi H, Seike M, Yoshimatsu H. Adiponectin protects LPS-induced liver injury through modulation of TNF-alpha in KK-Ay obese mice. Hepatology. 2004; 40(1):177-84.

[77] Housa D, Housova J, Vernerova Z, Haluzik M.   Adipocytokines and cancer.Physiol Res. 2006; 55(3):233-44.

[78] Kato H, Kashiwagi H, Shiraga M, Tadokoro S, Kamae T, Ujiie H, Honda S,Miyata S, Ijiri Y, Yamamoto J, Maeda N, Funahashi T, Kurata Y, Shimomura I,Tomiyama Y, Kanakura Y.   Adiponectin acts as an endogenous antithrombotic factor. Arterioscler Thromb Vasc Biol. 2006; 26(1):224-30.

[79] Holcomb IN, Kabakoff RC, Chan B, Baker TW, Gurney A, Henzel W, Nelson C, Lowman HB, Wright BD, Skelton NJ, Frantz GD, Tumas DB, Peale FV Jr, Shelton DL, Hebert CC. FIZZ1, a novel cysteine-rich secreted protein associated with pulmonary inflammation, defines a new gene family. EMBO J. 2000; 19(15):4046-55

[80] Rajala MW, Obici S, Scherer PE, Rossetti L. Adipose-derived resistin and gut-derived resistin-like molecule-beta selectively impair insulin action on glucose production. J Clin Invest. 2003;111(2):225-30.

[81] Gerstmayer B, Kusters D, Gebel S, Muller T, Van Miert E, Hofmann K, Bosio A. Identification of RELM gamma, a novel resistin-like molecule with a distinct expression pattern. Genomics. 2003; 81(6):588-95.

[82] Koerner A, Kratzsch J, Kiess W. Adipocytokines: leptin-the classical. Resistin- the controversical, adiponectin-the promising, and more to come. Best Pract Res Clin Endocrinol Metab 2005; 19: 525-546.

[83] Steppan CM, Bailey ST, Bhat S, Brown EJ, Banerjee RR, Wright CM, Patel HR, Ahima RS, Lazar MA. The hormone resistin links obesity to diabetes. Nature. 2001; 409(6818):307-12.

[84] Pang S, Le Y. Role of Resistin in inflammation and inflammation related diseases. Cell Mol Immunol, 2006; 3(1):29-34

[85] Bokarewa M, Nagaev I, Dahlberg L, Smith U, Tarkowski A. Resistin, an adipokine with potent proinflammatory properties. J Immunol. 2005; 174(9):5789-95.

[86] Lehrke M, Reilly MP, Millington SC, Iqbal N, Rader DJ, Lazar MA. An inflammatory cascade leading to hyperresistinemia in humans. PLoS Med. 2004; 1(2):e45.

[87] Harsch IA, Koebnick C, Wallaschofski H, Schahin SP, Hahn EG, Ficker JH,Lohmann T, Konturek PC. Resistin levels in patients with obstructive sleep apnoea syndrome--the link to subclinical inflammation? Med Sci Monit. 2004; 10(9):CR510-5.

[88] Reilly MP, Lehrke M, Wolfe ML, Rohatgi A, Lazar MA, Rader DJ. Resistin is an inflammatory marker of atherosclerosis in humans. Circulation. 2005; 111(7):932-9.

[89] Verma S, Li SH, Wang CH, Fedak PW, Li RK, Weisel RD, Mickle DA. Resistin promotes endothelial cell activation: further evidence of adipokine-endothelial interaction. Circulation. 2003; 108(6):736-40.

[90] Kawanami D, Maemura K, Takeda N, Harada T, Nojiri T, Imai Y, Manabe I, Utsunomiya K, Nagai R. Direct reciprocal effects of resistin and adiponectin on vascular endothelial cells: a new insight into adipocytokine-endothelial cell interactions. Biochem Biophys Res Commun. 2004; 314(2):415-9

[91] Burnett MS, Lee CW, Kinnaird TD, Stabile E, Durrani S, Dullum MK, Devaney JM, Fishman C, Stamou S, Canos D, Zbinden S, Clavijo LC, Jang GJ, Andrews JA,Zhu J, Epstein SE. The potential role of resistin in atherogenesis. Atherosclerosis.2005; 182(2):241-8.

[92] Senolt L, Housa D, Vernerova Z, Jirasek T, Svobodova R, Veigl D, Anderlova K, Muller-Ladner U, Pavelka K, Haluzik M. Resistin is abundantly present in rheumatoid arthritis synovial tissue,synovial fluid, and elevated serum resistin reflects disease activity. Ann Rheum Dis. 2006; [Epub ahead of print].

[93] Schaffler A, Ehling A, Neumann E, Herfarth H, Tarner I, Scholmerich J,Muller-Ladner U, Gay S. Adipocytokines in synovial fluid. JAMA. 2003; 290(13):1709-10.

[94] Fukuhara A, Matsuda M, Nishizawa M, Segawa K, Tanaka M, Kishimoto K, Matsuki Y, Murakami M, Ichisaka T, Murakami H, Watanabe E, Takagi T, Akiyoshi M, Ohtsubo T, Kihara S, Yamashita S, Makishima M, Funahashi T, Yamanaka S, Hiramatsu R,Matsuzawa Y, Shimomura I. Visfatin: a protein secreted by visceral fat that mimics the effects of insulin. Science. 2005; 307(5708):426-30.

[95] Jia SH, Li Y, Parodo J, Kapus A, Fan L, Rotstein OD, Marshall JC. Pre-B cell colony-enhancing factor inhibits neutrophil apoptosis in experimental inflammation and clinical sepsis. J Clin Invest. 2004; 113(9):1318-27.

[96] Moschen AR, Kaser A, Enrich B, Mosheimer B, Theurl M, Niederegger H, Tilg H.Visfatin, an adipocytokine with proinflammatory and immunomodulating properties.J Immunol. 2007 Feb 1; 178(3):1748-58.

[97] Tatemoto, K., Hosoya, M., Habata, Y., Fujii, R., Kakegawa, T., Zou, M. X., Kawamata, Y., Fukusumi, S., Hinuma, S., Kitada, C., et al., Isolation and characterization of a novel endogenous peptide ligand for the human APJ receptor. Biochem. Biophys. Res. Commun.1998; 251,471-476.

[98] Boucher, J., Masri, B., Daviaud, D., Gesta, S., Guigné, C., Mazzucotelli, A., Castan-Laurell, I., Tack, I., Knibiehler, B., Carpene, C., Audigier, Y., Saulnier-Blache, J. S., Valet, P. Apelin, a newly identified adipokine up-regulated by insulin and obesity. Endocrinology 2005; 146,1764-1771.

[99] Daviaud D, Boucher J, Gesta S, Dray C, Guigne C, Quilliot D, Ayav A, Ziegler O, Carpene C, Saulnier-Blache JS, Valet P, Castan-Laurell I. TNFalpha up-regulates apelin expression in human and mouse adipose tissue. FASEB J. 2006; 20(9):1528-30.

[100] Heinonen, M. V., Purhonen, A. K., Miettinen, P., Paakkonen, M., Pirinen, E., Alhava, E., Akerman, K., Herzig, K. H. Apelin, orexin-A and leptin plasma levels in morbid obesity and effect of gastric banding. Regul. Pept. 2005; 130:7-13.

[101] Xu, H., Barnes, G. T., Yang, Q., Tan, G., Yang, D., Chou, C. J., Sole, J., Nichols, A., Ross, J. S., Tartaglia, L. A., Chen, H. Chronic inflammation in fat plays a crucial role in the development of obesity-related insulin resistance. J. Clin. Invest. 2003; 112:1821-1830.

[102] K. Hida, J. Wada, J. Eguchi, H. Zhang, M. Baba, A. Seida, I. Hashimoto, T. Okada, A. Yasuhara, A. Nakatsuka, K. Shikata, S. Hourai, J. Futami, E. Watanabe, Y. Matsuki, R. Hiramatsu, S. Akagi, H. Makino and Y.S. Kanwar, Visceral adipose tissue-derived serine protease inhibitor: a unique insulin-sensitizing adipocytokine in obesity, Proc. Natl. Acad. Sci. USA 2005; 102: 10610–10615.

[103] Kloting N, Berndt J, Kralisch S, Kovacs P, Fasshauer M, Schon MR, Stumvoll M, Bluher M. Vaspin gene expression in human adipose tissue: association with obesity and type 2 diabetes.Biochem Biophys Res Commun. 2006; 339(1):430-6.

3

Estrogen Receptors in Glucose Homeostasis

Malin Hedengran Faulds and Karin Dahlman-Wright

Karolinska Institutet

Sweden

1. Introduction

Metabolic diseases affect more than 230 million people worldwide with an expectancy to increase to around 350 million in the coming 25 years. It is currently the fourth leading cause of death by disease. The metabolic syndrome refers to a group of interrelated metabolic abnormalities that include disturbed glucose homeostasis, insulin resistance (IR), increased body weight and abdominal fat accumulation, mild dyslipidemia and hypertension. Individuals with the metabolic syndrome have an increased risk of cardiovascular disease (CVD) and Type 2 diabetes (T2D).

Estrogens have traditionally been connected with female reproduction, however, the importance of these hormones in tissues outside of the reproductive system including the liver, bone, the cardiovascular system and brain have since been established (Gruber et al., 2002). Estrogen and the estrogen receptors (ERs) are well-known regulators of glucose homeostasis and several epidemiological and prospective studies associate estrogen to various aspects of the metabolic syndrome (Louet et al., 2004). Postmenopausal women develop visceral obesity, IR and are at high risk for T2D. Treatment of healthy postmenopausal women with estrogen has been shown to improve insulin sensitivity and to lower blood glucose (Crespo et al., 2002). Furthermore, hormone replacement therapy (HRT) in postmenopausal women with coronary artery disease was associated with a 35% reduction in the incidence of T2D (Kanaya et al., 2003). Male aromatase-deficient patients, as well as a male patient with loss of ERα function, display impaired glucose metabolism, IR and hyperinsulinemia (Zirilli, et al. 2008). In addition, the aromatase deficient patients showed impaired liver functions, hepatic steatosis, and altered lipid profile (Maffei, et al. 2004). Additional observations in rodents support the notion that estrogen mediates anti-diabetic effects. For example, female rodents are protected against hyperglycemia, unless they are ovariectomized, in spontaneous rodent models of T2D.

Studies in knock-out mouse models have shed light on the role of estrogen and its receptors in rodent obesity and glucose tolerance. Mice with functional knock-out of the aromatase enzyme (ArKO mice) are unable to synthesize endogenous estrogen and display an obese and insulin resistant phenotype (Fisher et al., 1998). A similar phenotype was observed in mice lacking ERα (ERαKO) but not in mice lacking ERβ (ERβKO), indicating that ERα is the major mediator for the estrogenic effects on insulin sensitivity and body weight (Heine et al., 2000). Although ERα appears to be more important in relation to body weight and insulin sensitivity, it remains possible that ERβ also contributes in this context, particularly in older mice and under specific metabolic conditions (Foryst-Ludwig et al., 2008).

2. Carbohydrate metabolism

Carbohydrate catabolism starts with digestion in the small intestine where monosaccharides derived from food are absorbed into the circulation. The most important carbohydrate is glucose, which is metabolized by most organisms. Circulating levels of glucose are controlled by two hormones; insulin and glucagon. When circulating levels of glucose are raised, insulin is secreted by the pancreatic β cells to stimulate glucose uptake in liver, muscles and white adipose tissue (WAT), where excess glucose is stored as glycogen by the process of glycogenesis. When blood glucose levels decrease, glucagon is secreted from the pancreatic α cells to stimulate the breakdown of glycogen to glucose through glycogenolysis (see figure 1).

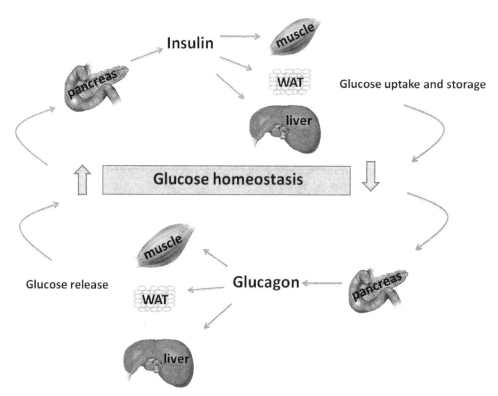

Fig. 1. **Regulation of glucose homeostasis.** In response to glucose excess, insulin is secreted by the pancreatic β cells to stimulate glucose uptake and storage in muscles, liver and white adipose tissue (WAT). When glucose levels decrease, glucagon is secreted to stimulate glucose release into circulation.

The β cells in the pancreatic islets of Langerhans release insulin in two phases. The first is a rapid response to increase blood glucose levels and the second phase is a slow release that is triggered independently of glucose. There are several substances apart from glucose known to stimulate insulin release, including amino acids from dietary proteins, acetylcholine released from vagus nerve endings, gastrointestinal hormones and glucose-dependent insulinotropic peptides (reviewed by (Kieffer et al., 1996)).

The hormone glucagon is secreted from the α cells in the pancreatic islets of Langerhans and promotes conversion of hepatic glycogen into glucose, which is subsequently released into the blood. The output of glucagon is triggered by low levels of circulating glucose (Nussey & Whitehead, 2001).

IR is a physiological condition where insulin is less effective in lowering circulating glucose. IR in muscle and WAT reduces glucose uptake whereas hepatic IR results in reduced glycogen synthesis and storage and a failure of insulin to suppress glucose production and subsequent release into the blood (reviewed by (Benito, 2011)). IR commonly refers to the reduced glucose lowering effects of insulin as described above. However, other functions of insulin are also affected. For example, IR in adipocytes results in reduced uptake of circulating lipids and increased hydrolysis of stored triglycerides, which leads to elevated levels of circulating free fatty acids (Savage et al., 2007). High plasma levels of insulin, glucose and lipids due to IR are major components of the metabolic syndrome, which could develop into T2D.

3. Estrogen signaling and estrogen receptors

Estrogens are sex steroids, which stem from the common pre-cursor cholesterol. The last step in the synthesis of estrogen from androgens is catalyzed by the P450 enzyme aromatase. The three major physiological estrogens include 17β-estradiol (E2), estrone (E1) and estriol. The major physiological estrogen in fertile females is E2, which has a similar affinity for both ERs. In addition, ERs are activated by a range of synthetic ligands including selective estrogen receptor modulators (SERMs) such as raloxifen and tamoxifen, the ERα selective agonist propyl-pyrazole-triol (PPT) and the ERβ-selective agonist diarylpropionitrile (DPN) (Heldring et al., 2007).

Estrogens exert their physiological effects through the two ER subtypes, ERα and ERβ, which are members of the superfamily of nuclear receptors. The human ESR1 gene, which is encoding for ERα, is located on the chromosome 6, at 6q25.1, and includes 8 exons. The ERβ encoding gene, ESR2, is located on chromosome 14 at 14q22–24. ERα is mainly expressed in reproductive tissues, kidney, bone, WAT and liver, while ERβ is expressed in the ovary, prostate, lung, gastrointestinal tract, bladder and the central nervous systems (CNS) (Matthews & Gustafsson, 2003).

Genetic associations have been described for polymorphisms of the ESR1 gene and several pathological conditions related to metabolism in general, including cardiovascular diseases, T2D, myocardial infarction, hypertension and venous thromboembolism (Schuit et al., 2004; Shearman et al., 2003; Yoshihara et al., 2009). Polymorphisms of the ESR1 gene can also affect lipoprotein metabolism (Lamon-Fava et al., 2010).

ESR2 polymorphisms have been associated with anorexia nervosa, bulimic disease and premature coronary artery disease (Eastwood et al., 2002; Nilsson et al., 2004; Peter et al., 2005). ERs share a common structure with the other members of the nuclear receptor family. The N-terminal A/B domain is the most variable region with less than 20% amino acid identity between the two ERs and confers subtype specific actions on target genes. This region harbors the activation function-1 (AF-1), which is ligand-independent and shows promoter- and cell-specific activities. The centrally located C-domain harbors the DNA binding domain (DBD), which is involved in DNA binding and receptor dimerization. This domain is highly conserved between ERα and ERβ with 97% amino acid identity. The D-domain is referred to as the hinge domain and displays low conservation between ERα and ERβ (30%). This domain has been shown to contain a nuclear localization signal. The C-terminal E-domain contains the ligand-binding domain (LBD) and the two subtypes display 56% conservation in this region. The LBD contains a hormone-dependent activation function (AF-2) and also includes functions responsible for ligand binding and receptor dimerization. The F-domain has less than 20% amino acid identity between the two ER subtypes and the functions of this domain remain undefined (Zhao et al., 2008).

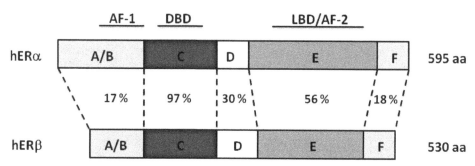

Fig. 2. **Structure and homology between human ERα and ERβ.** The A/B domain is referring to the ligand independent transcription activation function-1 (AF-1). The C domain is mediating DNA binding and the D domain represents the hinge domain, which harbors nuclear localization signals. The E domain is involved in ligand binding and contains the ligand dependent AF-2 function, which is involved in ligand binding. Depicted is also the homology in percent between the various domains between the two subtypes.

Like other nuclear receptors, ligand-bound ERs act as dimers to regulate transcriptional activation. Full transcriptional activity of the ERs is mediated through a synergistic action between the two activation domains, AF-1 and AF-2. Both ERα and ERβ contain a potent AF-2 function, but unlike ERα, ERβ seems to have a weaker corresponding AF-1 function and depends more on the ligand-dependent AF-2 for its transcriptional activation function (Dahlman-Wright et al., 2006). In their unliganded state, ERs are associated with protein complexes of heat shock proteins, which inhibit their functions.

The classical estrogen signaling occurs through a direct binding of ligand activated ER dimers to estrogen-responsive elements (EREs) in the regulatory regions of estrogen target genes followed by activation of the transcriptional machinery at the transcription start sites of regulated genes. Estrogen also modulates gene expression by a second mechanism in which ERs interact with other DNA bound transcription factors, such as activating protein-1 (AP-1) and stimulating protein-1 (Sp-1) to regulate gene expression, through a process referred to as transcription factor cross-talk. Estrogen may also elicit effects through non-genomic mechanisms, which involve the activation of downstream signaling cascades like protein kinase A (PKA), protein kinase C (PKC) and mitogen-activated protein (MAP) kinase via membrane-localized ERs.

Recently, an orphan G protein-coupled receptor (GPR) 30 in the cell membrane was reported to mediate non-genomic and rapid estrogen signaling (Revankar et al., 2005; Thomas et al., 2005). GPR30 is structurally unrelated to ERα and ERβ and the rapid effects from stimulation of this receptor include release of intracellular Ca^{2+} and subsequent activation of calcium-calmodulin-dependent kinases or activation of MAP kinase and phosphoinositide 3-kinase pathways. Human GPR30 is located on chromosome 7p22.3, and is composed of three exons. Exon3 constitutes the amino acid coding region of GPR30. Based on genetic linkage analysis, the region of the chromosome containing GPR30 is thought to be related to familial hypertensive disease in humans (Lafferty et al., 2000). The mRNA for GPR30 appears to be expressed in most tissues.

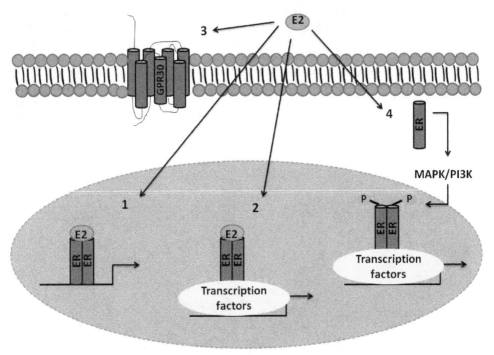

Fig. 3. **Estrogen signaling mechanisms.** I. Classical pathway involving activation of the ERs followed by DNA binding. II. Non-classical pathway involving interactions with transcription factors and subsequent indirect DNA binding. III. Non-genomic pathway involving GPR30. IV. Ligand-independent pathway involving kinase cascades and subsequent ER phosphorylation.

4. Estrogen signaling in glucose homeostasis

Estrogen and estrogen signaling have long been known to be important regulators of glucose homeostasis and are implicated in maintaining normal insulin sensitivity. Fluctuations in estrogen levels below the physiological range, as a consequence of menopause or ovariectomy, may promote IR and T2D. In humans, the most consistent effects of oral contraceptives or HRT are decreased levels of fasting plasma glucose and improved glucose tolerance. Absence of estrogen signaling in men, due to deficiency of the aromatase enzyme or ERα, results in impaired glucose metabolism. It has also been shown that polymorphisms in the ERα gene are associated with development of the metabolic syndrome and T2D (Yoshihara et al., 2009).

Estrogens further display inhibitory effects on maltase, sucrose and lactase activities in the intestine. Estrogen supplements have been shown to manifest a range of disaccharidase and lipase inhibitory actions that help to delay the absorption of dietary carbohydrates in the intestine, which will lead to suppression of the increased glucose levels observed after meals (Hamden et al., 2011).

Several rodent studies link estrogen to glucose regulatory effects. Female rodents are protected against hyperglycemia, unless they are ovariectomized, in spontaneous rodent models of T2D and ArKO mice display severe IR (Jones et al., 2000). ERα and ERβ have both been suggested to be involved in blood glucose homeostasis. ERαKO mice are insulin resistant and ERα has been shown to be involved in regulation of glucose metabolism by acting in different tissues including liver, skeletal muscle, adipose tissue, endocrine pancreas and the central nervous system (CNS) as depicted in figure 4. Although ERα appears to be more important in relation to body weight and insulin sensitivity, it remains possible that ERβ also contributes in this context, particularly in older mice and under specific metabolic conditions.

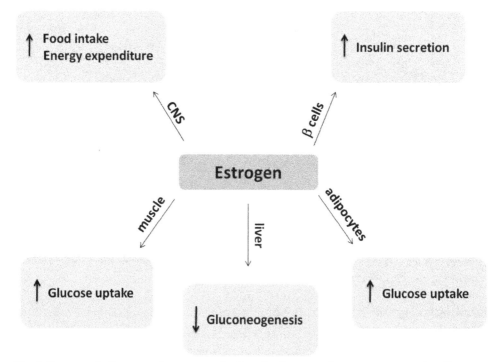

Fig. 4. **Estrogen influences glucose metabolism in the central nervous system (CNS), pancreatic β cells, muscles, liver and adipocytes.**

4.1 ERs and the role of the central nervous system in glucose homeostasis

The first finding supporting that the central nervous system (CNS) was involved in the regulation of glucose homeostasis was that ruptures in the fourth ventricle resulted in glucosuria. This initial study was followed by numerous other studies and it is now firmly established that the CNS regulates glucose homeostasis through the hormones insulin, leptin and glucagon-like peptide (GLP)-1, as well as by glucose and fatty acids (FA). A series of complex systems regulate energy homeostasis in order to keep energy levels and body weight stable (Miller, 1982). Glucose is the vital energy source for the brain. There are several glucose sensing neurons in the hypothalamus, which have been established to be essential components in the regulation of feeding behavior and hypoglycemic counter-regulatory responses (reviewed in (Marty et al., 2007)). The hypothalamus is subdivided into interconnecting nuclei, including the arcuate nucleus (ARC), paraventricular nucleus (PVN), ventromedial nucleus (VMN), dorsomedial nucleus (DMN) and lateral hypothalamic area (LHA) (Simpson et al., 2009). These central brain circuits receive signals from the periphery, which indicate satiety, energy levels and energy stores (Morton et al, 2006) and process these afferent signals to modulate food intake and energy expenditure.

The actions of insulin have also been shown to play a direct role in the CNS since neuron-specific insulin receptor deficient (NIRKO) mice develop mild IR and display elevated circulating insulin levels (Bruning et al., 2000). Injections of insulin directly into the third cerebral ventricle have been shown to suppress hepatic glucose production without effecting body weight or circulating levels of insulin (Obici et al., 2002). Further, inhibition of insulin or its downstream signaling pathway in the CNS, i.e. the insulin receptor and phosphatidylinositol-3 kinase (PI3K), impaired the ability of increased levels of insulin to suppress gluconeogenesis. Targeted deletion of insulin receptor expression selectively in the hypothalamus elicited IR in rats, which is in accordance with the results in NIRKO mice. These studies show that the CNS regulates glucose homeostasis through the action of insulin and requires intact insulin signaling pathways involving the binding of insulin to its receptor and subsequent activation of down-stream mediators.

Estrogen is known to be highly relevant for the regulation of satiety, energy expenditure and body weight. Ovariectomy and menopause are associated with increased food intake, which can be reversed with estrogen replacement therapy (Eckel, 2004; Tchernof et al., 2000). The anorectic effects of estrogen are partially mediated through actions in the hypothalamus as demonstrated by studies showing that direct E2 injections into the PVN area or the ARC/VMN of the hypothalamus effectively reduced food intake (Butera & Beikirch, 1989; Nunez et al., 1980). The same study also showed that the hypothalamic neurons, which regulate energy homeostasis, were affected by E2 administration. Energy homeostasis and feeding behavior controlled by the hypothalamus also follow the menstrual cycle and food intake in women varies across the cycle with the lowest daily food intake during the peri-ovulatory period when estrogen levels are peaking (Asarian & Geary, 2006).

ERα and ERβ are both expressed in the different areas of the hypothalamus (Gillies & McArthur, 2010). ERα appears to be the major mediator of the estrogenic effects on central regulation of body weight by estrogens but whether this is regulated by food intake or actions on energy expenditure is controversial. Total ERα knockout mice are obese with increased fat accumulation in the absence of increased food intake. Targeted disruption of ERα in the VMN areas in the hypothalamus of female mice leads to weight gain, increased visceral adiposity, hyperphagia, hyperglycemia and impaired energy expenditure (Musatov et al., 2007). ERβ knockout mice, on the other hand, display similar food consumption patterns as wild-type mice (Foryst-Ludwig et al., 2008).

4.2 ERs and the role of pancreatic β cells in glucose homeostasis

The endocrine pancreas is an adapting tissue with the capacity to quickly respond to variations in the metabolic status of the organism. The β cells in the islets of Langerhans readily adapt to peripheral IR by increasing their secretory response, as well as their cell mass. If β cells fail to compensate, blood glucose concentration will rise to pathological levels and frank T2D will develop.

Estrogenic effects on various physiological aspects of the islet of Langerhans have been known for a long time and estrogens are established regulators of pancreatic β cell functions. In humans, E2 reverses the effect of menopause on glucose and insulin metabolism, resulting in increased pancreatic insulin secretion, as well as improved insulin sensitivity (Brussaard et al., 1997; Stevenson et al., 1994). Plasma insulin levels are increased in pregnant rats in response to the increased levels of estrogen. Studies in mice have suggested that long-term exposure to E2 increased insulin content, insulin gene expression and insulin release without changing β cell mass. E2 has also been shown to acutely enhance glucose stimulated insulin secretion at physiological concentrations through the action of ERα both *in vitro* and *in vivo* (Alonso-Magdalena et al., 2008; Nadal et al., 1998).

ERα has been identified as the functional predominant receptor isoform in the murine pancreas. E2-dependent insulin release in cultured pancreatic islets was reduced in ERα-deficient mice, when compared to islets derived from either ERβ-deficient or wild-type mice (Alonso-Magdalena et al., 2008). Also, E2, acting mainly through ERα, has been shown to protect pancreatic β cells from apoptosis induced by oxidative stress in mice.

Even though ERα seems to be the dominant subtype to convey the estrogenic response in the pancreas, the role of ERβ might also be of importance. ERβ-deficient mice have been shown to display a mild islet hyperplasia and delayed first phase insulin release (Barros et al., 2009).

The membrane bound estrogen-responsive GPR30 is also expressed in rodent pancreas. Studies using adult female GPR30-deficient mice reveal that these mice do not exhibit E2-induced release of insulin, which is consistent with experiments using isolated pancreatic islet cells *in vitro* (Martensson et al., 2009). There are not any differences in expression of glucose-related genes, such as the glucose transporter (GLUT) 2 and glucokinase, in GPR30 knockout mice when compared with wild-type mice (Martensson et al., 2009). Thus, GPR30 may act as a regulator of insulin release after E2 stimulation. Consistent with this, GPR30 mRNA is expressed in secretory gland cells, which may indicate that GPR30 is involved in insulin secretion pathways (Levin & Weissman, 2009).

4.3 ERs and the role of the liver in glucose homeostasis

The liver is the largest organ in the body and possesses purifying and metabolizing functions. One of its most important tasks is to store glucose in the form of glycogen. The liver is capable of containing up to 10% of its volume as glycogen. The liver releases glycogen when nutrients are scarce. Liver glycogen is converted into circulating glucose in response to pancreatic signals; in hypoglycemic conditions glucagon is released to stimulate a release of hepatic glycogen. In a hyperglycemic state, the pancreas releases insulin to stimulate the liver to release less glucose. The maintenance of glucose homeostasis is depending on whole body glucose uptake and glucose production by glycogenolysis and gluconeogenesis in the liver.

Hepatic IR is impairment of insulin action in the liver, however, the mechanisms behind this is not completely elucidated. Hepatic IR is found in both obese non-diabetic, obese T2D patients and patients with non-alcoholic fatty livers. Early manifestations of hepatic IR are increased fasting gluconeogenesis.

Liver abnormalities are common outcomes of obesity-related IR. Hepatic steatosis is primarily caused by increased hepatic free fatty acids (FFA) released from insulin resistant adipocytes. Due to hepatic IR, hyperinsulinemia and hyperglycemia induce *de novo* lipogenesis. Fat accumulation in adipocytes is typically followed by fat deposition in the liver and skeletal muscle and by subsequent development of IR in these tissues. There are indications showing that obesity-related IR can cause fatty liver while, vice versa, excessive intra-hepatic fat accumulation may promote IR and weight gain.

Estrogens regulate liver glucose homeostasis mainly by acting via ERα as shown by studies in ERα-deficient mice. Euglycaemic-hyperinsulinaemic clamp analysis revealed that ERα deficiency was associated with a pronounced hepatic IR as determined by the inability of insulin to suppress liver glucose production (Bryzgalova et al., 2008). Global gene expression analysis of hepatic tissue isolated from ERα-deficient and control mice revealed that ERα-deficiency was associated with increased expression of key genes involved in hepatic lipid biosynthesis

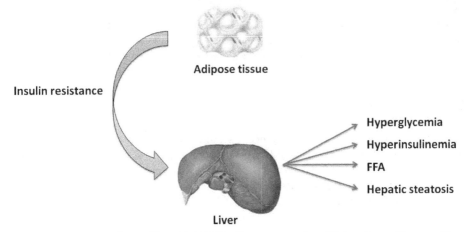

Fig. 5. **Schematic overview of hepatic IR.** The liver responds to IR in adipose tissue with increased release of glucose and free fatty acids (FFAs), as well as an increased accumulation of triglycerides, which will cause hyperinsulinemia and hepatic steatosis.

4.4 ERs and the role of skeletal muscle in glucose homeostasis

Skeletal muscle accounts for 40–60% of the human body mass and is the major site of glucose disposal, thereby regulating whole body glucose homeostasis. Insulin-stimulated disposal of circulating glucose is mediated through glucose transport across the muscle cell surface and this step is one of the rate-limiting steps for glucose clearance. Glucose crosses the plasma membranes and enters the skeletal muscle through the GLUT proteins by facilitated transport. Glucose clearance in response to postprandial insulin secretion is mainly mediated by skeletal muscle. The insulin signaling pathways inducing glucose uptake in skeletal muscle are well studied and involve insulin receptor, insulin receptor substrate (IRS), phosphatidylinositol-3 kinase (PI3-K) and AKT kinase subsequently leading to translocation of GLUT-4 to the cell membrane. IR in skeletal muscle is thought to be a primary defect in T2D (see fig. 6 for overview).

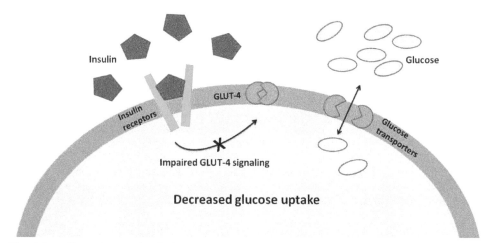

Fig. 6. **Insulin resistance in skeletal muscle cells.** When insulin binds to its receptors, translocation of GLUT-4 to the cell membrane is triggered and glucose can readily cross the cell membrane by facilitated transport and be stored in the skeletal muscles. Under insulin resistant states, the GLUT-4 signaling is impaired, leading to decreased glucose uptake by the muscles.

ERα and ERβ receptors seem to have opposing effects on the expression of GLUT-4 transporters. ERα was shown to induce and ERβ seems to inhibit GLUT-4 expression in skeletal muscle (Barros et al., 2006). Recent studies indicate that tamoxifen-treated ERα knockout mice displayed increased GLUT-4 expression in skeletal muscle, which indicates a pro-diabetogenic effect of ERβ (Barros et al., 2009). It appears that both ER isoforms determine the metabolic estrogen actions in skeletal muscle with ERα mediating protective actions and ERβ deleterious.

4.5 ERs and the role of adipose tissue in glucose homeostasis

Adipose tissue is formed by mature adipocytes, pre-adipocytes, immune cells, extracellular matrix and vascular endothelium. Under normal physiologic conditions, insulin concentrations control within a narrow range the balance between fatty acid storage as triglycerides and their release into the circulation during fasting state. Adipose tissue is very sensitive to insulin concentrations and insulin inhibits lipolysis at concentrations that are much lower than those needed to inhibit hepatic glucose production or stimulate muscle glucose uptake. Although insulin-dependent postprandial glucose disposal *in vivo* is believed to occur mainly by uptake into skeletal muscle, insulin-enhanced glucose uptake into adipose tissue also contributes to whole-body glucose homeostasis.

There are well-documented sex differences in the pathophysiology of obesity and metabolic disorders. Women tend to accumulate more subcutaneous fat whereas men accumulate more visceral fat (Bonds et al., 2006; Crespo et al., 2002; Nuutila et al., 1995). The prevalence of early IR and impaired glucose tolerance seem to be higher in men than in women.

E2 is considered an important regulator of adipose tissue development and lipid deposition in humans, rodents and other species. The deficiency of estrogen hormones after menopause or in experimental models, causes an increase in body mass and intra-abdominal adipose tissue leading to an android feature. The effects observed as a consequence of deficiency of sex steroids can be reversed by hormone replacement therapy.

Changes in adipose tissue distribution in women have been associated with increased risk of diseases and metabolic disturbances, including coronary artery disease, IR and glucose intolerance (Bonds et al., 2006). In obesity and T2D, there is a marked adipocyte resistance to the anti-lipolytic effects of insulin and the circulating FFA concentrations are typically elevated (Kissebah et al., 1976). Chronic over feeding induces metabolic stress and the adipocytes become hypertrophic and fail to proliferate and differentiate in a sufficient manner.

Sex hormone programming in animals has also been shown to affect adipose tissue. A single postnatal injection of estradiol benzoate resulted in the development of IR, increased adipose tissue mass and adipocyte size in adult female rats, suggesting that postnatal ER activation exerts strong programming effects on metabolic processes (Alexanderson et al., 2010).

Stromal cells from adipose tissue have been shown to locally produce estrogens (Simpson et al., 2009). It is well confirmed that there is a decrease in steroid hormone-binding globulins in obese states in both pre- and post-menopausal women. In post-menopausal women, there is a direct association between estrogen levels and body mass index (BMI) (Cleary & Grossmann, 2009; Lukanova et al., 2004). E2 is mainly produced by the adipocytes after menopause through conversion of androgens or estrone and this production is not regulated by feedback mechanisms (Siiteri, 1987). It is suggested that this adipose-derived E2 may participate in the ERα-mediated enrichment of insulin biosynthesis (Alonso-Magdalena et al., 2008) and in the induction of glucose stimulated insulin secretion to help the pancreatic β–cells adapt to the higher demand of insulin during obesity.

5. Concluding remarks

Lifestyle evolution and the higher intake of high calorie diets largely contribute to the worldwide growing incidence of metabolic diseases. In addition to the most common preventive strategy based on physical activity and reduced calorie intake, identification of new molecular targets able to limit the development of metabolic disturbances represents one of the most important public health challenges.

Estrogens have emerged as important regulators of glucose homeostasis during the last decades, corroborating data from clinical and experimental studies. Insulin sensitivity has been demonstrated to be higher in women before menopause than in age-matched men and postmenopausal women, which supports a beneficial effect of estrogens on insulin action and glucose homeostasis. It is also highly recognized that menopause promotes visceral fat accumulation and IR, which will ultimately lead to significantly higher risk of developing T2D. In addition, HRT has been reported to reverse the symptoms and to dampen the incidence of T2D in postmenopausal women by 21–35% compared to women not given HRT.

Effects of estrogen signaling on glucose homeostasis have been further demonstrated by studies showing that patients bearing genetic mutations and, thus, lack either ERα or aromatase expression, develop obesity, IR and impaired glucose tolerance. Genetically engineered mice models have confirmed these clinical observations, as ERα or aromatase gene deficiency similarly promotes several features of the metabolic syndrome. Taken together, ERα seems to play a protective role in insulin and glucose metabolism, with actions on the liver, adipose tissue, muscle and pancreatic β cells. In addition, ERα regulates food intake and energy expenditures through actions on the CNS. ERβ seems to have an opposing role with the potential to negatively influence insulin and glucose metabolism by impairing the function of adipose tissue and inhibiting the expression of GLUT4 in the muscle.

Established and novel ER subtype selective ligands are valuable tools for deciphering the specific roles of ERα and ERβ in physiology and disease. The development of novel treatment regimes for metabolic disease targeting ERα is hampered by the uterotrophic and mammotrophic effects of ERα with the major concern being the risk of developing hormone-dependent cancer. Further studies are needed to identify and develop novel compounds that target estrogen signaling in selective metabolic tissues but lack the mitogenic effects in others, like ovaries and the breast.

6. References

Alexanderson, C., Stener-Victorin, E., Kullberg, J., Nilsson, S., Levin, M., Cajander, S., et al. (2010) A single early postnatal estradiol injection affects morphology and gene expression of the ovary and parametrial adipose tissue in adult female rats. *J Steroid Biochem Mol Biol, 122*(1-3), 82-90.

Alonso-Magdalena, P., Ropero, A. B., Carrera, M. P., Cederroth, C. R., Baquie, M., Gauthier, B. R., et al. (2008). Pancreatic insulin content regulation by the estrogen receptor ER alpha. *PLoS One, 3*(4), e2069.

Asarian, L., & Geary, N. (2006). Modulation of appetite by gonadal steroid hormones. *Philos Trans R Soc Lond B Biol Sci, 361*(1471), 1251-1263.

Barros, R. P., Gabbi, C., Morani, A., Warner, M., & Gustafsson, J. A. (2009). Participation of ERalpha and ERbeta in glucose homeostasis in skeletal muscle and white adipose tissue. *Am J Physiol Endocrinol Metab, 297*(1), E124-133.

Barros, R. P., Machado, U. F., Warner, M., & Gustafsson, J. A. (2006). Muscle GLUT4 regulation by estrogen receptors ERbeta and ERalpha. *Proc Natl Acad Sci U S A, 103*(5), 1605-1608.

Benito, M. Tissue specificity on insulin action and resistance: past to recent mechanisms. (2011) *Acta Physiol (Oxf), 201*(3), 297-312.

Bonds, D. E., Lasser, N., Qi, L., Brzyski, R., Caan, B., Heiss, G., et al. (2006). The effect of conjugated equine oestrogen on diabetes incidence: the Women's Health Initiative randomised trial. *Diabetologia, 49*(3), 459-468.

Bruning, J. C., Gautam, D., Burks, D. J., Gillette, J., Schubert, M., Orban, P. C., et al. (2000). Role of brain insulin receptor in control of body weight and reproduction. *Science, 289*(5487), 2122-2125.

Brussaard, H. E., Gevers Leuven, J. A., Frolich, M., Kluft, C., & Krans, H. M. (1997). Short-term oestrogen replacement therapy improves insulin resistance, lipids and fibrinolysis in postmenopausal women with NIDDM. *Diabetologia, 40*(7), 843-849.

Bryzgalova, G., Lundholm, L., Portwood, N., Gustafsson, J. A., Khan, A., Efendic, S., et al. (2008). Mechanisms of antidiabetogenic and body weight-lowering effects of estrogen in high-fat diet-fed mice. *Am J Physiol Endocrinol Metab, 295*(4), E904-912.

Butera, P. C., & Beikirch, R. J. (1989). Central implants of diluted estradiol: independent effects on ingestive and reproductive behaviors of ovariectomized rats. *Brain Res, 491*(2), 266-273.

Cleary, M. P., & Grossmann, M. E. (2009). Minireview: Obesity and breast cancer: the estrogen connection. *Endocrinology, 150*(6), 2537-2542.

Crespo, C. J., Smit, E., Snelling, A., Sempos, C. T., & Andersen, R. E. (2002). Hormone replacement therapy and its relationship to lipid and glucose metabolism in diabetic and nondiabetic postmenopausal women: results from the Third National Health and Nutrition Examination Survey (NHANES III). *Diabetes Care, 25*(10), 1675-1680.

Dahlman-Wright, K., Cavailles, V., Fuqua, S. A., Jordan, V. C., Katzenellenbogen, J. A., Korach, K. S., et al. (2006). International Union of Pharmacology. LXIV. Estrogen receptors. *Pharmacol Rev, 58*(4), 773-781.

Eastwood, H., Brown, K. M., Markovic, D., & Pieri, L. F. (2002). Variation in the ESR1 and ESR2 genes and genetic susceptibility to anorexia nervosa. *Mol Psychiatry, 7*(1), 86-89.

Eckel, L. A. (2004). Estradiol: a rhythmic, inhibitory, indirect control of meal size. *Physiol Behav, 82*(1), 35-41.

Fisher, C. R., Graves, K. H., Parlow, A. F., & Simpson, E. R. (1998). Characterization of mice deficient in aromatase (ArKO) because of targeted disruption of the cyp19 gene. *Proc Natl Acad Sci U S A, 95*(12), 6965-6970.

Foryst-Ludwig, A., Clemenz, M., Hohmann, S., Hartge, M., Sprang, C., Frost, N., et al. (2008). Metabolic actions of estrogen receptor beta (ERbeta) are mediated by a negative cross-talk with PPARgamma. *PLoS Genet, 4*(6), e1000108.

Gillies, G. E., & McArthur, S. (2010) Estrogen actions in the brain and the basis for differential action in men and women: a case for sex-specific medicines. *Pharmacol Rev, 62*(2), 155-198.

Gruber, C. J., Tschugguel, W., Schneeberger, C., & Huber, J. C. (2002). Production and actions of estrogens. *N Engl J Med, 346*(5), 340-352.

Hamden, K., Jaouadi, B., Zarai, N., Rebai, T., Carreau, S., & Elfeki, A. (2011). Inhibitory effects of estrogens on digestive enzymes, insulin deficiency, and pancreas toxicity in diabetic rats. *J Physiol Biochem, 67*(1), 121-128.

Heine, P. A., Taylor, J. A., Iwamoto, G. A., Lubahn, D. B., & Cooke, P. S. (2000). Increased adipose tissue in male and female estrogen receptor-alpha knockout mice. *Proc Natl Acad Sci U S A, 97*(23), 12729-12734.

Heldring, N., Pike, A., Andersson, S., Matthews, J., Cheng, G., Hartman, J., et al. (2007). Estrogen receptors: how do they signal and what are their targets. *Physiol Rev, 87*(3), 905-931.

Jones, M. E., Thorburn, A. W., Britt, K. L., Hewitt, K. N., Wreford, N. G., Proietto, J., et al. (2000). Aromatase-deficient (ArKO) mice have a phenotype of increased adiposity. *Proc Natl Acad Sci U S A, 97*(23), 12735-12740.

Kanaya, A. M., Vittinghoff, E., Shlipak, M. G., Resnick, H. E., Visser, M., Grady, D., et al. (2003). Association of total and central obesity with mortality in postmenopausal women with coronary heart disease. *Am J Epidemiol, 158*(12), 1161-1170.

Kieffer, T. J., Heller, R. S., Unson, C. G., Weir, G. C., & Habener, J. F. (1996). Distribution of glucagon receptors on hormone-specific endocrine cells of rat pancreatic islets. *Endocrinology, 137*(11), 5119-5125.

Kissebah, A. H., Alfarsi, S., Adams, P. W., & Wynn, V. (1976). Role of insulin resistance in adipose tissue and liver in the pathogenesis of endogenous hypertriglyceridaemia in man. *Diabetologia, 12*(6), 563-571.

Lafferty, A. R., Torpy, D. J., Stowasser, M., Taymans, S. E., Lin, J. P., Huggard, P., et al. (2000). A novel genetic locus for low renin hypertension: familial hyperaldosteronism type II maps to chromosome 7 (7p22). *J Med Genet, 37*(11), 831-835.

Lamon-Fava, S., Asztalos, B. F., Howard, T. D., Reboussin, D. M., Horvath, K. V., Schaefer, E. J., et al. (2010). Association of polymorphisms in genes involved in lipoprotein metabolism with plasma concentrations of remnant lipoproteins and HDL subpopulations before and after hormone therapy in postmenopausal women. *Clin Endocrinol (Oxf), 72*(2), 169-175.

Levin, P. D., & Weissman, C. (2009). Obesity, metabolic syndrome, and the surgical patient. *Anesthesiol Clin, 27*(4), 705-719.

Louet, J. F., LeMay, C., & Mauvais-Jarvis, F. (2004). Antidiabetic actions of estrogen: insight from human and genetic mouse models. *Curr Atheroscler Rep, 6*(3), 180-185.

Lukanova, A., Lundin, E., Zeleniuch-Jacquotte, A., Muti, P., Mure, A., Rinaldi, S., et al. (2004). Body mass index, circulating levels of sex-steroid hormones, IGF-I and IGF-binding protein-3: a cross-sectional study in healthy women. *Eur J Endocrinol, 150*(2), 161-171.

Maffei, L., Murata, Y., Rochira, V., Tubert, G., Aranda, C., Vazquez, M., Clyne, C.D., Davis, S., Simpson, E.R. & Carani, C. (2004) Dysmetabolic syndrome in a man with a novel mutation of the aromatase gene: effects of testosterone, alendronate, and estradiol treatment. *J Clin Endocrinol Metab, 89*, 61-70.

Martensson, U. E., Salehi, S. A., Windahl, S., Gomez, M. F., Sward, K., Daszkiewicz-Nilsson, J., et al. (2009). Deletion of the G protein-coupled receptor 30 impairs glucose tolerance, reduces bone growth, increases blood pressure, and eliminates estradiol-stimulated insulin release in female mice. *Endocrinology, 150*(2), 687-698.

Marty, N., Dallaporta, M., & Thorens, B. (2007). Brain glucose sensing, counterregulation, and energy homeostasis. *Physiology (Bethesda), 22*, 241-251.

Matthews, J., & Gustafsson, J. A. (2003). Estrogen signaling: a subtle balance between ER alpha and ER beta. *Mol Interv, 3*(5), 281-292.

Miller, D. S. (1982). Factors affecting energy expenditure. *Proc Nutr Soc, 41*(2), 193-202.

Morton, G. J., Cummings, D. E., Baskin, D. G., Barsh, G. S., & Schwartz, M. W. (2006). Central nervous system control of food intake and body weight. *Nature, 443*(7109), 289-295.

Musatov, S., Chen, W., Pfaff, D. W., Mobbs, C. V., Yang, X. J., Clegg, D. J., et al. (2007). Silencing of estrogen receptor alpha in the ventromedial nucleus of hypothalamus leads to metabolic syndrome. *Proc Natl Acad Sci U S A, 104*(7), 2501-2506.

Nadal, A., Rovira, J. M., Laribi, O., Leon-quinto, T., Andreu, E., Ripoll, C., et al. (1998). Rapid insulinotropic effect of 17beta-estradiol via a plasma membrane receptor. *Faseb J, 12*(13), 1341-1348.

Nilsson, M., Naessen, S., Dahlman, I., Linden Hirschberg, A., Gustafsson, J. A., & Dahlman-Wright, K. (2004). Association of estrogen receptor beta gene polymorphisms with bulimic disease in women. *Mol Psychiatry, 9*(1), 28-34.

Nunez, A. A., Gray, J. M., & Wade, G. N. (1980). Food intake and adipose tissue lipoprotein lipase activity after hypothalamic estradiol benzoate implants in rats. *Physiol Behav, 25*(4), 595-598.

Nussey, S., & Whitehead, S. (2001).

Nuutila, P., Maki, M., Laine, H., Knuuti, M. J., Ruotsalainen, U., Luotolahti, M., et al. (1995). Insulin action on heart and skeletal muscle glucose uptake in essential hypertension. *J Clin Invest, 96*(2), 1003-1009.

Obici, S., Zhang, B. B., Karkanias, G., & Rossetti, L. (2002). Hypothalamic insulin signaling is required for inhibition of glucose production. *Nat Med, 8*(12), 1376-1382.

Peter, I., Shearman, A. M., Vasan, R. S., Zucker, D. R., Schmid, C. H., Demissie, S., et al. (2005). Association of estrogen receptor beta gene polymorphisms with left ventricular mass and wall thickness in women. *Am J Hypertens, 18*(11), 1388-1395.

Revankar, C. M., Cimino, D. F., Sklar, L. A., Arterburn, J. B., & Prossnitz, E. R. (2005). A transmembrane intracellular estrogen receptor mediates rapid cell signaling. *Science, 307*(5715), 1625-1630.

Savage, D. B., Petersen, K. F., & Shulman, G. I. (2007). Disordered lipid metabolism and the pathogenesis of insulin resistance. *Physiol Rev, 87*(2), 507-520.

Schuit, S. C., Oei, H. H., Witteman, J. C., Geurts van Kessel, C. H., van Meurs, J. B., Nijhuis, R. L., et al. (2004). Estrogen receptor alpha gene polymorphisms and risk of myocardial infarction. *Jama, 291*(24), 2969-2977.

Shearman, A. M., Cupples, L. A., Demissie, S., Peter, I., Schmid, C. H., Karas, R. H., et al. (2003). Association between estrogen receptor alpha gene variation and cardiovascular disease. *Jama, 290*(17), 2263-2270.

Siiteri, P. K. (1987). Adipose tissue as a source of hormones. *Am J Clin Nutr, 45*(1 Suppl), 277-282.

Simpson, K. A., Martin, N. M., & Bloom, S. R. (2009). Hypothalamic regulation of food intake and clinical therapeutic applications. *Arq Bras Endocrinol Metabol, 53*(2), 120-128.

Stevenson, J. C., Crook, D., Godsland, I. F., Collins, P., & Whitehead, M. I. (1994). Hormone replacement therapy and the cardiovascular system. Nonlipid effects. *Drugs, 47 Suppl 2,* 35-41.

Tchernof, A., Poehlman, E. T., & Despres, J. P. (2000). Body fat distribution, the menopause transition, and hormone replacement therapy. *Diabetes Metab, 26*(1), 12-20.

Thomas, P., Pang, Y., Filardo, E. J., & Dong, J. (2005). Identity of an estrogen membrane receptor coupled to a G protein in human breast cancer cells. *Endocrinology, 146*(2), 624-632.

Yoshihara, R., Utsunomiya, K., Gojo, A., Ishizawa, S., Kanazawa, Y., Matoba, K., et al. (2009). Association of polymorphism of estrogen receptor-alpha gene with circulating levels of adiponectin in postmenopausal women with type 2 diabetes. *J Atheroscler Thromb, 16*(3), 250-255.

Zhao, C., Dahlman-Wright, K., & Gustafsson, J. A. (2008). Estrogen receptor beta: an overview and update. *Nucl Recept Signal, 6*, e003.

Zirilli, L., Rochira, V., Diazzi, C., Caffagni, G., & Carani, C. (2008) Human models of aromatase deficiency. *J Steroid Biochem Mol Biol, 109*, 212-218.

4

Glucokinase as a Glucose Sensor in Hypothalamus - Regulation by Orexigenic and Anorexigenic Peptides

Carmen Sanz, Isabel Roncero, Elvira Alvarez,
Verónica Hurtado and Enrique Blázquez
*University Complutense of Madrid. Medical School and CIBERDEM,
Department of Cellular Biology and Department of Biochemistry and Molecular Biology,
Spain*

1. Introduction

Glucose homeostasis requires hormonal and neural mechanisms in an attempt to get a normal functioning of the brain and of peripheral tissues. Blood glucose levels must be maintained within a physiological range depending of feeding and hormonal status, having the alterations of normoglycemic levels deleterious consequences. Hypothalamus plays a major role on feeding behaviour and energy homeostasis. It contains the called "satiety centre" and "hunger centre" located in ventromedial (VMH) and lateral hypothalamus (LH) respectively. These brain areas, besides others, may be altered by metabolic signals, such as changes in the electrical activity of neurons by direct application of glucose or by modifications of blood glucose levels. In this regard, glucose activates or inhibits neuronal activity, and both responses suggest the presence of glucose sensors in these brain areas.

Glucose sensors are molecular designs responsible for detecting and measuring glucose concentrations in the extracellular space. Thus, glucose sensor are presents in gut, endocrine pancreatic cells, portal vein, central nervous system and rare neuroendocrine cells, and they are responsible to avoid marked blood glucose oscillations, which permit to maintain glucose homeostasis.

First evidence of the existence of a glucose sensor system was reported in pancreatic beta-cells (Matschinsky 1990), constituted by glucokinase (GK). GK catalyses glucose phosphorylation with low afffinity and it is not inhibited by its product (glucose-6-phosphate), which allows increased glucose utilization as its concentration rises. Due to GK properties, the glucose catabolism rate is proportional to glucose levels in the extracellular space and for that reason GK is the major contributor to glucose sense, since catalyses the rate-limiting step of glucose catabolism. Interestingly, glucose transporter isoform 2 (GLUT-2) also with a high Km for glucose transport, has a different role since glucose transport occurs in both directions of the beta-cell membrane and glucose transport is 100-fold higher that the rates of glucose metabolism.

Our previous findings (Alvarez et al., 1996; Navarro et al., 1996) indicating the presence of GK together with GLUT-2 and glucagon-like peptide-1 receptor (GLP-1R) in the same cells of hypothalamic areas implied in the control of feeding behaviour, suggest that a glucose sensor system may be present in those structures as discussed in the section 3.

GLP-1, together with others peptides, such as leptin, insulin, GLP-2, are anorexigenic peptides that acts in hypothalamic areas contributing to generate a state of satiety. By the contrary peptides orexigenic such as neuropeptide Y (NPY), orexin, galanin, ghrelin, etc, contribute to increase food intake. These effects may be the results of an accurate molecular crosstalk between the cells which secrete these peptides and the glucose sensing cells.

The importance of GK in the hypothalamic glucose sensing and its relation with anorexigenic and orexigenic peptides are discussed in this chapter.

2. Brain glucose sensor

Glucose is needed as an energy substrate but also as a signaling molecule in several processes. Glucoregulatory mechanisms are of primary functional concern to provide a continued glucose supply to the central neurons system and to face metabolic needs of peripheral tissues. Alterations of normoglycemic levels have deleterious consequences that increase the morbidity and mortality rates of the population.

In the 1950's, the glucostatic hypothesis (Mayer 1953) postulated that glucose receptors exist in the hypothalamus and possibly in other central and peripheral regions involved in the regulation of food intake. Thus, glucose balance should be tightly regulated and taking into account the pancreatic glucose sensor concept, it would be reasonable to suggest the existence of a similar system in the brain that might modulate feeding behaviour and the release of counteregulatory hormones that defend against hypoglycemia. We proposed (Alvarez et al., 1996; Navarro et al., 1996) that the hypothalamus senses plasma glucose levels in a similar fashion to beta-cells, causing changes in the expression and secretion of neuropeptides (Yang et al., 2004). Our findings indicated that GK mRNA and protein are coexpressed together with GLUT-2 in the hypothalamus of human and experimental animals, mainly in areas involved in the control of food intake such as VMH and LH (Navarro et al., 1996; Roncero et al., 2000). Taking into account these studies, it have been addressed central role of GK as glucose sensor, reinforced by GLUT-2, the K^+_{ATP} channel subunits SUR1 and SUR2, as well as Kir6.2, in central glucose sensing (Jordan et al., 2010).

By analogy with the beta-cell, the general idea is that the glucose metabolism and variations in ratio ATP/ADP are the keys for neural sensing of glucose. However the ATP metabolism is a general mechanism for any electrical response, while neurons produce specific electrical responses. Others authors have proposed relationship between neuronal glucose-sensing and electrical responses (Figure 1). These hypothesis include electrogenic glucose entry, the existence of specific non-transporting detectors of extracellular glucose or glucose receptors and the possibility that glial cells would be responsible of glucose changes detection.

An example of electrogenic glucose entry to neuron is the mediated by the sodium–glucose co-transporters (SGLTs), where glucose is directly coupled to Na$^+$ ion movement. That entry is directly conditioned by extracellular glucose concentration. This mechanism is used in the secretion of GLP-1 by intestinal cells in response to glucose (Gribble et al., 2003) and in the excitability of glucose-response neurons of VMH and arcuate nucleus (ARC) (Yang et al., 1999) that will comment below.

Diez-Sampedro suggest the existence of a "glucose receptor" that mediates the changes in electrical activitiy (Diez-Sampedro et al., 2003). Thus, in some peripheral neurons, have been identified a glucose transporter protein (SGLT3/SLC5A4) that not transport glucose into the cell, instead, this protein acted as a sensing receptor, converting elevations of extracellular glucose into Na⁺-dependent depolarization of the membrane (Figure 1).

An additional hypothesis (Pellerin & Magistretti 2004) is that astrocytes could be the primary physiological detectors of extracellular glucose changes. This model proposed that rise in extracellular glucose induce glial lactate production which is transported from glia and into the neurons by lactate transporter (MCT1) and trigger the depolarization and excitation of neurons by closing the K^+_{ATP} channels (Burdakov & Ashcroft 2002) (Figure 1).

2.1 Glucose-inhibited (GI) and glucose-excited (GE) neurons

Claude Bernard showed the earliest evidence that the brain is involved in glycemic control since the lesion of the hypothalamus in dog, induced hyperglycemia (Bernard 1849). Later, Jean Mayer (Mayer 1953) proposed that hypothalamic cells could monitor plasma glucose variations and postulated that these cells transduced variations of glucose concentrations into electrical or chemical signals that control feeding behavior. Electrophysiological studies carried out in hypothalamic slices, demonstrated the existence of neurons able to modulate their firing activity in response to changes in extracellular glucose levels (Anand et al., 1964). These are glucose-excited (GE; previously called glucose-responsive) neurons, which increase their firing rate with elevation of glucose concentrations in extracellular, or glucose-inhibited (GI; previously called glucose-sensitive) neurons, which are activated by a decrease in extracellular glucose concentration or by cellular glucoprivation (Routh 2002; Yang et al., 2004).

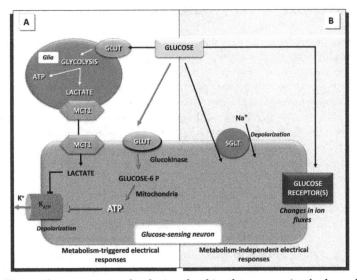

Fig. 1. Signalling pathways proposed to be involved in glucose sensing by hypothalamic neurons. A) Signalling pathways of glucose-metabolism-triggered electrical responses for neural sensing of glucose. Red lines indicate the canonical pathways share with beta-cell. Other signalling pathways could be mediate by previous glucose metabolization to lactate by glial cells. B) Pathways that triggers glucose metabolism-independent electrical responses. These pathways involved electrogenic glucose entry through sodium-glucose cotransporters (SGLT) or the presence of glucose receptors

Although both types of neurons are widely distributed in the brain, they are highly present in regions involved in the control of energy homeostasis and food intake such as hypothalamic nuclei and the brain stem (Adachi et al., 1995). Additionally it has been recently reported a novel glucose-sensing region in the medial amygdalar nucleus (Zhou et al., 2010).

The existence of glucose-regulated neurons has been studied by intravenous or intracerebroventricular injections of 2-deoxyglucose or 5-thio-glucose and posterior electrophysiological recordings or by the detection c-fos-like immunoreactivity (which is highly expressed in activated neurons). Using these approaches, responsive neurons have been found in the VMH, paraventricular (PVN) and LH, ARC, parabrachial nucleus (PBN), nucleus tractus solitarius (NTS), area postrema (AP), dorsal motor nucleus of the vagus (DMNX), and the region of the basolateral medulla (BLM) (Ritter & Dinh 1994; Dallaporta et al., 1999).

2.2 Electrophysiological pattern

Diverse signalling pathways are involved in the modulation of the electrical activity of hypothalamic neurons by glucose. On the one hand, glucose could alter neuronal electrical activity acting as energy substrate by influencing energy metabolism inside neuron and glia cells (Figure 1). On the other hand glucose could be considerer as an extracellular signalling messenger that could trigger specific glucose receptors controlling the membrane ion fluxes. Other possibility could be that glucose itself can be transported by electrogenic transporters (Figure 1). Which of these general mechanisms is dominant in different glucose-sensing neurons remains to be determined.

The mechanisms regulating GE cells have been more thoroughly understood and were assumed to employ a beta-cell glucosensing strategy. Thus, glucose enters the beta-cell via GLUT-2, facilitating its diffusion down a concentration gradient. Then GK phosphorylates glucose allowing for its entry into the glycolytic pathway that leads to an increase in the ATP. The consequent increase in the cytosolic ATP/ADP concentration ratio then closes the K^+_{ATP} channels. In the beta-cell, these channels are made up of Kir6.2/SUR1 subunits (Ashcroft & Rorsman 2004). Since open K^+_{ATP} channels generate hyperpolarization of the beta-cell and so dampen its excitability, their closure results in decreasing potassium outflow and depolarization with increased electrical activity. Actually, GK are the key glucose-sensing features of this scheme because they ensure that changes in extracellular glucose levels within the physiological range are converted to proportional changes in electrical excitability. This is due to the low affinity for glucose of GK, unlike the more ubiquitously expressed hexokinase I, and that GK is not inhibited by its product, glucose-6-phosphate.

The functional importance of GK in GE neurons was studied by pharmacological inhibition which decreased neuronal activity. *In vitro* studies on primary VMH cultures have shown that selective downregulation of GK leads to selective loss of glucose sensing and a decrease in cellular ATP concentration corresponding with an increase in K^+_{ATP} channel activation (Dunn-Meynell et al., 2002; Kang et al., 2006). This supports the model that inhibition of GK, in at least a proportion of GE neurons, reduces ATP production causing K^+_{ATP} channel opening and cell hyperpolarization. Recent findings indicate that although elements of canonical model used in beta-cell, are functional in some hypothalamic cells, this pathway is not universally essential for excitation of glucose-sensing neurons by glucose. In rats and humans, the expression of GLUT-2, GK (Navarro et al., 1996; Roncero et al., 2000) and Kir6.2 was found in some but not all GE neurons (Kang et al., 2004) and were also present in non-glucose-sensing neurons (Lynch et al., 2000). For example, glucose-induced excitation of ARC neurons was recently reported in mice lacking Kir6.2, and no significant increases in cytosolic ATP levels could be detected in hypothalamic neurons after changes in extracellular glucose. Thus, the molecular support for the idea that all GE neurons rely on the beta-cell tools to sense glucose is currently inconclusive and possible alternative glucose-sensing strategies could include electrogenic glucose entry, glucose-induced release of glial lactate, and extracellular glucose receptors (Pellerin & Magistretti 2004; Burdakov et al., 2005).

Much less is known about GI neurons and whether these neurons follow the same glucose sensing strategy remains unclear (Burdakov & Lesage 2010). It has been proposed to involve reduction in the depolarizing activity of the Na^+/K^+ pump, or activation of a hyperpolarizing Cl⁻ current. Although it has been suggested that the metabolic model of glucose sensing applies to GI neurons, there is convincing evidence for metabolism-independent neuronal glucose sensing in GI neurons. As it has been mentioned, Kang group's (Kang et al., 2004) showed that some but not all glucose sensing neurons of the VMN express GK and SUR1, suggesting that other regulatory mechanisms must control glucose sensing in some of these neurons. Furthermore, Gonzalez et al (Gonzalez et al., 2009), used direct electrophysiological measurements of glucose sensing orexin neurons to show that metabolism independent glucose sensing exists in GI neurons. They found that GK inhibitors do not block glucose sensing in these neurons. However, despite the evidence for metabolism-independent as well as dependent glucose sensing mechanisms, the nature of the glucose sensing machinery in GI neurons remains unclear.

2.3 Hypothalamic distribution of GE and GI neurons

Hypothalamic glucose-sensing neurons comprise subgroups of cells in PVN, LH, ARC, VMH hypothalamic regions, and can be either electrically inhibited or excited by elevations in extracellular glucose (Anand et al., 1964; Oomura et al., 1969; Routh 2002; Wang et al., 2004). The distribution of GE glucose response neurons in the hypothalamus are confinated mostly to the VMH, ARC, and PVN (Dunn-Meynell et al., 1998; Silver & Erecinska 1998; Wang et al., 2004). However, GI neurons are found mainly in the LH (Oomura et al., 1974), median ARC, and PVN.

There are two major subpopulations of neurons in the ARC of the hypothalamus implicated in the control of feeding. One population contains pro-opiomelanocortin (POMC) and α-melanocyte-stimulating hormone (α-MSH) that are anorexigenic peptides and inhibits food intake. The second population of neurons contains agouti-related protein (AgRP) and neuropeptide Y (NPY) orexigenic peptides that stimulate food intake (Cone et al., 2001). GI neurons are present in the VMN in the ARC and in the LH and partly overlap with the orexigenic NPY/AgRP and possibly orexin neurons. GE neurons correspond in part to POMC neurons in the VMN and possibly in the ARC and POMC neurons in the LH (Mountjoy & Rutter 2007).

2.4 Effect of glucose concentrations on the brain glucose sensors

Some of the glucose-sensing neurons in the LH, ARC and VMH hypothalamic regions electrically respond to changes in glucose within the physiological ranges of glucose (Wang et al., 2004; Burdakov et al., 2005; Song & Routh 2005). As a general rule, the extracellular concentration of glucose in the brain is 10–30% of that in the blood (Silver & Erecinska 1998). During euglycemia, brain glucose levels are 0.7-2.5 mM, and may be reached 5mM under severe plasma hyperglycemia. On the other hand, plasma hypoglycaemia can cause the brain glucose to fall to 0.2-0.5 mM. Changes in plasma glucose corresponding to meal-to-meal fluctuation (about 5–8mM) (Silver & Erecinska 1994) lead to changes in glucose concentration in the brain that it is expected to be in the range between 1 and 2.5mM (Routh 2002). It is also noteworthy that glucose-sensing neurons located near regions with a reduced blood–brain barrier for example, the median eminence region that neighbors the hypothalamic ARC (Elmquist et al., 1999), may be exposed to a much higher glucose concentrations than other brain cells, even approaching those present in the plasma. If this is the case, for glucose-sensing neurons of the ARC, high glucose concentrations (greater than 5 mM) may well comprise a physiologically relevant stimulus (Fioramonti et al., 2004) . In this way, it has been described in the ARC, the presence of GE and GI neurons responsive to glucose over either a low (0–5 mM) or a high glucose concentration range (5–20 mM); the latter are referred to as high GE (HGE) or high GI (HGI) neurons, respectively (Fioramonti et al., 2004; Penicaud et al., 2006).

More details about the effect of glucose oscillations in the glucose sensor GK will be discussed in the section 4 of this chapter.

3. Glucokinase as part of a hypothalamic glucose sensor system

GK is a member of the hexokinase family (ATP:D-hexose 6-phosphotransferase, EC 2.7.1.1) that catalyses the phosphorylation of glucose to glucose 6-phosphate. Hexokinases I, II and III have a high affinity for glucose, with low Km (Michaelis constant) values in the micromolar range. GK or hexokinase type IV has a low affinity for glucose; it is not inhibited by physiological concentrations of glucose 6-phosphate, and has a molecular mass of about 50 kDa (Iynedjian 1993)

For years, the liver and the pancreatic islets were considered to be the only tissues in which GK activity could be detected. Later on, GK mRNAs of appropriate sizes were found in the corticotroph anterior pituitary cell line AtT-20, in rat pituitaries (Hughes et al., 1991) and in brain and intestine of the rat, but no enzyme activity was reported in neither (Jetton et al., 1994; Alvarez et al., 1996; Navarro et al., 1996). However, Roncero et al 2000 described that GK gene expression in rat brain gave rise to a protein of 52 kDa, with a high Km phosphorylating activity. Brain GK showed kinetic properties similar to those previously reported for the enzyme of hepatic or pancreatic islet origin. It has a high apparent Km for glucose (8.9–15 mM) and displays no product inhibition by glucose 6-phosphate. The contribution of GK to the total glucose phosphorylating activity was 40–19% in different cerebral regions, measured with a radiometric assay, and of 25–14% as determined by a spectrophotometric method.

The presence of tissue-specific promoters in the GK gen allows differential regulation. The upstream promoter, now rightly called neuro-endocrine promoter to distinguish it from the hepatic promoter (Iynedjian et al., 1996; Levin et al., 2004), is functional in beta-cells and in the brain (Magnuson & Shelton 1989; Roncero et al., 2000), while the downstream promoter is used only in liver . GK levels in beta-cells appear to be controlled by glucose, probably through a post-transcriptional mechanism (Iynedjian 1993; Matschinsky et al., 1993). In contrast, the liver-specific promoter is mainly affected by insulin and glucagon, which explains the extraordinary transcriptional regulation by the nutritional state (Iynedjian 1993).

The short-term regulation of GK activity involves several mechanisms: Long-chain fatty acyl-CoAs have been shown to be allosteric competitive inhibitors in vitro of the liver enzyme (Tippett & Neet 1982) and human beta-cell GK (Moukil et al., 2000). Glucose regulates the activity of GK through a "mnemonic" mechanism, which increases the activity of liver GK in the presence of high levels of glucose and decreases it when the glucose level is low (Cornish-Bowden & Storer 1986). GK activity in the liver is also regulated by the GK regulatory protein (GKRP), which behaves as a competitive inhibitor of GK. In the presence of fructose 6-phosphate GKRP binds to GK and inhibits its activity, whereas fructose 1-phosphate prevents the formation of the complex GKRP-GK (Van Schaftingen 1989). GKRP is not only a protein that binds and inactivates GK, but also regulates the translocation of GK between the cytoplasm and the nucleus. When glycogenolysis and/or gluconeogenesis are activated, the concentration of fructose 6-phosphate increases in the liver and produces the inhibition of GK, which facilitates the release of glucose by the liver. When carbohydrates are present in the diet, fructose is phosphorylated to fructose-1 phosphate, which favours glucose utilization by the liver (Agius & Peak 1993; Toyoda et al., 1995; Shiota et al., 1999). Thus, in the liver, the subcellular translocation of GK regulates the enzyme activity in accordance with the metabolic needs of the cells. It is therefore accepted that translocation of GK to the nucleus at low glucose concentrations needs GKRP as an anchoring protein that allows transport through the nuclear pore complex. However, it is unclear whether the nuclear export of GK requires GKRP. In pancreatic islets, GK activity may also be regulated by a protein, in a similar way to that described in hepatocytes (Malaisse et al., 1990).

Subsequent research has also identified several GK binding proteins that could act as cytoplasmic binding proteins. They include a dual-specificity protein phosphatase, the glucokinase-associated phosphatase (Munoz-Alonso et al., 2000), and the bifunctional enzyme 6-phosphofructo-2-kinase/fructose-2,6-bisphosphatase (Baltrusch et al., 2001). Other studies indicate that a minor fraction of GK and GKRP may be integrated in a multienzyme complex, including the pro-apoptotic protein BAD, and become associates with mitochondria in hepatocytes (Arden et al., 2006). These data suggest the existence of different pools of cytoplasmic GK with specialized metabolic functions (Arden et al., 2006). It has also been reported that AMP-activated protein kinase (AMPK) inhibits GK translocation from the nucleus.

In pancreatic beta-cells GK is considered to be a true glucose sensor (Matschinsky 1990) involved in glucose-dependent insulin release. The GK glucose sensor concept is supported by the fact that GK mutations are responsible for some types of maturity-onset diabetes of the young-2 (MODY-2) (Vionnet et al., 1992) and for persistent hyperinsulinaemic hypoglycaemia in infancy (PHHI) (Christesen et al., 2002). In addition, as noted above, targeted disruption of the GK gene in the beta-cells of mice produces severe alterations in insulin release (Grupe et al., 1995).

3.1 Expression, activity and localization of hypothalamic GK and glucokinase regulatory protein (GKRP) in the hypothalamus

Several brain areas, such as the LH and VMH and the dorsomedial medulla oblongata, including the NTS and the motor nucleus of the vagus, modulate glucose homeostasis in the liver and pancreas (Oomura & Yoshimatsu 1984). As previously cited, glucose is mainly excitatory in the VMH and inhibitory in the LH and NTS (Oomura & Yoshimatsu 1984), suggesting the presence of glucose sensors in neurons of these brain areas. Indeed, stimulation of glucoreceptors present in the neurons of the VMH, promotes the release of the counter-regulatory hormones, catecholamines and glucagon, which defend the organism against glucopenia (Borg et al., 1995).

Our findings, indicate that GLUT-2, GK and GLP-1R are expressed in the same cells of the rat and human hypothalamus (Alvarez et al., 1996) (Figure 2), and are located in areas involved in the regulation of energy homeostasis, feeding behaviour and glucose metabolism. It is noteworthy that in the brain, GLP-1 contributes to reducing food intake (Navarro et al., 1996; Turton et al., 1996), and the co-localization of those three components in hypothalamic neurons suggests that a glucose sensor system may be involved in the transduction of signals required to produce a state of satiety.

As we previously cited, GK activity may also be regulated by GKRP, acting in accordance with the metabolic needs of the cells (Van Schaftingen et al., 1984; Shiota et al., 1999; Roncero et al., 2004). Interestingly, we reported the coexpression of GK and GKRP in both rat and human brains (Roncero et al., 2000; Alvarez et al., 2002; Roncero et al., 2004), as well as GKRP interacting with GK in the presence of fructose-6-phosphate, which suggests that both are active and both may participate in the glucosensing process in the central nervous system (Alvarez et al., 2002).

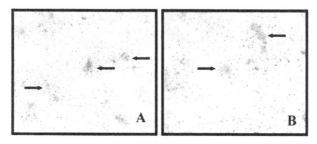

Fig. 2. In situ hybridization histochemistry of GLP-1R and GLUT-2 or GK mRNAs. **A** double-labeling of GLP-1R and GLUT-2 mRNAs in the VMH. **B** Double-labeling of GLP-1R and GK mRNAs in the VMH. Silver grains indicate the localization of either GLUT-2 or GK mRNAs. Blue reaction product indicates labelling of GLP-1R mRNAs. (Microphotographs suministrated by Dr. J. Chowen)

GK and GKRP have been found in foetal pancreas and liver (Vandercammen & Van Schaftingen 1993; Garcia-Flores et al., 2002). Also in foetal hypothalamus GK mRNA was present in day 18 of development (Sutherland et al., 2005). Our result concluded that GK and GKRP were functionally active before birth in the rat brain. Both proteins colocalised in the same cells of hypothalamus and the cerebral cortex of 21-day-old foetuses (F-21) (Roncero et al., 2009) (Figure 3).

The presence of GK mRNA was confirmed in approximately 50% of GE and GI neurons in the VMH. Some of these neurons also contained mRNAs for subunits of K^+_{ATP} channels (Kang et al., 2004). The use of specific small interfering RNA (siRNA) to knock-down GK in primary cultures of neurons from the rat VMH, abolished the responses to glucose (Kang et al., 2006). Together, these findings supported the idea that GK was the glucose sensor of at least a fraction of VMH neurons, functioning as the rate determining enzyme of glucose metabolism and controlling neuronal excitability. In the VMH, GK mRNA was shown to be expressed in neurons synthesizing POMC and NPY/AgRP, which play critical roles in neural pathways involved in the regulation of food intake and energy expenditure.

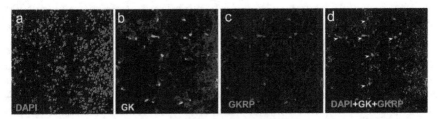

Fig. 3. GK and GKRP detection in the hypothalamus. Inmunofluorescent detection of GK (green b) or GKRP (red c) proteins in VMH from twenty-one-day old foetuses. Nuclear staining (a) was carried out in blue with 4,6-diamid-o-2-phenylindole (DAPI). The arrows (d) indicate the double positive cells for GK and GKRP.

4. Regulation of hypothalamic GK by glucose or regulatory peptides

The glucose-sensing neurons have receptors for orexigenic and anorexigenic neuropeptides that may modulate feeding behaviour through a glucose sensor system (Schuit et al., 2001).

The effects of orexigenic and anorexigenic peptides and glucose on GK gene expression were tested (Sanz et al., 2007) in GT1-7 immortalized hypothalamic neurons, which are glucose-sensing cells (Lee et al., 2005) able to respond to glucose deprivation or high-glucose levels, as well as having intrinsic GK activity. Neither the promoter activity of the GK gene in transfected GT1-7 cells nor the endogenous GK gene expression were modified by the action of different concentrations of glucose or GLP-1, leptin, or NPY in the extracellular space. However, GK enzyme activities were modified by these peptides.

Using hypothalamic slices in culture, instead cell line, which it is a better physiological model, the effect of glucose orexigenic and anorexigenic peptides on GK activities in VMH and LH areas were assayed. In the VMH there was a tendency for GK activities to increase as glucose rose in the extracellular media and high-GK activity was found at lower glucose concentrations in the LH. These findings could reflect a different type of behavior for the GE and GI neurons located in the VMH and the LH, when challenged by different concentrations of glucose. This would be in agreement with the tendency of GK activity to increase with rises in glucose in the range of 0.5–20 mM that was reported in the VMH (Sanz et al., 2007), while neurons in LH were not excited by the higher concentrations of glucose but by lower concentrations of this hexose, as happens with GK activities (Sanz et al., 2007). The observed changes in GK activity in response to glucose in certain hypothalamic areas suggest that such activity would not only be tissue-specific but also even cell-specific in defined brain areas. Interestingly, GK activities were thus significantly lower in LH than in VMH at high glucose concentrations, but this effect was reversed by the presence of insulin. This distinctive response observed in LH at high glucose may be related to different functional activities of these two areas, rather than to other kind of effects. The data obtained in these studies indicate a different response to glucose levels in the VMH and LH and also that some orexigenic and anorexigenic peptides might modulate GK activities in neurons of these areas. Additionally, it suggests that in most of the cases modifications of hypothalamic GK occur at the enzyme activity level rather than in transcriptional expression.

5. Role of hypothalamic GK on the control of feeding behaviour and body weight

Coexpression of GLUT-2, GK and GKRP in areas involved in feeding behaviour (Roncero et al., 2000; Roncero et al., 2004) might play a role in glucose sensing, in which GK and GKRP made possible a real sensor activity. Furthermore the effects of anorexigenic and orexigenic peptides through its receptors in this system should facilitate the transduction of signals required to produce a state of satiety. In fact, we have reported experimental evidences that GLP-1 is an anorexigenic peptide and controls the glucose metabolism in the human hypothalamus areas involved in the regulation of feeding behaviour (Alvarez et al., 2005) (Navarro et al., 1996).

5.1 Anorexigenic and orexigenic peptides

Early suggestions that hypothalamus plays a major role on feeding behaviour and energy homeostasis were obtained after brain lesion and stimulation studies. Remembering these observations, such as electrical stimulation of VMH suppress food intake and that bilateral lesions of these structures induce hyperphagia and obesity, VMH was named as the satiety centre, while alterations of LH induced the opposite set of responses and thus was called the hunger centre. Also, the dorsomedial medulla oblongata, including the NTS and the motor nucleus of the vagus, are implied in these processes. Now, we know the existence of specific subpopulations of neurons involved in energy homeostasis that are included in neuronal pathways with anorexigenic and orexigenic biomolecules (table 1), that generate integrated responses to afferent stimuli related to modifications in metabolites or in fuels storage.

The VMH is the responsible for integrating peripheral signals of nutrient status and adiposity. For example, the ARC contains neurons secreting the NPY and POMC. These neuropeptides have opposite effects on energy homeostasis, since NPY increases food intake and inhibit energy expenditure, while POMC exerts the contrary effects (Adage et al., 2001). Other studies suggest that some VMH neurons are GABAergic, although there is not a clear relationship to glucose-sensing capacity. More recent findings show that most VMH neurons express the protein steroidogenic factor-1 (SF-1) and that SF-1-positives neurons have key roles in glucose homeostasis (Tong et al., 2007; Tsuneki et al., 2010). The LH cells contain the peptides orexins/hypocretins, which are not expressed anywhere else in the brain (de Lecea et al., 1998; Sakurai et al., 1998). Lack of orexin/hypocretin produces hypophagia and late onset obesity among others effects (Hara et al., 2001).

A number of peptidic hormones, previously thought to be specific to the gastroenteropancreatic system and later found also in the mammalian brain, have been shown to modulate appetite, energy, and body weight. They play these physiological effects together with other biomolecules such as NPY, opioid peptides, galanin, vasopressin, and GHRH (Bray 1992). Thus, feeding behaviour is controlled by the antagonist effects of anorexigenic and orexigenic biomolecules. The complex mechanisms underlying the abundance of such variety of feeding behaviour-modulating substances can be understood on the basis of, the specific role for each molecule as a regulatory mechanism in energy balance status, the specifity of macronutrient intake (carbohydrate, fat or proteins) and meal size control, and the shifts in feeding behaviour related to hormonal status, gender, age, and circadian rhythms (Leibowitz 1992).

It is accepted that cells of several hypothalamic nuclei detect circulating satiety signals and transmit this information to other brain areas. Anorexigenic and orexigenic biomolecules are located in VMH, LH, PVN and ARC interacting one to others in a way that they may induce a characteristic feeding behaviour. Thus, peptide Y (Y3-36) is released from gastrointestinal tract postprandially, and acts on NPY Y_2 receptor in the ARC to inhibit feeding with a "long-term" effect (Batterham et al., 2002). On the contrary, other satiety signals induced by gut-brain peptides such as GLP-1, GLP-2 and CCK produced (Navarro et al., 1996; Turton et al., 1996; Rodriquez de Fonseca et al., 2000; Tang-Christensen et al., 2000) a "short-term" effect, while insulin and leptin (Batterham et al., 2002) inhibit the appetite by increasing the formation of POMC and reducing NPY action. In addition, ghrelin a peptide released by the stomach is stimulated before the meals to facilitate NPY action (Coiro et al., 2006).

ANOREXIGENIC		OREXIGENIC
CART	Leptin	AGRP
CCK	α-MSH	Galanin
CRH	Neurotensin	Ghrelin
GLP-1	Oxytocin	MCH
GHRH	Pro-opiomelanocortin	Noradrenaline
GLP-2	Peptide Y (Y 3-36)	NPY
IL-1β	TRH	Opioid peptides
Insulin	Serotonin	Orexin A and B
	Urocortin	

Table 1. Anorexigenic and orexigenic biomolecules implied in the control of feeding behaviour.

Intracerebroventricular or subcutaneous administration of GLP-1 produced a marked reduction of food intake and water ingestion. Exendin-4, proved to be a potent agonist of GLP-1R also decreased both food and water intake in a dose-dependent manner, while exendin (9-39) considered as an antagonist of the GLP-1R, reversed the inhibitory effects of GLP-1 or exendin-4 (Navarro et al., 1996; Turton et al., 1996; Rodriguez de Fonseca et al., 2000). Additionally, icv administration of GLP-1 to mice and rats produced a marked decrease of food intake but not of water ingestion. Surprisingly, this effect was avoided by the administration of exendin (9-39) (Tang-Christensen et al., 2000) .

5.2 Hypothalamic slices as a physiological model for the study of hypothalamic regulation by glucose and peptides

Some hypothalamic neuronal cell models have been generated from embryonic and adult animals to carry out molecular genetic analysis of hypothalamic neuronal function. Some examples are the GT1-7 and N1E-115 cell lines or the recently hypothalamic neuronal cell models generated by Belsham´s group (Dalvi et al., 2011). However, the use of organotypic slice cultures is an approach with many advantages. A broad range of studies shows that organotypic cultures retain many in vivo characteristics as regards, neuronal morphology, cellular and anatomical relations and network connections (Sundstrom et al., 2005). The advantages of the slices culture are the isolated and well defined environment of the in vitro preparations and in this way several brain areas have been studied (hippocampus, cerebellum, cortex, striatum, brain stem structures, spinal cord, retina and hypothalamus).

For these reasons, these cultures are increasingly been used as models to investigate mechanisms and treatment strategies for neurodegenerative disorders or exposure to neurotoxic compounds (Kristensen et al., 2003), traumatic brain injury (TBI) (Morrison et al., 2006) and neurogenesis (Lossi et al., 2009). Hypothalamic slices have also been frequently used for electrophysiological studies developed in vitro to evaluate the firing rate of specific neurons located in VMH and LH (Yang et al., 1999)

Most hypothalamic organotypic slice cultures have been derived from neonatal animals. In fact, slices of developing brain tissue can be grown for several weeks as so called organotypic slice cultures (Noraberg et al., 2005), but also adult rats have been used. In this sense our group have used short-term hypothalamic slices cultures, obtained from adult rat, to test the effect of different peptides on the gene expression and enzymatic activity in the VMH and LH areas (Sanz et al., 2007; Sanz et al., 2008). Thus, the hypothalamic organotypic cultures are a useful model for the study of the physiological effect of some peptides on specific hypothalamic nuclei, which could be dissected after the treatment and analyzed by enzymatic, molecular, biochemical or histological procedures.

5.3 Interactions between anorexigenic peptides and cerebral glucose metabolism in humans

By previous studies we know that GLP-1 is an anorexigenic peptide. The proglucagon gene is expressed mainly in the brainstem and hypothalamus, through a mRNA transcript identical to that produced in pancreas and intestine (Drucker & Asa 1988), which permits the formation of glucagon-related peptides in the brain. Furthermore, the hypothalamus and brainstem are the areas with the highest concentration of GLP-1 and its receptors (Uttenthal et al., 1992), suggesting that this peptide has a local function, as well as a more remote signalling role. The expression of GLP-1R gene gives rise to a protein with effects on the selective release of neurotransmitters (Mora et al., 1992), appetite and fluid homeostasis, as well as serves as a signal to reduce food intake (Navarro et al., 1996; Turton et al., 1996; Rodriquez de Fonseca et al., 2000). Also, the coexpression of GLP-1R with those of GLUT-2 and GK in the same cells suggest that these proteins play a role in glucose sensing (Navarro et al., 1996). A further step was to evaluate the GLP-1 effect on cerebral-glucose metabolism in control subjects by positron emission tomography (PET), using 2-F-18 deoxy-D-glucose (FDG). PET is an imaging technology in which compounds labelled with positron-emitting radioisotopes serve as molecular probes to identify and determine biochemical processes in vivo.

We used (Alvarez et al., 2005) intravenously injected FDG to trace the transport and phosphorylation of glucose in brain. FDG-6-phosphate is the end product of the process of glucose metabolism and it is not a substrate for subsequent metabolic reactions then it is retained in the cell proportionately to the rate of glycolysis. The activity measured reflects FDG transport and phosphorylation by the cells and, in the case of the hypothalamus and brainstem which contains cells expressing GLUT-2 and GK, may provide some information about brain glucose sensing.

PET imaging was sensitive to GLP-1 administration (Figure 4). Thus, this peptide significantly reduced cerebral glucose metabolism in the hypothalamus and brainstem as compared with the data obtained in normal control subjects without GLP-1 administration. These changes can be explained in terms of this peptide can enter the brain by binding to blood barrier-free organs such as the subfornical organ and the area postrema (Orskov et al., 1996). Also, it could be transported into the brain through the choroid plexus, which has a high density of GLP-1 receptors.

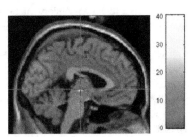

Fig. 4. PET of glucose metabolism in brains of human controls subjects, i.v. perfused with or without GLP-1 (0.75 pmol/Kg body weight for 30 minutes). The differences between both tests were of 6 months, and were projected on sagittal normalized brain MRI. PET imaging was sensitive to the peptide administration. Thus GLP-1 significantly reduced (p<0.001) cerebral glucose metabolism in the hypothalamus and brainstem as compared with the data obtained in normal control subjects without peptide administration.

Using PET technology we observed that iv administration of GLP-1 produced a significant reduction in carbohydrate metabolism in selective areas of the brain, including the hypothalamus and brainstem, both areas involved in feeding behaviour. Thus, the accumulation of FDG-6-phosphate into the cells serves to assess the facilitated transport and hexokinase phosphorylation of glucose, which, in the case of hypothalamus and brainstem cells containing GLUT-2 and GK, might facilitate the glucose-sensing process. These findings are of interest because glucoreceptive sites controlling food intake and blood glucose have been found in the medulla oblongata and mesencephalon of the rat (Ritter et al., 2000), in addition to those reported in the hypothalamus. Also, GLP-1 is expressed in human brain, and it most likely mediates the effect of GLP-1 on glucose metabolism in selective areas of hypothalamus and brainstem; it may also facilitate the process of glucose sensing in these areas. Because the reduced number of neurons involved in glucose sensing (Oomura et al., 1969; Ashford et al., 1990) , approximately 40% of cells in the VMH and 30% of cells in the LH, PET imaging offers a good procedure for identifying these cell signals in vivo more accurately compared with the more commonly used in vitro procedures.

These findings provide first evidences of the action of an anorexigenic peptide on glucose metabolism in the hypothalamus and brainstem, and might explain the satiety–induced effects of peripheral or central administration of GLP-1 and the central alterations produced by the iv administration of the peptide. Furthermore, open new doors for studying the effects of other regulatory peptides in subjects under control and pathophysiological situations.

6. Others hypothalamic metabolic sensors: AMPK structure and regulation

AMP-activated protein kinase (AMPK) functions as a cellular energy sensor being activated during energy depletion. The kinase is mainly activated by an increase AMP/ATP ratio. Activation of AMPK regulates a large number of downstream targets stimulating ATP-generating, catabolic pathways and inhibiting anabolic pathways (Hardie et al., 1998; Rutter et al., 2003).

AMPK is a heterotrimeric serine/threonine kinase consisting of a catalytic α-subunit encoded by 2 genes (α1 or α2), a β-subunit encoded by 2 genes (β1, β2) and a regulatory γ-subunit encoded by 3 genes (γ1, γ2, γ3). Different isoforms and alternative splicing of some mRNAs encoding these subunits, give rise to large variety of heterotrimeric combinations (Hardie 2007; Viollet et al., 2009). It is known that some tissues can express several types of AMPK complexes.

AMPK can be regulated by an allosteric mechanism, through AMP binding to γ subunit, and by covalent phosphorylation at Thr^{172} located in the kinase domain of the α-subunit. The level of phosphorylation is also regulated by AMP through stimulation of upstream kinases and by inhibition of dephosphorylation by protein phosphatases. One of the identified upstream kinases of AMPK is the tumor-suppressor (Liver Kinase B1: LKB1). In neural and endothelial cells AMPK may be also activated by rises in cytosolic Ca^{2+} concentration. The calmodulin-dependent protein kinase kinase (CaMKK) can also activate AMPK by phosphorylation of Thr^{172}.

The AMPK is able to detect changes in cellular energy state that occur in response to variations in nutrient concentrations. Any cellular or metabolic stress that reduces ATP production or accelerates ATP consumption will increase the ratio of the ADP/ATP, which will be amplified by the action of adenylate kinase resulting in increased AMP/ATP with consequent activation of AMPK. Once activated, AMPK first directly affects the activity of key enzymes of glucose metabolism and fatty acids and at a second more long term regulates transcriptional control of the main elements involved in these metabolic pathways. The net result of the activation of AMPK will restore energy balance inhibiting anabolic pathways responsible for the synthesis of macromolecules. (Figure 5)

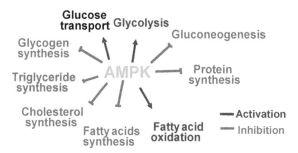

Fig. 5. AMPK regulation of downstream metabolic events. AMPK restores energy balance by activation of processes that produce energy and inhibition of those that consume energy.

6.1 Role of AMPK in hypothalamic glucose sensing

AMPK is broadly expressed throughout the brain with a mainly neuronal distribution (Turnley et al., 1999). Hypothalamic AMPK has been proposed to play a role in the central regulation of food intake and energy balance. In this way, fasting increases and re-feeding decreases AMPK activity in various hypothalamic nuclei (Minokoshi et al., 2004). Several studies have demonstrated that hypothalamic AMPK is regulated by blood glucose levels. Peripheral or central hyperglycaemia inhibits AMPK in several hypothalamic nuclei. Insulin-induced hypoglycaemia and inhibition of intracellular glucose utilization through the administration of 2-deoxyglucose both increased hypothalamic AMPK activity and food intake.

The use of catalytic subunit of AMPK knockout mice (AMPKα1$^{-/-}$ and AMPKα2$^{-/-}$) indicated that AMPKα1$^{-/-}$ mice has no metabolic alterations, whereas AMPKα2$^{-/-}$ mice showed insulin-resistance characterized by impaired insulin stimulated whole-body glucose utilization and skeletal muscle glycogen synthesis and reduced insulin secretion. However, they showed no apparent changes in body weight and food intake (Viollet et al., 2009).

In the last years AMPK has been proposed as a cellular energy sensor that is able to assemble many regulatory signals and nutritional environmental changes, also involved in maintaining whole body energy balance (Hardie et al., 2006). Regulation of AMPK activity in hypothalamic areas involved in the control of feeding behaviours have been also described as a mechanism to detect nutritional variations including glucose levels (Mountjoy & Rutter 2007). Neurons implied in the control of food intake have as well glucose sensor that respond to fluctuations in extracellular glucose levels.

In general most cells will express glucose transporters that have high affinity for glucose; therefore ATP synthesis by glucose metabolism only stops when glucose levels are pathologically low. However, cells that have a glucose sensor mechanism, express GLUT-2 and GK. The presence of these proteins of high Km for transport and metabolism of glucose will allow that ATP synthesis decreases when decreases the concentration of glucose in the physiological range and this allows that in these cells the AMPK can be activated by low levels of glucose and inhibited by high glucose levels in the physiological range.

The hypothalamic AMPK role has been studied in vivo by expression of AMPK mutants: Inhibition of hypothalamic AMPK suppresses neuronal NPY/AgRP signalling and inhibit food intake. However, elevated AMPK increases NPY/AgRP expression, food intake and body weight (Minokoshi et al., 2004).

The role of AMPK in the two major subpopulations of neurons involved in the regulation of feeding was later analyzed by knock out of AMPKα2 in specific neurons of mice. The results showed that genetic deletion of AMPKα2 in hypothalamic POMC neurons (POMC AMPKα2-KO) developed obesity. However, AMPKα2 specifically knocked in AgRP neurones (AgRP AMPKα2-KO) exhibited an age-related lean phenotype (Claret et al., 2007). Those mice do not respond to changes in extracellular glucose. The unexpected results suggest that absence of AMPK in orexigenic AgRP neurons reduced body weight, whereas lack of AMPK in anorexigenic POMC neurons increased body weight. These results suggest a role for AMPK as a common glucose-sensor in these neurons (Claret et al., 2007). It is important to emphasize that GE neurons do not overlap completely with POMC neurons in the ARC while the GI neurons do not completely overlap with NPY/AgRP neurons. Those findings indicated the complexity of the functions of hypothalamic AMPK.

6.2 Regulation by orexigenic and anorexigenic peptides

Several reports indicate that AMPK is also regulated by several orexigenic and anorexigenic signals (Minokoshi et al., 2004). Thus, hypothalamic AMPK activity was inhibited in ARC and PVN by anorexigenic peptides as leptin and insulin by contrast, orexigenic peptides (ghrelin) increased specifically α2AMPK activity

In other hand, other studies reported AMPK-independent pathways. The effect of leptin were maintained in POMC α2AMPK-KO neurons and insulin depolarised AgRP neurons in AgRP α2AMPK-KO (Claret et al., 2007). The different results may be explained, in addition to the different techniques and experimental setups, by the presence of distinct subpopulations of GE and GI neurons with different neuropeptide phenotypes, responses to hormonal stimuli and, in some cases, different glucose-sensing mechanisms.

The downstream pathways of AMPK in the hypothalamus may involve the acetyl-CoA carboxylase (ACC)-malonyl-CoA-carnitine palmitoyltransferase 1 (CPT1) pathway and the

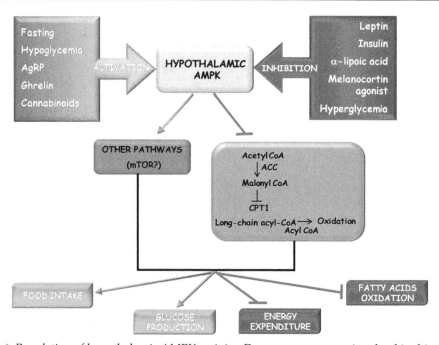

Fig. 6. Regulation of hypothalamic AMPK activity. Downstream targets involved in this signaling pathway. Several orexigenic and anorexigenic peptides regulate AMPK activity. Some of downstream targets of AMPK in the hypothalamus: ACC, acetyl-CoA carboxylase; CPT1, carnitine palmitoyltransferase 1. The effect of AMPK on the mammalian target of rapamycin (mTOR) pathway has not been directly proved in the hypothalamus.

mammalian target of rapamycin (mTOR) pathway. Activation of ACC, as a consequence of AMPK inhibition, would lead to increased intracellular malonyl-CoA levels, which would inhibit mitochondrial CPT1 and fatty acid oxidation.

The mTOR is another possible target of AMPK (Figure 6). AMPK inhibits mTOR signalling, thereby suppressing protein synthesis, which is an important pathway by which AMPK conserves cellular energy. The mTOR signalling pathway plays a crucial role in the regulation of food intake and body weight in the hypothalamus (Cota et al., 2006; Ropelle et al., 2008). The mTOR is colocalized with AgRP/NPY and POMC neurons in the ARC (Perrin et al., 2004). Fasting downregulates mTOR signalling, whereas re-feeding activates it.

Interestingly, hypothalamic AMPK also mediates the counter-regulatory response to hypoglycaemia, increasing the release of peripheral hormones such as corticosterone, catecholamines and glucagon (Han et al., 2005; McCrimmon et al., 2006). Thus AMPK is not only a peripheral or a central mediator, but also a key enzyme in coordinating the interaction between peripheral and central energy regulation.

It is generally accepted that in peripheral organs, fuel overabundance alters the activity of metabolic sensors (decreased AMPK and increased the mTOR and its down-stream target the S6Kinase (p70S6K)) causing insulin resistance (Kola et al., 2005).

AMPK and mTOR activity respond to changes in glucose and other nutrients in hypothalamic centres involved in control of feeding and deregulation of this signalling pathways might be implied in the develop of obesity and diabetes type 2. GLP-1 treatment to type 2 diabetic subjects normalizes fasting levels of blood glucose and decreases glucose levels after ingestion of a meal (Niswender 2010). GLP-1 is able to induce several effects that contribute to feeding behaviour. Preliminary data from our laboratory also suggest that, at least some of those effects, might mediate through regulation of AMPK and p70S6K in VMH and LH.

7. Conclusions

Glucoregulatory mechanisms are of primary functional concern to provide a continued glucose supply to the central nervous system and to face metabolic needs of peripheral tissues. Glucose sensors are molecular designs that accurately measure glucose concentrations in the extracellular space facilitating the mechanisms need to maintain glucose homeostasis. GK might be responsible of glucose sensing in some of hypothalamic GE and GI neurons (VMH, LH ARC, PVN and dorsomedial nucleus). GK properties of high-Km phosphorylation of glucose and that it is not inhibited by glucose-6-phosphate, enable that glucose catabolism be proportional to glucose levels in the extracellular space. Also, the functional coexpression of GK with GLUT-2, GKRP and GLP-1R in hypothalamic areas implied in feeding behaviour, could orchestrate regulatory signals to maintain body weight and energy balance. Glucose, orexigenic and anorexigenic peptides contribute to control GK, as well as other energetic sensors such as AMPK. The effect of nutrients occurs on GK and AMPK enzyme activities as required by a short-term response and in a distinctive pattern between VMH and LH. Also, GLP-1 produced a significant reduction of glucose metabolism in selective areas of human brain including hypothalamus and brainstem, both areas involved in feeding behaviour. These findings open new doors for studying the effects of others regulatory peptides in subjects under control and pathophysiological situations. In summary, this chapter has shown a view of the complexity of the network of regulatory signals, where GK, AMPK and regulatory peptides are involved, leading to an optimal energy balance and body weight.

8. Acknowledgment

This work was supported by the CIBER de Diabetes y Enfermedades Metabólicas Asociadas (CIBERDEM) of the Instituto de Salud Carlos III, Madrid, Spain; by grants from the Ministerio de Ciencia e Innovación, Fondo de Investigaciones Sanitarias, Spain and from the Fundación de Investigación Médica Mutua Madrileña, Spain and from Complutense University of Madrid-Santander Bank, Spain.

9. References

Adachi, A.; Kobashi, M. & Funahashi, M. (1995). Glucose-responsive neurons in the brainstem. *Obes Res,* Vol.3 Suppl 5, (Dec), pp. 735S-740S.
Adage, T.; Scheurink, A. J.; de Boer, S. F.; de Vries, K.; Konsman, J. P.; Kuipers, F.; Adan, R. A.; Baskin, D. G.; Schwartz, M. W. & van Dijk, G. (2001). Hypothalamic, metabolic, and behavioral responses to pharmacological inhibition of CNS melanocortin signaling in rats. *J Neurosci,* Vol.21, No.10, (May 15), pp. 3639-3645.

Agius, L. & Peak, M. (1993). Intracellular binding of glucokinase in hepatocytes and translocation by glucose, fructose and insulin. *Biochem J*, Vol.296 (Pt 3), (Dec 15), pp. 785-796.

Alvarez, E.; Martinez, M. D.; Roncero, I.; Chowen, J. A.; Garcia-Cuartero, B.; Gispert, J. D.; Sanz, C.; Vazquez, P.; Maldonado, A.; de Caceres, J.; Desco, M.; Pozo, M. A. & Blazquez, E. (2005). The expression of GLP-1 receptor mRNA and protein allows the effect of GLP-1 on glucose metabolism in the human hypothalamus and brainstem. *J Neurochem*, Vol.92, No.4, (Feb), pp. 798-806.

Alvarez, E.; Roncero, I.; Chowen, J. A.; Thorens, B. & Blazquez, E. (1996). Expression of the glucagon-like peptide-1 receptor gene in rat brain. *J Neurochem*, Vol.66, No.3, (Mar), pp. 920-927.

Alvarez, E.; Roncero, I.; Chowen, J. A.; Vazquez, P. & Blazquez, E. (2002). Evidence that glucokinase regulatory protein is expressed and interacts with glucokinase in rat brain. *J Neurochem*, Vol.80, No.1, (Jan), pp. 45-53.

Anand, B. K.; Chhina, G. S.; Sharma, K. N.; Dua, S. & Singh, B. (1964). Activity of Single Neurons in the Hypothalamic Feeding Centers: Effect of Glucose. *Am J Physiol*, Vol.207, (Nov), pp. 1146-1154.

Arden, C.; Baltrusch, S. & Agius, L. (2006). Glucokinase regulatory protein is associated with mitochondria in hepatocytes. *FEBS Lett*, Vol.580, No.8, (Apr 3), pp. 2065-2070.

Ashcroft, F. & Rorsman, P. (2004). Type 2 diabetes mellitus: not quite exciting enough? *Hum Mol Genet*, Vol.13 Spec No 1, (Apr 1), pp. R21-31.

Ashford, M. L.; Boden, P. R. & Treherne, J. M. (1990). Glucose-induced excitation of hypothalamic neurones is mediated by ATP-sensitive K+ channels. *Pflugers Arch*, Vol.415, No.4, (Jan), pp. 479-483.

Baltrusch, S.; Lenzen, S.; Okar, D. A.; Lange, A. J. & Tiedge, M. (2001). Characterization of glucokinase-binding protein epitopes by a phage-displayed peptide library. Identification of 6-phosphofructo-2-kinase/fructose-2,6-bisphosphatase as a novel interaction partner. *J Biol Chem*, Vol.276, No.47, (Nov 23), pp. 43915-43923.

Batterham, R. L.; Cowley, M. A.; Small, C. J.; Herzog, H.; Cohen, M. A.; Dakin, C. L.; Wren, A. M.; Brynes, A. E.; Low, M. J.; Ghatei, M. A.; Cone, R. D. & Bloom, S. R. (2002). Gut hormone PYY(3-36) physiologically inhibits food intake. *Nature*, Vol.418, No.6898, (Aug 8), pp. 650-654.

Bernard, C. (1849). Chiens rendus diabetiquex. *Compt End Soc Biol*, Vol.1, pp. 60

Borg, W. P.; Sherwin, R. S.; During, M. J.; Borg, M. A. & Shulman, G. I. (1995). Local ventromedial hypothalamus glucopenia triggers counterregulatory hormone release. *Diabetes*, Vol.44, No.2, (Feb), pp. 180-184.

Bray, G. A. (1992). Peptides affect the intake of specific nutrients and the sympathetic nervous system. *Am J Clin Nutr*, Vol.55, No.1 Suppl, (Jan), pp. 265S-271S.

Burdakov, D. & Ashcroft, F. M. (2002). Shedding new light on brain metabolism and glial function. *J Physiol*, Vol.544, No.Pt 2, (Oct 15), pp. 334.

Burdakov, D. & Lesage, F. (2010). Glucose-induced inhibition: how many ionic mechanisms? *Acta Physiol (Oxf)*, Vol.198, No.3, (Mar), pp. 295-301.

Burdakov, D.; Luckman, S. M. & Verkhratsky, A. (2005). Glucose-sensing neurons of the hypothalamus. *Philosophical Transactions of the Royal Society B: Biological Sciences,* Vol.360, No.1464, (December 29, 2005), pp. 2227-2235.

Claret, M.; Smith, M. A.; Batterham, R. L.; Selman, C.; Choudhury, A. I.; Fryer, L. G.; Clements, M.; Al-Qassab, H.; Heffron, H.; Xu, A. W.; Speakman, J. R.; Barsh, G. S.; Viollet, B.; Vaulont, S.; Ashford, M. L.; Carling, D. & Withers, D. J. (2007). AMPK is essential for energy homeostasis regulation and glucose sensing by POMC and AgRP neurons. *J Clin Invest,* Vol.117, No.8, (Aug), pp. 2325-2336.

Coiro, V.; Saccani-Jotti, G.; Rubino, P.; Manfredi, G.; Melani, A. & Chiodera, P. (2006). Effects of ghrelin on circulating neuropeptide Y levels in humans. *Neuro Endocrinol Lett,* Vol.27, No.6, (Dec), pp. 755-757.

Cone, R. D.; Cowley, M. A.; Butler, A. A.; Fan, W.; Marks, D. L. & Low, M. J. (2001). The arcuate nucleus as a conduit for diverse signals relevant to energy homeostasis. *Int J Obes Relat Metab Disord,* Vol.25 Suppl 5, (Dec), pp. S63-67.

Cornish-Bowden, A. & Storer, A. C. (1986). Mechanistic origin of the sigmoidal rate behaviour of rat liver hexokinase D ('glucokinase'). *Biochem J,* Vol.240, No.1, (Nov 15), pp. 293-296.

Cota, D.; Proulx, K.; Smith, K. A.; Kozma, S. C.; Thomas, G.; Woods, S. C. & Seeley, R. J. (2006). Hypothalamic mTOR signaling regulates food intake. *Science,* Vol.312, No.5775, (May 12), pp. 927-930.

Christesen, H. B.; Jacobsen, B. B.; Odili, S.; Buettger, C.; Cuesta-Munoz, A.; Hansen, T.; Brusgaard, K.; Massa, O.; Magnuson, M. A.; Shiota, C.; Matschinsky, F. M. & Barbetti, F. (2002). The second activating glucokinase mutation (A456V): implications for glucose homeostasis and diabetes therapy. *Diabetes,* Vol.51, No.4, (Apr), pp. 1240-1246.

Dalvi, P. S.; Nazarians-Armavil, A.; Tung, S. & Belsham, D. D. (2011). Immortalized Neurons for the Study of Hypothalamic Function. *American Journal of Physiology - Regulatory, Integrative and Comparative Physiology,* Vol., pp.

Dallaporta, M.; Himmi, T.; Perrin, J. & Orsini, J. C. (1999). Solitary tract nucleus sensitivity to moderate changes in glucose level. *Neuroreport,* Vol.10, No.12, (Aug 20), pp. 2657-2660.

de Lecea, L.; Kilduff, T. S.; Peyron, C.; Gao, X.; Foye, P. E.; Danielson, P. E.; Fukuhara, C.; Battenberg, E. L.; Gautvik, V. T.; Bartlett, F. S., 2nd; Frankel, W. N.; van den Pol, A. N.; Bloom, F. E.; Gautvik, K. M. & Sutcliffe, J. G. (1998). The hypocretins: hypothalamus-specific peptides with neuroexcitatory activity. *Proc Natl Acad Sci U S A,* Vol.95, No.1, (Jan 6), pp. 322-327.

Diez-Sampedro, A.; Hirayama, B. A.; Osswald, C.; Gorboulev, V.; Baumgarten, K.; Volk, C.; Wright, E. M. & Koepsell, H. (2003). A glucose sensor hiding in a family of transporters. *Proc Natl Acad Sci U S A,* Vol.100, No.20, (Sep 30), pp. 11753-11758.

Drucker, D. J. & Asa, S. (1988). Glucagon gene expression in vertebrate brain. *J Biol Chem,* Vol.263, No.27, (Sep 25), pp. 13475-13478.

Dunn-Meynell, A. A.; Rawson, N. E. & Levin, B. E. (1998). Distribution and phenotype of neurons containing the ATP-sensitive K+ channel in rat brain. *Brain Research,* Vol.814, No.1-2, pp. 41-54.

Dunn-Meynell, A. A.; Routh, V. H.; Kang, L.; Gaspers, L. & Levin, B. E. (2002). Glucokinase is the likely mediator of glucosensing in both glucose-excited and glucose-inhibited central neurons. *Diabetes,* Vol.51, No.7, (Jul), pp. 2056-2065.

Elmquist, J. K.; Elias, C. F. & Saper, C. B. (1999). From lesions to leptin: hypothalamic control of food intake and body weight. *Neuron,* Vol.22, No.2, (Feb), pp. 221-232.

Fioramonti, X.; Lorsignol, A.; Taupignon, A. & Penicaud, L. (2004). A new ATP-sensitive K+ channel-independent mechanism is involved in glucose-excited neurons of mouse arcuate nucleus. *Diabetes,* Vol.53, No.11, (Nov), pp. 2767-2775.

Garcia-Flores, M.; Zueco, J. A.; Arenas, J. & Blazquez, E. (2002). Expression of glucose transporter-2, glucokinase and mitochondrial glycerolphosphate dehydrogenase in pancreatic islets during rat ontogenesis. *Eur J Biochem,* Vol.269, No.1, (Jan), pp. 119-127.

Gonzalez, J. A.; Reimann, F. & Burdakov, D. (2009). Dissociation between sensing and metabolism of glucose in sugar sensing neurones. *J Physiol,* Vol.587, No.Pt 1, (Jan 15), pp. 41-48.

Gribble, F. M.; Williams, L.; Simpson, A. K. & Reimann, F. (2003). A novel glucose-sensing mechanism contributing to glucagon-like peptide-1 secretion from the GLUTag cell line. *Diabetes,* Vol.52, No.5, (May), pp. 1147-1154.

Grupe, A.; Hultgren, B.; Ryan, A.; Ma, Y. H.; Bauer, M. & Stewart, T. A. (1995). Transgenic knockouts reveal a critical requirement for pancreatic beta cell glucokinase in maintaining glucose homeostasis. *Cell,* Vol.83, No.1, (Oct 6), pp. 69-78.

Han, S. M.; Namkoong, C.; Jang, P. G.; Park, I. S.; Hong, S. W.; Katakami, H.; Chun, S.; Kim, S. W.; Park, J. Y.; Lee, K. U. & Kim, M. S. (2005). Hypothalamic AMP-activated protein kinase mediates counter-regulatory responses to hypoglycaemia in rats. *Diabetologia,* Vol.48, No.10, (Oct), pp. 2170-2178.

Hara, J.; Beuckmann, C. T.; Nambu, T.; Willie, J. T.; Chemelli, R. M.; Sinton, C. M.; Sugiyama, F.; Yagami, K.; Goto, K.; Yanagisawa, M. & Sakurai, T. (2001). Genetic ablation of orexin neurons in mice results in narcolepsy, hypophagia, and obesity. *Neuron,* Vol.30, No.2, (May), pp. 345-354.

Hardie, D. G. (2007). AMP-activated/SNF1 protein kinases: conserved guardians of cellular energy. *Nat Rev Mol Cell Biol,* Vol.8, No.10, (Oct), pp. 774-785.

Hardie, D. G.; Carling, D. & Carlson, M. (1998). The AMP-activated/SNF1 protein kinase subfamily: metabolic sensors of the eukaryotic cell? *Annu Rev Biochem,* Vol.67, pp. 821-855.

Hardie, D. G.; Hawley, S. A. & Scott, J. W. (2006). AMP-activated protein kinase--development of the energy sensor concept. *J Physiol,* Vol.574, No.Pt 1, (Jul 1), pp. 7-15.

Hughes, S. D.; Quaade, C.; Milburn, J. L.; Cassidy, L. & Newgard, C. B. (1991). Expression of normal and novel glucokinase mRNAs in anterior pituitary and islet cells. *J Biol Chem,* Vol.266, No.7, (Mar 5), pp. 4521-4530.

Iynedjian, P. B. (1993). Mammalian glucokinase and its gene. *Biochem J,* Vol.293 (Pt 1), (Jul 1), pp. 1-13.

Iynedjian, P. B.; Marie, S.; Wang, H.; Gjinovci, A. & Nazaryan, K. (1996). Liver-specific enhancer of the glucokinase gene. *J Biol Chem*, Vol.271, No.46, (Nov 15), pp. 29113-29120.

Jordan, S. D.; Konner, A. C. & Bruning, J. C. (2010). Sensing the fuels: glucose and lipid signaling in the CNS controlling energy homeostasis. *Cell Mol Life Sci*, Vol.67, No.19, (Oct), pp. 3255-3273.

Kang, L.; Dunn-Meynell, A. A.; Routh, V. H.; Gaspers, L. D.; Nagata, Y.; Nishimura, T.; Eiki, J.; Zhang, B. B. & Levin, B. E. (2006). Glucokinase is a critical regulator of ventromedial hypothalamic neuronal glucosensing. *Diabetes*, Vol.55, No.2, (Feb), pp. 412-420.

Kang, L.; Routh, V. H.; Kuzhikandathil, E. V.; Gaspers, L. D. & Levin, B. E. (2004). Physiological and molecular characteristics of rat hypothalamic ventromedial nucleus glucosensing neurons. *Diabetes*, Vol.53, No.3, (Mar), pp. 549-559.

Kola, B.; Hubina, E.; Tucci, S. A.; Kirkham, T. C.; Garcia, E. A.; Mitchell, S. E.; Williams, L. M.; Hawley, S. A.; Hardie, D. G.; Grossman, A. B. & Korbonits, M. (2005). Cannabinoids and ghrelin have both central and peripheral metabolic and cardiac effects via AMP-activated protein kinase. *J Biol Chem*, Vol.280, No.26, (Jul 1), pp. 25196-25201.

Kristensen, B. W.; Noer, H.; Gramsbergen, J. B.; Zimmer, J. & Noraberg, J. (2003). Colchicine induces apoptosis in organotypic hippocampal slice cultures. *Brain Res*, Vol.964, No.2, (Feb 28), pp. 264-278.

Lee, K.; Li, B.; Xi, X.; Suh, Y. & Martin, R. J. (2005). Role of neuronal energy status in the regulation of adenosine 5'-monophosphate-activated protein kinase, orexigenic neuropeptides expression, and feeding behavior. *Endocrinology*, Vol.146, No.1, (Jan), pp. 3-10.

Leibowitz, S. F. (1992). Neurochemical-neuroendocrine systems in the brain controlling macronutrient intake and metabolism. *Trends Neurosci*, Vol.15, No.12, (Dec), pp. 491-497.

Levin, B. E.; Routh, V. H.; Kang, L.; Sanders, N. M. & Dunn-Meynell, A. A. (2004). Neuronal glucosensing: what do we know after 50 years? *Diabetes*, Vol.53, No.10, (Oct), pp. 2521-2528.

Lossi, L.; Alasia, S.; Salio, C. & Merighi, A. (2009). Cell death and proliferation in acute slices and organotypic cultures of mammalian CNS. *Prog Neurobiol*, Vol.88, No.4, (Aug), pp. 221-245.

Lynch, R. M.; Tompkins, L. S.; Brooks, H. L.; Dunn-Meynell, A. A. & Levin, B. E. (2000). Localization of glucokinase gene expression in the rat brain. *Diabetes*, Vol.49, No.5, (May 1, 2000), pp. 693-700.

Magnuson, M. A. & Shelton, K. D. (1989). An alternate promoter in the glucokinase gene is active in the pancreatic beta cell. *J Biol Chem*, Vol.264, No.27, (Sep 25), pp. 15936-15942.

Malaisse, W. J.; Malaisse-Lagae, F.; Davies, D. R.; Vandercammen, A. & Van Schaftingen, E. (1990). Regulation of glucokinase by a fructose-1-phosphate-sensitive protein in pancreatic islets. *Eur J Biochem*, Vol.190, No.3, (Jul 5), pp. 539-545.

Matschinsky, F.; Liang, Y.; Kesavan, P.; Wang, L.; Froguel, P.; Velho, G.; Cohen, D.; Permutt, M. A.; Tanizawa, Y.; Jetton, T. L. & et al. (1993). Glucokinase as pancreatic beta cell glucose sensor and diabetes gene. *J Clin Invest,* Vol.92, No.5, (Nov), pp. 2092-2098.

Matschinsky, F. M. (1990). Glucokinase as glucose sensor and metabolic signal generator in pancreatic beta-cells and hepatocytes. *Diabetes,* Vol.39, No.6, (Jun), pp. 647-652.

Mayer, J. (1953). Glucostatic Mechanism of Regulation of Food Intake. *New England Journal of Medicine,* Vol.249, No.1, pp. 13-16.

McCrimmon, R. J.; Fan, X.; Cheng, H.; McNay, E.; Chan, O.; Shaw, M.; Ding, Y.; Zhu, W. & Sherwin, R. S. (2006). Activation of AMP-activated protein kinase within the ventromedial hypothalamus amplifies counterregulatory hormone responses in rats with defective counterregulation. *Diabetes,* Vol.55, No.6, (Jun), pp. 1755-1760.

Minokoshi, Y.; Alquier, T.; Furukawa, N.; Kim, Y. B.; Lee, A.; Xue, B.; Mu, J.; Foufelle, F.; Ferre, P.; Birnbaum, M. J.; Stuck, B. J. & Kahn, B. B. (2004). AMP-kinase regulates food intake by responding to hormonal and nutrient signals in the hypothalamus. *Nature,* Vol.428, No.6982, (Apr 1), pp. 569-574.

Mora, F.; Exposito, I.; Sanz, B. & Blazquez, E. (1992). Selective release of glutamine and glutamic acid produced by perfusion of GLP-1 (7-36) amide in the basal ganglia of the conscious rat. *Brain Res Bull,* Vol.29, No.3-4, (Sep-Oct), pp. 359-361.

Morrison, B., 3rd; Cater, H. L.; Benham, C. D. & Sundstrom, L. E. (2006). An in vitro model of traumatic brain injury utilising two-dimensional stretch of organotypic hippocampal slice cultures. *J Neurosci Methods,* Vol.150, No.2, (Jan 30), pp. 192-201.

Moukil, M. A.; Veiga-da-Cunha, M. & Van Schaftingen, E. (2000). Study of the regulatory properties of glucokinase by site-directed mutagenesis: conversion of glucokinase to an enzyme with high affinity for glucose. *Diabetes,* Vol.49, No.2, (Feb), pp. 195-201.

Mountjoy, P. D. & Rutter, G. A. (2007). Glucose sensing by hypothalamic neurones and pancreatic islet cells: AMPle evidence for common mechanisms? *Exp Physiol,* Vol.92, No.2, (Mar), pp. 311-319.

Munoz-Alonso, M. J.; Guillemain, G.; Kassis, N.; Girard, J.; Burnol, A. F. & Leturque, A. (2000). A novel cytosolic dual specificity phosphatase, interacting with glucokinase, increases glucose phosphorylation rate. *J Biol Chem,* Vol.275, No.42, (Oct 20), pp. 32406-32412.

Navarro, M.; Rodriquez de Fonseca, F.; Alvarez, E.; Chowen, J. A.; Zueco, J. A.; Gomez, R.; Eng, J. & Blazquez, E. (1996). Colocalization of glucagon-like peptide-1 (GLP-1) receptors, glucose transporter GLUT-2, and glucokinase mRNAs in rat hypothalamic cells: evidence for a role of GLP-1 receptor agonists as an inhibitory signal for food and water intake. *J Neurochem,* Vol.67, No.5, (Nov), pp. 1982-1991.

Niswender, K. (2010). Diabetes and obesity: therapeutic targeting and risk reduction - a complex interplay. *Diabetes Obes Metab,* Vol.12, No.4, (Apr), pp. 267-287.

Noraberg, J.; Poulsen, F. R.; Blaabjerg, M.; Kristensen, B. W.; Bonde, C.; Montero, M.; Meyer, M.; Gramsbergen, J. B. & Zimmer, J. (2005). Organotypic hippocampal slice cultures for studies of brain damage, neuroprotection and neurorepair. *Curr Drug Targets CNS Neurol Disord,* Vol.4, No.4, (Aug), pp. 435-452.

Oomura, Y.; Ono, T.; Ooyama, H. & Wayner, M. J. (1969). Glucose and osmosensitive neurones of the rat hypothalamus. *Nature,* Vol.222, No.5190, (Apr 19), pp. 282-284.

Oomura, Y.; Ooyama, H.; Sugimori, M.; Nakamura, T. & Yamada, Y. (1974). Glucose inhibition of the glucose-sensitive neurone in the rat lateral hypothalamus. *Nature,* Vol.247, No.439, (Feb 1), pp. 284-286.

Oomura, Y. & Yoshimatsu, H. (1984). Neural network of glucose monitoring system. *J Auton Nerv Syst,* Vol.10, No.3-4, (May-Jun), pp. 359-372.

Orskov, C.; Poulsen, S. S.; Moller, M. & Holst, J. J. (1996). Glucagon-like peptide I receptors in the subfornical organ and the area postrema are accessible to circulating glucagon-like peptide I. *Diabetes,* Vol.45, No.6, (Jun), pp. 832-835.

Pellerin, L. & Magistretti, P. J. (2004). Neuroenergetics: calling upon astrocytes to satisfy hungry neurons. *Neuroscientist,* Vol.10, No.1, (Feb), pp. 53-62.

Penicaud, L.; Leloup, C.; Fioramonti, X.; Lorsignol, A. & Benani, A. (2006). Brain glucose sensing: a subtle mechanism. *Curr Opin Clin Nutr Metab Care,* Vol.9, No.4, (Jul), pp. 458-462.

Perrin, C.; Knauf, C. & Burcelin, R. (2004). Intracerebroventricular infusion of glucose, insulin, and the adenosine monophosphate-activated kinase activator, 5-aminoimidazole-4-carboxamide-1-beta-D-ribofuranoside, controls muscle glycogen synthesis. *Endocrinology,* Vol.145, No.9, (Sep), pp. 4025-4033.

Ritter, S. & Dinh, T. T. (1994). 2-Mercaptoacetate and 2-deoxy-D-glucose induce Fos-like immunoreactivity in rat brain. *Brain Res,* Vol.641, No.1, (Mar 28), pp. 111-120.

Ritter, S.; Dinh, T. T. & Zhang, Y. (2000). Localization of hindbrain glucoreceptive sites controlling food intake and blood glucose. *Brain Res,* Vol.856, No.1-2, (Feb 21), pp. 37-47.

Rodriguez de Fonseca, F.; Navarro, M.; Alvarez, E.; Roncero, I.; Chowen, J. A.; Maestre, O.; Gomez, R.; Munoz, R. M.; Eng, J. & Blazquez, E. (2000). Peripheral versus central effects of glucagon-like peptide-1 receptor agonists on satiety and body weight loss in Zucker obese rats. *Metabolism,* Vol.49, No.6, (Jun), pp. 709-717.

Roncero, I.; Alvarez, E.; Chowen, J. A.; Sanz, C.; Rabano, A.; Vazquez, P. & Blazquez, E. (2004). Expression of glucose transporter isoform GLUT-2 and glucokinase genes in human brain. *J Neurochem,* Vol.88, No.5, (Mar), pp. 1203-1210.

Roncero, I.; Alvarez, E.; Vazquez, P. & Blazquez, E. (2000). Functional glucokinase isoforms are expressed in rat brain. *J Neurochem,* Vol.74, No.5, (May), pp. 1848-1857.

Roncero, I.; Sanz, C.; Alvarez, E.; Vazquez, P.; Barrio, P. A. & Blazquez, E. (2009). Glucokinase and glucokinase regulatory proteins are functionally coexpressed before birth in the rat brain. *J Neuroendocrinol,* Vol.21, No.12, (Dec), pp. 973-981.

Ropelle, E. R.; Pauli, J. R.; Fernandes, M. F.; Rocco, S. A.; Marin, R. M.; Morari, J.; Souza, K. K.; Dias, M. M.; Gomes-Marcondes, M. C.; Gontijo, J. A.; Franchini, K. G.; Velloso, L. A.; Saad, M. J. & Carvalheira, J. B. (2008). A central role for neuronal AMP-activated protein kinase (AMPK) and mammalian target of rapamycin (mTOR) in high-protein diet-induced weight loss. *Diabetes,* Vol.57, No.3, (Mar), pp. 594-605.

Routh, V. H. (2002). Glucose-sensing neurons: Are they physiologically relevant? *Physiology & Behavior*, Vol.76, No.3, pp. 403-413.

Rutter, G. A.; Da Silva Xavier, G. & Leclerc, I. (2003). Roles of 5'-AMP-activated protein kinase (AMPK) in mammalian glucose homoeostasis. *Biochem J*, Vol.375, No.Pt 1, (Oct 1), pp. 1-16.

Sakurai, T.; Amemiya, A.; Ishii, M.; Matsuzaki, I.; Chemelli, R. M.; Tanaka, H.; Williams, S. C.; Richardson, J. A.; Kozlowski, G. P.; Wilson, S.; Arch, J. R.; Buckingham, R. E.; Haynes, A. C.; Carr, S. A.; Annan, R. S.; McNulty, D. E.; Liu, W. S.; Terrett, J. A.; Elshourbagy, N. A.; Bergsma, D. J. & Yanagisawa, M. (1998). Orexins and orexin receptors: a family of hypothalamic neuropeptides and G protein-coupled receptors that regulate feeding behavior. *Cell*, Vol.92, No.4, (Feb 20), pp. 573-585.

Sanz, C.; Roncero, I.; Vazquez, P.; Navas, M. A. & Blazquez, E. (2007). Effects of glucose and insulin on glucokinase activity in rat hypothalamus. *J Endocrinol*, Vol.193, No.2, (May), pp. 259-267.

Sanz, C.; Vazquez, P.; Navas, M. A.; Alvarez, E. & Blazquez, E. (2008). Leptin but not neuropeptide Y up-regulated glucagon-like peptide 1 receptor expression in GT1-7 cells and rat hypothalamic slices. *Metabolism*, Vol.57, No.1, (Jan), pp. 40-48.

Schuit, F. C.; Huypens, P.; Heimberg, H. & Pipeleers, D. G. (2001). Glucose sensing in pancreatic beta-cells: a model for the study of other glucose-regulated cells in gut, pancreas, and hypothalamus. *Diabetes*, Vol.50, No.1, (Jan), pp. 1-11.

Shiota, C.; Coffey, J.; Grimsby, J.; Grippo, J. F. & Magnuson, M. A. (1999). Nuclear import of hepatic glucokinase depends upon glucokinase regulatory protein, whereas export is due to a nuclear export signal sequence in glucokinase. *J Biol Chem*, Vol.274, No.52, (Dec 24), pp. 37125-37130.

Silver, I. A. & Erecinska, M. (1994). Extracellular glucose concentration in mammalian brain: continuous monitoring of changes during increased neuronal activity and upon limitation in oxygen supply in normo-, hypo-, and hyperglycemic animals. *J Neurosci*, Vol.14, No.8, (Aug), pp. 5068-5076.

Silver, I. A. & Erecinska, M. (1998). Glucose-induced intracellular ion changes in sugar-sensitive hypothalamic neurons. *J Neurophysiol*, Vol.79, No.4, (Apr), pp. 1733-1745.

Song, Z. & Routh, V. H. (2005). Differential effects of glucose and lactate on glucosensing neurons in the ventromedial hypothalamic nucleus. *Diabetes*, Vol.54, No.1, (Jan), pp. 15-22.

Sundstrom, L.; Morrison, B., 3rd; Bradley, M. & Pringle, A. (2005). Organotypic cultures as tools for functional screening in the CNS. *Drug Discov Today*, Vol.10, No.14, (Jul 15), pp. 993-1000.

Sutherland, V. L.; McReynolds, M.; Tompkins, L. S.; Brooks, H. L. & Lynch, R. M. (2005). Developmental expression of glucokinase in rat hypothalamus. *Brain Res Dev Brain Res*, Vol.154, No.2, (Feb 8), pp. 255-258.

Tang-Christensen, M.; Larsen, P. J.; Thulesen, J.; Romer, J. & Vrang, N. (2000). The proglucagon-derived peptide, glucagon-like peptide-2, is a neurotransmitter involved in the regulation of food intake. *Nat Med*, Vol.6, No.7, (Jul), pp. 802-807.

Tippett, P. S. & Neet, K. E. (1982). An allosteric model for the inhibition of glucokinase by long chain acyl coenzyme A. *J Biol Chem*, Vol.257, No.21, (Nov 10), pp. 12846-12852.

Tong, Q.; Ye, C.; McCrimmon, R. J.; Dhillon, H.; Choi, B.; Kramer, M. D.; Yu, J.; Yang, Z.; Christiansen, L. M.; Lee, C. E.; Choi, C. S.; Zigman, J. M.; Shulman, G. I.; Sherwin, R. S.; Elmquist, J. K. & Lowell, B. B. (2007). Synaptic glutamate release by ventromedial hypothalamic neurons is part of the neurocircuitry that prevents hypoglycemia. *Cell Metab*, Vol.5, No.5, (May), pp. 383-393.

Toyoda, Y.; Miwa, I.; Satake, S.; Anai, M. & Oka, Y. (1995). Nuclear location of the regulatory protein of glucokinase in rat liver and translocation of the regulator to the cytoplasm in response to high glucose. *Biochem Biophys Res Commun*, Vol.215, No.2, (Oct 13), pp. 467-473.

Tsuneki, H.; Wada, T. & Sasaoka, T. (2010). Role of orexin in the regulation of glucose homeostasis. *Acta Physiol (Oxf)*, Vol.198, No.3, (Mar), pp. 335-348.

Turnley, A. M.; Stapleton, D.; Mann, R. J.; Witters, L. A.; Kemp, B. E. & Bartlett, P. F. (1999). Cellular distribution and developmental expression of AMP-activated protein kinase isoforms in mouse central nervous system. *J Neurochem*, Vol.72, No.4, (Apr), pp. 1707-1716.

Turton, M. D.; O'Shea, D.; Gunn, I.; Beak, S. A.; Edwards, C. M.; Meeran, K.; Choi, S. J.; Taylor, G. M.; Heath, M. M.; Lambert, P. D.; Wilding, J. P.; Smith, D. M.; Ghatei, M. A.; Herbert, J. & Bloom, S. R. (1996). A role for glucagon-like peptide-1 in the central regulation of feeding. *Nature*, Vol.379, No.6560, (Jan 4), pp. 69-72.

Uttenthal, L. O.; Toledano, A. & Blazquez, E. (1992). Autoradiographic localization of receptors for glucagon-like peptide-1 (7-36) amide in rat brain. *Neuropeptides*, Vol.21, No.3, (Mar), pp. 143-146.

Van Schaftingen, E. (1989). A protein from rat liver confers to glucokinase the property of being antagonistically regulated by fructose 6-phosphate and fructose 1-phosphate. *Eur J Biochem*, Vol.179, No.1, (Jan 15), pp. 179-184.

Van Schaftingen, E.; Bartrons, R. & Hers, H. G. (1984). The mechanism by which ethanol decreases the concentration of fructose 2,6-bisphosphate in the liver. *Biochem J*, Vol.222, No.2, (Sep 1), pp. 511-518.

Vandercammen, A. & Van Schaftingen, E. (1993). Species and tissue distribution of the regulatory protein of glucokinase. *Biochem J*, Vol.294 (Pt 2), (Sep 1), pp. 551-556.

Viollet, B.; Athea, Y.; Mounier, R.; Guigas, B.; Zarrinpashneh, E.; Horman, S.; Lantier, L.; Hebrard, S.; Devin-Leclerc, J.; Beauloye, C.; Foretz, M.; Andreelli, F.; Ventura-Clapier, R. & Bertrand, L. (2009). AMPK: Lessons from transgenic and knockout animals. *Front Biosci*, Vol.14, pp. 19-44.

Vionnet, N.; Stoffel, M.; Takeda, J.; Yasuda, K.; Bell, G. I.; Zouali, H.; Lesage, S.; Velho, G.; Iris, F.; Passa, P. & et al. (1992). Nonsense mutation in the glucokinase gene causes early-onset non-insulin-dependent diabetes mellitus. *Nature*, Vol.356, No.6371, (Apr 23), pp. 721-722.

Wang, R.; Liu, X.; Hentges, S. T.; Dunn-Meynell, A. A.; Levin, B. E.; Wang, W. & Routh, V. H. (2004). The regulation of glucose-excited neurons in the hypothalamic arcuate nucleus by glucose and feeding-relevant peptides. *Diabetes,* Vol.53, No.8, (Aug), pp. 1959-1965.

Yang, X. J.; Kow, L. M.; Funabashi, T. & Mobbs, C. V. (1999). Hypothalamic glucose sensor: similarities to and differences from pancreatic beta-cell mechanisms. *Diabetes,* Vol.48, No.9, (Sep), pp. 1763-1772.

Yang, X. J.; Kow, L. M.; Pfaff, D. W. & Mobbs, C. V. (2004). Metabolic pathways that mediate inhibition of hypothalamic neurons by glucose. *Diabetes,* Vol.53, No.1, (Jan), pp. 67-73.

Zhou, L.; Podolsky, N.; Sang, Z.; Ding, Y.; Fan, X.; Tong, Q.; Levin, B. E. & McCrimmon, R. J. (2010). The Medial Amygdalar Nucleus: A Novel Glucose-Sensing Region That Modulates the Counterregulatory Response to Hypoglycemia. *Diabetes,* Vol.59, No.10, (October 1, 2010), pp. 2646-2652.

5

Expression of Neuropeptide Y of GIFT Tilapia (*Oreochromis sp.*) in Yeast *Pichia Pastoris* and Its Stimulatory Effects on Food Intake and Growth

Guangzhong Wang, Caiyun Sun, Haoran Lin and Wensheng Li*

State Key Laboratory of Biocontrol,
Institute of Aquatic Economic Animals and
Guangdong Provincial Key Laboratory for Aquatic Economic Animals,
School of Life Sciences, Sun Yat-Sen University, Guangzhou,
P. R. China

1. Introduction

Neuropeptide Y (NPY) , a peptide with 36 amino acid residues which was first isolated from porcine brain (Tatemoto et al., 1982), is most highly expressed in the hypothalamic arcuate nucleus (ARC) (Lin et al., 2004). NPY is a member of the NPY family which consists of NPY, peptide YY (PYY), pancreatic polypeptide (PP) and peptide Y (PY)(Cerda-Reverter and Larhammar, 2000a). There are three NPY-related peptides were expressed in fish. They are NPY, peptide YY and peptide Y(Cerda-Reverter et al., 2000b; Sundstrom et al., 2008). Currently, NPY peptides or cDNA sequences have been obtained from many fish species including catfish, goldfish, sea bass, Atlantic cod, flounder, rainbow trout, zebrafish(Volkoff, 2006). As other low molecular weight secreted peptide, NPY is synthesized as larger peptide precursor which consists of a hydrophobic signal peptide, the mature peptide, the amidation-proteolytic site, and the carboxy-terminal extended peptide (Cerda-Reverter and Larhammar, 2000a). A partial cDNA coding for the mature peptide of NPY of tilapia (red tilapia, *Oreochromis sp.*) has been cloned and reported. The size of the sequence is of 192bp, which encodes a 28 a.a. signal peptide and the 36 a.a. mature peptide, while the sequence encoding carboxy-terminal extension aside the C-terminal of mature peptide has not been reported yet (Carpio et al., 2006).

NPY is well known to be involved in many physiological functions, such as cardiovascular regulation, affective disorder, memory retention, neuroendocrine control and feeding in mammals(Pedrazzini, 2004). In fact, NPY has been considered as the most potent orexigenic peptide in mammals (Halford et al., 2004; Kalra et al., 1999; Valassi et al., 2008; Woods et al., 1998). Many studies have proved that NPY is also an important energy metabolism regulator of vertebrates. When fed with a high-carbohydrate diet; diabetic rats exhibit increased gene expression of the NPY in the hypothalamic ARC, and high-fat diet suppressed NPY expression(Chavez et al., 1998). Intraventricular administration of NPY has been shown to enhance carbohydrate and fat utilization in rats which leads to a significant increase in energy consumption and body weight (Kiris GA, 2007). NPY executes these functions mainly through its receptor Y1, Y2 and Y5 (Aldegunde and Mancebo, 2006; Pedrazzini et al., 2003).

NPY is one of the most highly conserved neuroendocrine peptides in vertebrates(Blomqvist et al., 1992). The NPY peptides of fish species also showed remarkable sequence homology with mammals, suggesting the similar functions of NPY in fish and mammals(Cerda-Reverter et al., 2000b; Sundstrom et al., 2005).As its mammalian counterpart, NPY is also a very important regulator of food intake and energy metabolism in fish(Volkoff, 2006; Volkoff et al., 2005). For example, both central and peripheral injections of mammalian or fish NPY significantly stimulated food intake in a dose dependent manner in goldfish (Lopez-Patino et al., 1999; Narnaware et al., 2000). NPY mRNA levels increased substantially a few hours before feeding goldfish, which was fed at fixed time, and then declined after feeding; Fasting could also upgrade the expression of goldfish NPY, while re-feeding restored the NPY mRNA levels (Narnaware and Peter, 2001a). In addition, NPY expression was regulated by high glucose or high fat diet but not affected by the protein composition of food (Narnaware and Peter, 2002). The relationship between NPY and feeding promotion were also found in other fish species. Ventricle injection with porcine NPY significantly promoted the feeding of rainbow trout within 2-3 hours(Aldegunde and Mancebo, 2006). Brain NPY mRNA level of Atlantic cod changed before and after diet, and reached the highest level at feeding time(Kehoe and Volkoff, 2007). The short-term changes of NPY level were all related to temporary feeding regulation. Similar to mammals, NPY is a long-term energy metabolism regulation factor, long-term treatment of NPY could also significantly change the growth and feeding behavior of fish species. Recombinant protein expressed in *Escherichia coli.* of tilapia NPY significantly promoted the growth and food intake of tilapia by injection(Carpio et al., 2006). Immersion bath with the same prokaryotic expression of NPY three times a week significantly increased the body weight and body length of catfish (Carpio Y, 2007). NPY either administered by i.p. injection or through feed stimulated food intake as well as growth of *Oreochromis niloticus* (Kiris GA, 2007).

Yeast has been used in food and feed additive production for a long time. Because of the lower toxicity and higher environmental security, the yeast culture supernatant of yeast expression system for foreign genes expression can be directly used as feed of animal without purification. In addition to the advantages of molecular and genetic manipulations sharing with *Saccharomyces*, *Pichia pastoris* has higher protein expression efficiency and is easier for high-density fermentation. Moreover, as a eukaryote, *Pichia pastoris* has advantages in post-translational processing of higher eukaryotic expression systems such as protein processing, protein folding, and posttranslational modification that *E. Coli.* systems can not carry out, while being as easy to manipulate as *E. Coli* or *Saccharomyces cerevisiae.* It is faster, easier, and lower cost than other eukaryotic expression systems and generally gives higher expression levels. *Pichia pastoris* itself secrete little proteins into the culture medium, such facilities the secretion and purification of recombinant proteins. In addition, single or multiple copies of foreign genes were easy to integration into the genome of *Pichia pastoris* in specific site, which makes the recombinant strains to be genetically stable. These features make *Pichia* a very useful protein expression system suitable for industrial production (Faber et al., 1995; Romanos et al., 1992).

Treating fish with hormones or peptides to induce the food intake and growth by injections is definitely not a realistic method in aquaculture because they would require expensive,

Expression of Neuropeptide Y of GIFT Tilapia (Oreochromis sp.) in Yeast Pichia Pastoris and Its Stimulatory
Effects on Food Intake and Growth

77

time-consuming injection in individual fish. To feed fish with capsules or feed containing agonists/antagonists of appetite-regulating factors might represent a viable solution (Gelineau, 2001; Volkoff et al., 2010). Previous experiments have shown that trout fed with CCK antagonists eat significantly more than their mean daily intake on the other days of the experiment (Gelineau, 2001). Tilapia, commonly known as the African carp, belongs to *Perciformes, Perciformes Suborder, Cichlidae*. Now, tilapia is one of the most important fish species used in aquaculture in the world. Because of its low cost, tilapia has been thought as the 21st century protein for poor people. In the present study, under purpose of developing new environmental friendly feed additives for fish, we isolated the ORF of NPY from GIFT tilapia and established the *Pichia* strains of pPICZαA-TiNPY1-X-33 and pPICZαA-TiNPY2-X-33 to express recombinant NPY proteins. Administration of the purified NPY to GIFT tilapia showed that long-term treatment of the recombinant peptide can stimulate food intake, promote growth and reduce feed conversion ratio. Moreover, this recombinant peptide obviously stimulated pituitary GH mRNA expression, while inhibit NPY and orexin mRNA expressions in hypothalamus.

2. Material and methods

2.1 Animals
All fish used in the present experiment are GIFT Strain tilapia (*Oreochromis niloticus*), and were obtained from local Panyu tilapia breeding fishery of Guangzhou, China. A male tilapia with body weight of 1.5kg was used for molecular cloning of NPY cDNA. Juvenile fish with the body weight ranging from 65 to 80g were selected for NPY feeding experiments. Since the tilapia at this stage was "prepubertal" and sexual dimorphism was not apparent, fish of mixed sexes were used for in vivo study. All fish were kept alive in well aerated freshwater under a 12L:12D photoperiod at 26 to 28°C. Fish for feeding experiment were cultured in a 150L tank with the density of 12 fish per tank and were acclimated to a constant flow of filtered water for two weeks before the feeding experiment. During the acclimation period, all fish were fed with normal extruded floating pellets twice a day. After finish the experiment, all fish were sacrificed by anesthesia in 0.05% MS222 (Sigma, St. Louis, MO) followed by spinosectomy according to the regulation of animal use at Sun Yat-Sen University.

2.2 Reagents and test substrates
TRIzol reagent, DNAse I, SuperScript II, T/A clone TM PCR Product Cloning Kit, Platinum Taq DNA Polymerase, Zeocin, and Real-time PCR Master Mix (SYBR Green) were purchased from Invitrogen (Carlsbad, CA). E.Z.N.A Gel Extraction Kit and E.Z.N.A Plasmid Extraction Kit were obtained from Omega Bio-Tek (USA). Anti-Neuropeptide Y Rabbit pAb was purchased from Calbiochem (U.S.A). Sheep anti-rabbit secondary antibody IgG-HRP was purchased from Boster Biological Engineering Co., Ltd., (China). His•Bind Columns was bought from Novagen (USA). Trpton, Yeast extract and Dextrose were purchased from OXIOID (Britain). The membrane of PVDF (0.2μm) was obtained from Pall life sciences (U.S.A). Protein Marker is BIO-RAD kaleidoscope Prestained Standards.

2.3 Molecular cloning of GIFT tilapia NPY
Specific primers for amplification of tilapia NPY cDNA were designed based on the reported NPY sequence of red tilapia (GenBank Accession No. AY779047). The forward

primer was F1 (5'-ATGCATCCTAACTTGGTGAGC-3') and the reverse primer was R1 (5'-GGCCACGCGTCGACTAGTAC-3', AUAP). PCR was performed using the RT sample prepared from the hypothalamus as the template to pull out GIFT NPY cDNA. Briefly, total RNA was extracted from the hypothalamus of GIFT tilapia using TRIzol®reagent method. 1µg total RNA was reverse transcribed to first strand cDNA by SuperScript First-Strand Synthesis System for RT-PCR (Invitrogen) and Oligo(dT)12-18 primer (Invitrogen Adapter Primer). 5µl of the above 20µl reverse transcription reaction mixture was used to amplify a NPY fragment with the size of 650 bp, which include the open reading frame (ORF) and the 3' untranslation region. The total volume of PCR reaction is 100µl containing with 0.5µl Platinum Taq DNA Polymerase and the corresponding PCR buffer, 200 µM of each dNTP, 30 µM $MgCl_2$ and 200 pmole of F1 and AUAP primers. PCR reactions were conducted for 36 cycles with the denaturation at 94 °C for 15 sec, annealing at 53°C for 15 sec and extension at 72°C for 1 min. The PCR products were size-fractionated in 1.5% agarose gel and purified by using E.Z.N.A® Gel Extraction Kit. The purified PCR product was then ligated into cloning T plasmid vector (pTZ57R/T plasmid vector). The recombinant pTZ57R/T vector was transformed into DH5a (Escherichia coli), after screening and identification, plasmids of positive colonies were extracted using E.Z.N.A® Plasmid Extraction Kit and sequenced using M13F primer.

2.4 Construction of pPICZaA-TiNPY1and pPICZaA-TiNPY2 expression vectors

Three gene specific primers for amplification of the mature peptide of tilapia NPY were designed based on the sequence obtained to establish two different expression vectors. A forward primer (F2: 5'-CGGCCTCGAGAAAAGAGAGGCTGAAGCTTACCCAGTGAA ACCA-3') contains an *Xho* I site and the sequence encoding partial signal peptide which could be digested by *Xho* I on yeast secretory expression vector pPICZαA(Invitrogen). The reverse primers were R2 (5'-TGCTCTAGATACCTCTGTCTTGT-3') which contains an *Xba* I site and R3 (5'-TGATCTAGATCAATGATGATGATGATGATGATACCTCTGTCTTGT-3'). Besides the *Xba* I site, R3 also contains the sequence encoding 6× his tag and a stop codon. Using the NPY cDNA we obtained as template, two fragments with the size of 201bp (NPY1) and 226bp (NPY2) were amplified by using primer pairs of F2/R2 and F2/R3, respectively. PCR reactions were conducted for 36 cycles with the denaturation at 94 °C for 15 sec, annealing at 65°C for 15 sec and extension at 72°C for 30 sec. The PCR products were size-fractionated in 1.5% agarose gel and purified by using E.Z.N.A® Gel Extraction Kit. The purified PCR product and *Pichia pastoris* expression vector pPICZαA were digested by *Xho* I and *Xba* I, respectively. After purification, the digested PCR products were ligated with the linearized pPICZαA. After sequencing confirmation, two recombinant expression vectors, pPICZαA-TiNPY1 and pPICZαA-TiNPY2, were established. The NPY gene of interest is cloned in frame with a C-terminal peptide containing the c-myc epitope and a polyhistidine (6× His) tag as in pPICZαA- TiNPY1, or with only the polyhistidine (6× His) tag as in pPICZαA- TiNPY2. The recombinant NPY proteins are expressed as fusions to an N-terminal signal peptide, a-factor secretion signal of the *Saccharomyces cerevisiae*. Both vectors would give high expression level of the interest gene in *Pichia pastoris* when induced by methanol.

2.5 Establishment of *Pichia X-33* strains of pPICZαA-TiNPY1 and pPICZαA-TiNPY2

The competent cells of *Pichia X-33* strain were prepared according to the manual of the Easyselect™ Pichia Expression Kit (Invitrogen). Two recombinant expression vectors of pPICZαA-TiNPY1 and pPICZαA-TiNPY2 were linearized by the digestion of PmeI (NEB) within the 5'AOX 1 region and then transformed into the competent cell of *Pichia X-33* by electroporation. The linearized pPICZαA-TiNPY1 or pPICZαA-TiNPY2 was directly integrated within the 5´ AOX1 region of Pichia host genome (*Pichia X-33* strain purchased from Invitrogen) by gene insertion. The two transformation mixtures were respectively spread onto YPDS plates (Yeast Extract Peptone Dextrose Medium), which contained 1% yeast extract, 2% peptone, 2% dextrose (glucose), 1 M sorbitol, 2% agar and 200 µg/ml Zeocin™(or 100 µg/ml Zeocin, and then screening on 200/500/1000 µg/ml Zeocin YPDS for multi-copy integrants). These plates then were incubated at 28-30°C for about 4 days until the positive single colonies of *Pichia X-33* were observed. In a parallel study, the PICZαA blank vectors were introduced into the competent cells of *Pichia X-33* strain and which acts as a negative control. At this point, two recombinant *Pichia X-33* strains were constructed, they were pPICZαA-TiNPY1-X-33 and pPICZαA-TiNPY2-X-33 , which could express recombinant TiNPY1 (tilapia NPY mature peptide with a C-terminal peptide containing the c-myc epitope and 6× His tag, total 58 a.a.) or TiNPY2 (tilapia NPY mature peptide with only the 6× His tag, total 42 a.a.) respectively.

2.6 Induction of recombinant protein expression of TiNPY1 and TiNPY2
Single colonies of genetically engineered *Pichia pastoris* strains pPICZαA-Ti NPY1-X-33, pPICZαA-TiNPY2-X-33 and pPICZαA-X-33 (as a negative control NC$_0$) were picked and cultured in 5ml BMGY medium(1% yeast extract, 2% peptone, 100 mM potassium phosphate, pH 6.0, 1.34% YNB, 4x10^{-5}% biotin, 1% glycerol) at 30°C in a shaking incubator (250rpm)for 24h. When the OD600 of the culture is within the range from 4.0 to 6.0, 200µl culture of each colony was stocked in 15% glycerol at -80 °C.

The remained cells were harvested by centrifuging at 1500 g for 5 minutes at 4°C. Discard the supernatant and resuspend the cell pellet into BMMY medium (1% yeast extract, 2% peptone, 100 mM potassium phosphate, pH 6.0, 1.34% YNB, 4x10^{-5}% biotin, 0.5% methanol) to induce NPY protein expression at 28-30°C with the shaking speed of 250rpm. The media of one of PICZαA-TiNPY1-X-33 or pPICZαA-TiNPY2-X-33 was not be replaced and maintained in BMGY medium to act as negative control of NC$_1$ and NC$_2$.

1ml cultures of each tube were sampled and cultured in BMMY medium with 0.5% methanol to maintain induction every 24 hours. In a parallel study, instead of replacing the culture medium, one culture of PICZαA-TiNPY1-X-33 or pPICZαA-TiNPY2-X-33 remained to be cultured in BMGY and act as negative control of NC$_1$ and NC$_2$. Sampled cultures were centrifuged to collect supernatant respectively, and the supernatants were stored at -20°C or directly concentrated and analyzed by Tricine-SDS-PAGE gel and western blot. The expressed recombinant protein by pPICZαA-TiNPY1-X-33 and pPICZαA-TiNPY2-X-33 were named TiNPY1 and TiNPY2.

2.7 Analysis of recombinant NPY proteins by Tricine-SDS-PAGE and western blot
The harvested supernatants with recombinant proteins were concentrated and analyzed by Tricine-SDS-PAGE gel electrophoresis according to the standard procedure. Samples were first run under 50V for 1h and then change the voltage to 75V for another 1h. After electrophoresis, the gel was stained with Coomassie blue for 20 min, and then analyzed whether the recombinant proteins TiNPY1 (with a molecular weight about 6.9KD) and TiNPY2 (with a molecular weight about 5.1KD) were present or not.

After analysis by Tricine- SDS-PAGE gel electrophoresis, samples induced with different time were analyzed by western blot. After separation by Tricine-SDS-PAGE gel electrophoresis, proteins were electro-transferred from the gel to a PVDF membrane. The recombinant protein was recognized with a rabbit polyclonal antibody against porcine NPY (purchased from Calbiochem Corporation, USA) with a dilution of 1:1000, which was recognized by sheep anti-rabbit secondary antibody IgG-HRP (purchased from Boster Biological Engineering Co., Ltd., China). Western blot results were detected by chemiluminescence detection system.

2.8 Expression kinetics of NPY
Since the protein banding patterns of TiNPY1 and TiNPY2 in supernatant were varying with different induction time, it is necessary to study the kinetics of NPY expression. In the present study, NPY1 expression was taken as a model to study the relationship of induction time and TiNPY1 protein expression pattern. Four colonies of pPICZαA-TiNPY1-X-33 were used to express recombinant protein of NPY. The supernatants were harvested for Tricine-SDS-PAGE gel electrophoresis and western blot at the time point of 12h, 24h and 48h after 0.5% methanol induction.

2.9 Purification of the recombinant NPY proteins
Since Recombinant protein TiNPY1 and TiNPY2 were conjugated with 6× His tag, His•Bind Column (NOVAGEN) could be used to purify these proteins. pH of supernatants of methanol-induced culture were adjusted to 7.9 by NaOH and then all samples were loaded into the His•Bind Column which was equilibrated with 15ml binding buffer(0.5 M NaCl, 20mM Tris-HCl, 5mM imidazole, pH 7.9) before use. The column was washed by 10ml wash buffer (0.5M NaCl, 60mM imidazole, 20mM Tris-HCl, pH 7.9) to remove unbound proteins. The recombinant protein was eluted by elute buffer with different concentration of imidazole (150/250/500mM imidazole, 0.5M NaCl, 20mM Tris-HCl, pH 7.9).Each fraction was eluted with one milliliter elution. Tricine-SDS-PAGE gel electrophoresis was conducted to analyze the purification with comparisons of before and after purified supernatants.

2.10 Sequencing of N-terminal amino acid of NPY
The purified TiNPY1 protein bands were electro-transferred from the gel to a PVDF membrane, and the sequencing of N-terminal amino acid of TiNPY1 was performed by using Sequencing instrument PROCISE491 (Applied Biosystemes Company, USA) with EDMEN degradation method.

2.11 Diet preparation and feeding experiment with juvenile tilapia
Five different diets for feeding experiments were prepared by homogeneously spraying three kinds of yeast culture supernatants directly onto the surface of ordinary commercial extruded floating feed. The concentrations of the recombinant proteins of NPY1 in three diets are 0.15, 0.3 and 0.6μg TiNPY1/g feed, respectively. A diet contains the recombinant protein TiNPY2 to a level of 0.3μg TiNPY2/g feed. A diet without any addition of recombinant protein acts as a negative control feed. All diets were stored at −20 °C before use.
After finishing two week's acclimation, 180 fish of GIFT Strain tilapia, with a body weight ranging from 60 to 80g (73.09±3.58 g) and length ranging from 12.0 to 14.0cm were randomly

assigned to 15 aquariums and 12 fish were cultured in an aquarium. All 15 aquariums were divided into five groups with three aquariums (three replicates, n=12) per group. One group was fed with a kind of diet. Group1, 2, 3 were fed with diets containing 0.15, 0.3 and 0.6µg TiNPY1/g feed, respectively. Group 4 took the control feed and group 5 was fed with 0.3µg TiNPY2/g feed. The feeding experiment was taken for 50 days. All fishes were cultured at 28 °C under a 12 L: 12D photoperiod. Fish were fed with the pellet feed two times daily to satiation at 09:00 and 18:00 (animals didn't take any feed within one hour after the beginning of feeding). The remained feeds were removed one hour after each feeding operation and dried to calculate food intake of fish in each tank. Every 10 days, all fish in each aquarium were caught and dried briefly with towel, and then the weight for each fish was measured. The fish were not fed with anything within 24h before measurement. The body length of each fish was also measured at the beginning and the end of feed experiment. The whole feeding experiment lasted for 50 days.

After finishing the feeding experiment, all fish were sacrificed and their tissues were removed for the following experiments: pituitaries and hypothalamuses were used for RNA extraction and RT-PCR; Livers and all guts were weighed to determine the hepatosomatic index (HSI) and visceral body weight, which were calculated as 100× liver weight/body weight and 100× gut weight/body weight. The mRNA expression of growth hormone (GH), NPY and orexin were detected by using Real-time PCR technique. Fish dorsal white muscle of each group was sampled for moisture, crude protein and total lipid content were analyzed according to the method of Kjeldahl (AOAC, 1984) and Soxhlet extraction method, respectively.

2.12 Data transformation and statistical analysis

For feeding experiment, feeding conversion ratio (SGR) was calculated in terms of the number of grams of feed that are used to produce one gram of whole fish. For real-time PCR measurement of GH, NPY and orexin mRNA, 18S mRNA acts as an internal control to normalized with mRNA of the target gene. Data were presented as means ± SEM and analyzed with one-way ANOVA followed by Fisher's Least Significance Difference (LSD) test. Differences between groups were considered as significant at $P < 0.05$.

3. Results

3.1 Molecular cloning of cDNA encoding the NPY of GIFT tilapia and construction of the expression vectors of pPICZaA-TiNPY1and pPICZaA-TiNPY2

The ORF and 3′ untranslation region (UTR) of GIFT tilapia NPY was cloned (Fig.1). The partial cDNA of NPY is 659bp in size with a 359bp 3′UTR and 300bp ORF encoding a 99 a.a. precursor protein. A putative signal peptide of 28 a.a. is located in the N-terminal of NPY. And a 36 a.a. mature peptide is highly conserved with that of human NPY (89% identity). The remained 35 a.a. is the C-terminal of NPY.

Two different expression vectors of GIFT tilapia were established and they were named as pPICZaA-TiNPY1 and pPICZaA-TiNPY2 (Fig.2) The insert size of pPICZaA-TiNP1 is 201bp which encodes 36 a.a. NPY mature peptide and a C-terminal peptide with a c-myc epitope and a polyhistidine (6× His) tag. The insert size of pPICZaA-TiNPY2 is 226bp which encodes NPY mature peptide and a polyhistidine (6× His) tag.

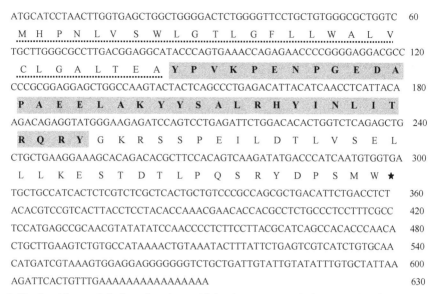

ATGCATCCTAACTTGGTGAGCTGGCTGGGGACTCTGGGGTTCCTGCTGTGGGCGCTGGTC 60
  M H P N L V S W L G T L G F L L W A L V

TGCTTGGGCGCCTTGACGGAGGCATACCCAGTGAAACCAGAGAACCCCGGGGAGGACGCC 120
  C L G A L T E A **Y P V K P E N P G E D A**

CCCGCGGAGGAGCTGGCCAAGTACTACTCAGCCCTGAGACATTACATCAACCTCATTACA 180
P A E E L A K Y Y S A L R H Y I N L I T

AGACAGAGGTATGGGAAGAGATCCAGTCCTGAGATTCTGGACACACTGGTCTCAGAGCTG 240
R Q R Y G K R S S P E I L D T L V S E L

CTGCTGAAGGAAAGCACAGACACGCTTCCACAGTCAAGATATGACCCATCAATGTGGTGA 300
  L L K E S T D T L P Q S R Y D P S M W ★

TGCTGCCATCACTCTCGTCTCGCTCACTGCTGTCCCGCCAGCGCTGACATTCTGACCTCT 360

ACACGTCCGTCACTTACCTCCTACACCAAACGAACACCACGCCTCTGCCCTCCTTTCGCC 420

TCCATGAGCCGCAACGTATATATCCAACCCCTCTTCCTTACGCATCAGCCACACCCAACA 480

CTGCTTGAAGTCTGTGCCATAAAACTGTAAATACTTTATTCTGAGTCGTCATCTGTGCAA 540

CATGATCGTAAAGTGGAGGAGGGGGGGTCTGCTGATTGTATTGTATATTTGTGCTATTAA 600

AGATTCACTGTTTGAAAAAAAAAAAAAAAAAA 630

Fig. 1. Nucleotides and deduced amino acid (a.a.) sequence of tilapia NPY. The a.a. sequence underlined with the black dotted line is the predicted signal peptide. The mature peptide of NPY is highlight in grey box.

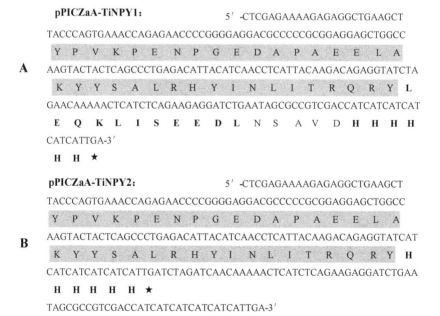

pPICZaA-TiNPY1:   5′-CTCGAGAAAAGAGAGGCTGAAGCT

TACCCAGTGAAACCAGAGAACCCCGGGGAGGACGCCCCCCGCGGAGGAGCTGGCC
  Y P V K P E N P G E D A P A E E L A

A   AAGTACTACTCAGCCCTGAGACATTACATCAACCTCATTACAAGACAGAGGTATCTA
  K Y Y S A L R H Y I N L I T R Q R Y L

GAACAAAAACTCATCTCAGAAGAGGATCTGAATAGCGCCGTCGACCATCATCATCAT
  E **Q** **K** **L** **I** S E E **D** N S A V D **H** **H** **H** **H**

CATCATTGA-3′
  H **H** ★

pPICZaA-TiNPY2:   5′-CTCGAGAAAAGAGAGGCTGAAGCT

TACCCAGTGAAACCAGAGAACCCCGGGGAGGACGCCCCCCGCGGAGGAGCTGGCC
  Y P V K P E N P G E D A P A E E L A

B   AAGTACTACTCAGCCCTGAGACATTACATCAACCTCATTACAAGACAGAGGTATCAT
  K Y Y S A L R H Y I N L I T R Q R Y **H**

CATCATCATCATCATTGATCTAGATCAACAAAAACTCATCTCAGAAGAGGATCTGAA
  H **H** **H** **H** **H** ★

TAGCGCCGTCGACCATCATCATCATCATCATTGA-3′

Fig. 2. Nucleotide and deduced amino acid sequences of NPY1 (A) and NPY2 (B) that were subcloned into pPICZaA to establish the expression vectors. The mature peptide of NPY is highlight in grey box, and the "H" in bold are 6XHis tags.

3.2 Establishment of the recombinant *Pichia X-33* stains of PICZαA-TiNPY1 and pPICZαA-TiNPY2

To get the high-yield strains of recombinant TiNPY1 and TiNPY2 produced by engineered *Pichia pastoris*, pPICZaA-TiNPY1 and pPICZaA-TiNPY2 were introduced into *Pichia X-33* strains by electroporation, respectively. After selection by using different concentration of Zeocin, the strains with the integration of TiNPY1, TiNPY2 and pPICzaA blank vector into the genome of *Pichia pastoris* X-33(Fig.3) were selected for our study. These strains with high Zeocin-resistance were named as pPICZαA-TiNPY1-X-33, pPICZαA-TiNPY2-X-33 and pPICZαA-X-33. pPICZαA-TiNPY1-X-33 can express a 58 a.a. peptide with 36 a.a. NPY mature peptide and a C-terminal peptide containing the c-myc epitope and 6× His tag, while the strain of pPICZαA-TiNPY1-X-33 can express a 42 a.a. peptide with NPY mature peptide and a 6× His tag.

3.3 Expression of recombinant NPY1 and NPY2 in *Pichia X-33* stains

To study the expression pattern of recombinant NPY1 and NPY2 in *Pichia pastoris* , pPICZαA-TiNPY1-X-33, pPICZαA-TiNPY2-X-33 were induced by using 5% methanol with the time points of 24h, 48h and 72h. The results of SDS-PAGE and Commassie blue staining of recombinant NPY at different times of methanol induction showed that six clones of each recombinant strain of pPICZαA-TiNPY1-X-33 and pPICZαA-TiNPY2-X-33 could express tilapia TiNPY1and TiNPY2, respectively. For pPICZαA-TiNPY2-X-33 after 24h methanol induction, in addition to a band with the size of 5-6KD was observed in all six colonies,

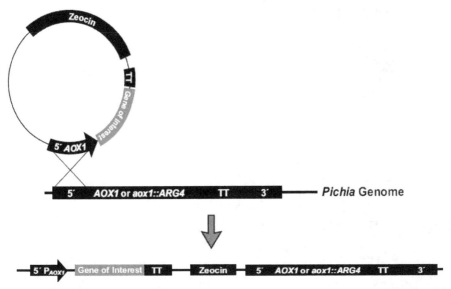

Fig. 3. Integration of TiNPY1, TiNPY2 and pPICza-A blank vector into the genome of Pichia pastoris X-33. The pPICzaA blank vector, pPICzaA-TiNPY-1 and pPICzaA-TiNPY-2 were transformed into Pichia pastoris X-33 by electroporation. After selection by using different concentration of Zeocin, three colonies of Pichia pastoris X-33 with high Zeocin resistance and high copy number were obtained, namely pPICZaA-TiNPY1-X-3, pPICZaA-TiNPY2-X-33 and pPICZaA-X-33.

there is a band with the size of 6-7KD expressed in colonies 1,2,3 and 4(Fig.4). After 48h induction, the band with the size of 5-6KD is still appear in all six colonies, but the expression level of the band is significantly lower than that of 24h-induction, while a band with a small size (2-4KD) was observed in all colonies(Fig.5). All bands almost disappeared except for colony 3 after methanol induction for 72h (Fig.6). Among the six colonies, only colony 3 has a stable expression pattern when induced by 5% methanol for 24h to 72h. Similar phenomenon was also observed in the strain of pPICZαA-TiNPY1-X-33. All six colonies selected expressed a peptide with the size of 7-9KD after 24h induction(Fig.4), but when the induction time increased to 48h, the band observed is about 5-6KD(Fig.5) and this band is still the major band after induction for 72h (Fig.6). In a parallel study, the pPICZαA - X-33 with methanol induction acts as negative control (NC0). The stains of pPICZαA-TiNPY1-X-33 and pPICZαA-TiNPY2-X-33 without methanol induction were also employed as negative controls (NC1 and NC2). No matter how long of the induction time, there is no band was present in the three negative controls.

Western blot was carried out to test the immunological characteristics of recombinant TiNPY1 and TiNPY2. These proteins were size-fractionated in 10% SDS-PAGE and transblotted onto the PVDF membrane. The recombinant proteins were recognized by a

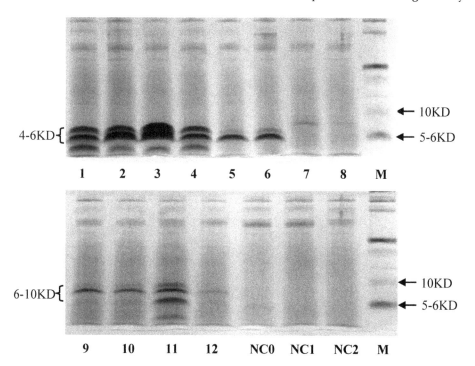

Fig. 4. SDS-PAGE detection of the expression of TiNPY1 and TiNPY2 after methanol induction for 24 hours.1-6:TiNPY2; 7-12:TiNPY1; NC0: pPICZaA-X-33 blank vector (negative control); NC1: pPICZaA-TiNPY1-X-33 without induction; NC2: pPICZaA-TiNPY2-X-33 without induction; M: protein marker. The size of TiNPY1 and TiNPY 2 is 6-9KD and 4-6KD, respectively.

Expression of Neuropeptide Y of GIFT Tilapia (Oreochromis sp.) in Yeast Pichia Pastoris and Its Stimulatory
Effects on Food Intake and Growth

85

rabbit polyclonal antibody against porcine NPY at a dilution 1:1000, which was recognized by sheep anti-rabbit secondary antibody IgG-HRP. 1µg of synthesized tilapia NPY with a molecular weight of 4.104KD was used as a positive control. The size of the NPY is smaller than both TiNPY1 and TiNPY2 because it lacks conjugated tags. The protein concentration of TiNPY1 and TiNPY2 in culture supernatants, when up-scale expressed in 1L shake-flask , were determined by scanning densitometry of dyed Tricine-SDS-PAGE gel and compared with the positive control (Fig.7,A). Western blot results showed that different from the SDS-PAGE detection that all colonies selected expressed the recombinant TiNPY1, only four colonies (No.2, 3, 4 and 6) were recognized by NPY antibodies (Fig.7,B). For TiNPY-2, SDS-PAGE showed that two of three colonies examined express two kinds of NPY with the molecular weight of 6-7KD and 5-6KD, while colony 3 only expressed the band with the size of 5-6KD (Fig.8,A). All these bands could be recognized by NPY antibody (Fig.8, B).

3.4 Time course study of the recombinant protein expression of TiNPY1
As the size and number of specific protein bands of TiNPY1 and TiNPY2 in supernatant were varying with different induction time, the expression kinetics of NPY1 was performed by inducing the expression of four pPICZaA-TiNPY1-X-33 colonies which came from the

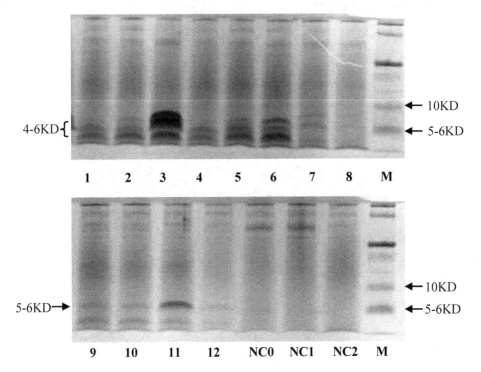

Fig. 5. SDS-PAGE detection of the expression of TiNPY1 and TiNPY2 after methanol induction for 48 hours.1-6:TiNPY2; 7-12:TiNPY1; NC0: pPICZaA-X-33 blank vector (negative control); NC1: pPICZaA-TiNPY1-X-33 without induction; NC2: pPICZaA-TiNPY2-X-33 without induction; M: protein marker. The size of TiNPY1 and TiNPY2 is 5-6KD and 4-6KD, respectively.

same colony (Fig.4, colony 11) and could express recombinant protein TiNPY1 efficiently. Tricine-SDS-PAGE result showed that when induced by methanol for 12h and 24h, the recombinant protein that pPICZαA-TiNPY1-X-33 expressed is about 10-12KD and 7-9KD. With the induction time increased to 48h, the molecular weight of TiNPY1 decreased to 6-7KD (Fig.9). Western blot result demonstrated that NPY antibody could only recognize the two protein bands induced by methanol for 12h as well as 24h. While after 48h induction, nothing could be observed in the membrane and two bands appeared before were missing, (Fig.10).

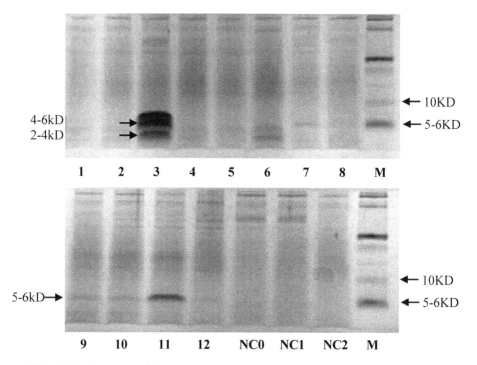

Fig. 6. SDS-PAGE detection of the expression of TiNPY1 and TiNPY2 after methanol induction for 72 hours. 1-6:TiNPY2; 7-12:TiNPY1; NC0: pPICZaA-X-33 blank vector (negative control); NC1: pPICZaA-TiNPY1-X-33 without induction; NC2: pPICZaA-TiNPY2-X-33 without induction; M: protein marker. The size of TiNPY1 and TiNPY2 is 5-6KD and 2-4kD, 4-6KD, respectively.

3.5 Purification of the recombinant tilapia NPY and sequencing of its N-terminal amino acid

As TiNPY1 and TiNPY2 were conjugated with 6× His tag, they could be purified with His•Bind Column by affinity chromatography. Samples from each fraction were size-fractionated by Tricine-SDS-PAGE with comparisons of supernatants before and after purification (Fig.11 and 12). The binding of the fusion recombinant proteins to the His•Bind Column (Ni-NTA column) was highly efficient as seen in Fig.11 (TiNPY1) and Fig.12 (TiNPY2). All of the three protein bands of TiNPY1 induced by methanol for 24 hours (Fig.

11) and two bands of TiNPY2 induced for 12 hours (Fig. 12) were eluted by 150mM imidazole. During the process of purification of TiNPY2, wash buffer was checked after washing to confirm that there were no recombinant proteins were washed out.

Two protein bands with larger molecular weight of TiNPY1 were purified and the 1-8th amino acids of their N-terminal were sequenced by instrument PROCISE491 (Applied Biosystemes Company, USA) with EDMEN degradation method. There are three kinds of proteins with different N-terminal a.a. (1-8th) were observed in the band with the largest molecular weight of TiNPY1. The protein with the N-terminal of N-EAYPVKPE is the major form which occupies 60-70% of TiNPY1. Proteins with the N-terminal of N-EAEAYPVK and N-YPVKPENP constitute of 20-30% and 5-10% of TiNPY1, respectively. The second band of TiNPY1 protein consists of two proteins with N-terminal of N-YPVKPENP (above 90%) and N-VKPENPGE (minority).

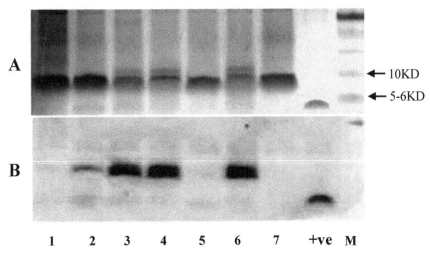

Fig. 7. SDS-PAGE to detect the expression of TiNPY1 (A) and western blot to confirm the immunological activity of recombinant TiNPY1. Samples (No.1-7) used in these experiments are recombinant TiNPY1 expressed by PICZaA-TiNPY1-X-33 after induction for different time. The synthesized tilapia NPY without His tags was used as positive control (4.104KD); M: protein marker

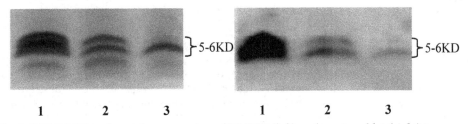

Fig. 8. SDS-PAGE to detect the expression of TiNPY2 (left) and western blot (right) to confirm the immunological activity of recombinant TiNPY2. Samples (No.1-3) used in these experiments are recombinant TiNPY2 expressed by PICZaA-TiNPY2-X-33.

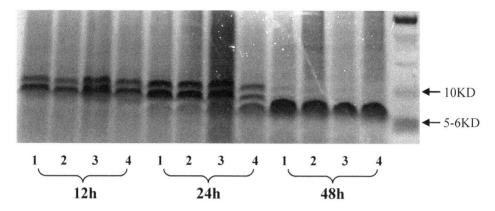

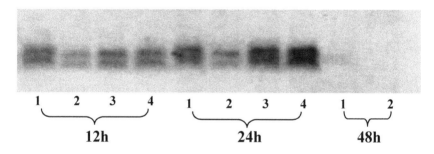

Fig. 9. Time course study of TiNPY1 expression induced by methanol. Four single colonies of pPICZaA-TiNPY1-X-33 with stable expression of TiNPY were used in the experiment. After induction of the expression by 0.5% methanol for 12h, 24h and 48h, the samples were harvested for SDS-PAGE.

Fig. 10. Time course study of TiNPY1 expression by Western blot. The same samples used in SDS-PAGE study were used in this experiment. Two samples of 48h were the sample 3 and 4 in SDS-PAGE, respectively. Only TiNPY1 expressed after 12h and 24h induction were recognized by polyclonal antibody of NPY.

3.6 Effects of recombinant TiNPY on food intake and growth of the juveniles of GIFT tilapia

The results of in vivo study showed that the recombinant proteins of NPY could significantly stimulated food intake and body growth of GIFT tilapia. Compared to the control group (group 4), the percentages of average body weight increased in the group fed with 0.15μgTiNPY1/g feed (group 1), 0.3μgTiNPY1/g feed (group 2) or 0.6μgTiNPY1/g feed (group 3) were 29.65%, 32.11% and 12.60%, respectively. And the body weight of tilapia fed with 0.3μgTiNPY2/g feed was increased to 43.05% which gained the highest growth speed. The specific growth rates (SGR) and the final mean body lengths of all experimental groups [group 1 ($P<0.001$), group 2 ($P<0.001$), group 3 ($P<0.05$) and group 5 ($P<0.001$)] were significantly higher than the control group (group 4) after 50 days (Table 1). There were no obvious difference in initial mean weight of the 5 groups, but after 50 days' experiment, the final mean weight of group 1, group 2 and group 5 were significantly higher than group 4

Expression of Neuropeptide Y of GIFT Tilapia (Oreochromis sp.) in Yeast Pichia Pastoris and Its Stimulatory
Effects on Food Intake and Growth

89

by 15.31% (P<0.001), 16.59% (P<0.001) and 22.45% (P<0.001), respectively. The final mean weight of group 3 was 6.29% higher than the control group but with no significant difference (Table 1 and Fig.13). The possible detrimental effects of high levels of NPY on tilapia were studied through evaluation of HSI and gut weight ratio. No significant difference was found between groups fed with recombinant tilapia NPY and control group (Table 1). In the present study, we also analyzed the contents of moisture, crude protein, total lipid and ash of the dorsal white muscle of tilapia in each groups and no significant differences were observed except for the lipid content of group 5 compared to the control (P<0.01) (Table 2).

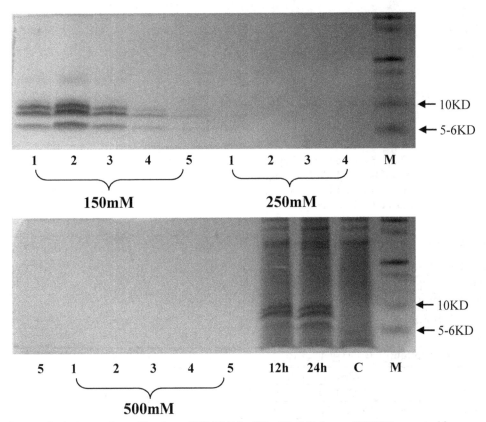

Fig. 11. Isolation and purification of TiNPY1 by His•Bind Column. TiNPY1 secreted by pPICZaA-TiNPY1-X-33 were isolated by His•Bind Column, and then were eluted by different concentration of imidazole (150mM, 250mM and 500mM). M: protein Marker; C: yeast culture supernatant flowing through His•Bind column; 12h and 24h: yeast culture supernatant induct for 12 and 24 hours.

After 50 days' feeding experiment, food consumptions in group 1 (0.15μgTiNPY1/g feed), 2 (0.3μgTiNPY1/g feed) and 5 (0.3μgTiNPY2/g feed) were significantly higher than the control group by18.03% (P<0.01), 20.80 %(P<0.01) and 30.22% (P<0.001) respectively, but there was no obvious difference between group3 (0.6μgTiNPY1/g feed) and control group (table 1). Consistent with the results of food consumption, feed conversion ratio (SGR) of group1 (1.72±0.017), group2 (1.73±0.017) and group5 (1.73±0.031) were significantly lower than the control group which with a FCR of 1.89±0.02. Again, no apparent distinction was observed between group3 and control group in FCR (Table 1 and Fig 14)

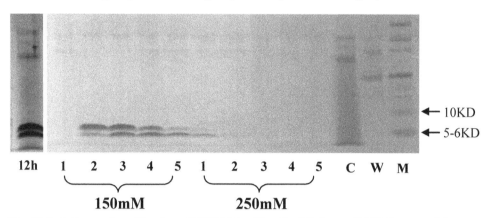

Fig. 12. Isolation and purification of TiNPY2 by His•Bind Column. TiNPY2 secreted by pPICZaA-TiNPY2-X-33 were isolated by His•Bind Column, and then eluted by different concentration of imidazole (150mM, 250mM). M: protein Marker; C: yeast culture supernatant flowing through His•Bind column; W: washing buffer. 12h: yeast culture supernatant induced for 12 hour.

Treatment	Group 1	Group 2	Group 3	Group 4	Group 5
Initial MBW(g)	72.94±0.49[a]	72.88±0.11[a]	73.03±0.30[a]	73.69±0.41[a]	72.94±0.27[a]
Final MBW(g)	181.78±1.77[c]	183.80±2.56[c]	167.56±6.12[a]	157.64±2.64[a]	193.04±3.82[c]
Initial MBL(cm)	13.01±0.06[a]	13.00±0.01[a]	12.99±0.06[a]	13.04±0.07[a]	13.00±0.07[a]
Final MBL(cm)	17.45±0.10[bc]	17.69±0.07[c]	17.32±0.10[b]	17.02±0.11[a]	17.69±0.07[c]
SGR	1.83±0.023[c]	1.85±0.027[c]	1.66±0.075[b]	1.52±0.037[a]	1.95±0.036[c]
Feed comsuption(g)	187.84±3.32[bc]	192.26±4.91[c]	174.13±5.26[b]	159.15±6.45[a]	207.24±2.94[c]
FCR	1.72±0.017[b]	1.73±0.017[b]	1.85±0.065[a]	1.89±0.020[a]	1.73±0.031[b]
HSI	2.92±0.088[a]	2.76±0.072[a]	2.85±0.103[a]	2.90±0.101[a]	2.81±0.080[a]
Gut weight ratio	7.61±0.27[a]	7.61±0.26[a]	7.58±0.20[a]	7.74±0.23[a]	7.71±0.07[a]

Table 1. Summary of the indexes related to the growth and feeding of tilapia treated with TiNPY1 and TiNPY2. Values are means ± SEM of three replicates, n=12 per replicate. Values with different superscripts are significantly different from each other (b indicated P <0.05 or c indicated P <0.001). MBW means body weight; MBL means body length; SGR (%/d) = (lnWt-lnW0)/d×100, Wt: final weights (g), W0: initial weights (g), d: experimental days; FCR = feed consumption (g)/fish weight gain (g); HIS=liver weight (g)/body weight (g); gut weight ratio= gut weight (g)/body weight (g). Group 1, 2, 3 were fed with 0.15, 0.3, 0.6μgTiNPY1/g feed; Group 4 fed with negative control diet; group 5 fed with 0.3μgTiNPY2/g feed.

Expression of Neuropeptide Y of GIFT Tilapia (Oreochromis sp.) in Yeast Pichia Pastoris and Its Stimulatory
Effects on Food Intake and Growth

91

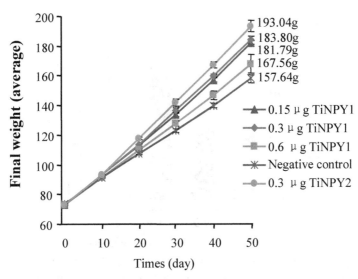

Fig. 13. Average individual body weight of tilapia fed with TiNPY1 or TiNPY2 in different days. Values are means ± SEM of three replicates (n=12 per replicate). The group fed with control diet acts as negative control.

Index	Group 1	Group 2	Group 3	Group 4	Group 5
Water (%)	76.40±0.31[a]	76.56±0.21[a]	76.34±0.20[a]	76.29±0.037[a]	76.48±0.20[a]
Protein (%)	21.10±0.36[a]	21.06±0.27[a]	21.15±0.15[a]	21.17±0.09[a]	21.11±0.13[a]
Lipid (%)	0.84±0.05[ab]	0.88±0.06[ab]	0.82±0.12[ab]	0.72±0.12[a]	0.98±0.05[b]
Ash (%)	1.35±0.05[a]	1.35±0.01[a]	1.36±0.02[a]	1.41±0.07[a]	1.33±0.04[a]

Table 2. White muscle composition of tilapia fed with TiNPY1 and TiNPY2 after 50 days. Values are means ± SEM of three replicates (n=12 per replicate). Values with different superscripts are significantly different from each other (P<0.05). Group 1, 2, 3 were fed with 0.15, 0.3, 0.6µgTiNPY1/g feed, respectively; Group 4 was fed with control diet and acts as a negative control. Group 5 was fed with 0.3µgTiNPY2/g feed.

3.7 Regulation of recombinant TiNPY on mRNA expressions of growth hormone, NPY and orexin in GIFT tilapia

Using real-time PCR technique, the effects of recombinant TiNPY on mRNA expressions of GH, NPY and orexin of tilapia were investigated. The results showed that 0.3µgTiNPY2/g feed could significantly stimulate pituitary GH mRNA expression. In contrast to TiNPY2, 0.15 and 0.3µgTiNPY1/g feed obviously inhibited GH mRNA expression and 0.6µgTiNPY1/g feed showed no effect on GH mRNA level (Fig.15).NPY and orexin are potent stimulators of food intake in teleosts and mainly expressed in hypothalamus of vertebrates. In this experiment, our study showed that 0.3µgTiNPY2/g feed significantly reduced mRNA expression of NPY as well as orexin and only 0.15 µgTiNPY1/g feed has similar inhibitory effect on NPY mRNA level (Fig.16 and 17). While 0.3, 0.6µgTiNPY1/g feed showed no effect on NPY mRNA expression (Fig.16) and all treatments of TiNPY1 haven't any obvious effect on orexin mRNA level (Fig.17).

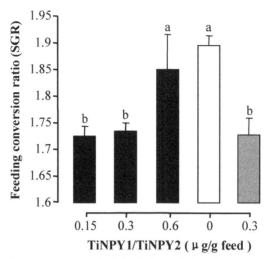

Fig. 14. Average feed conversion ratio (FCR) of tilapia fed with TiNPY1 (0.15, 0.3 and 0.6 µg/g feed, black columns) and TiNPY2 (0.3µg/g feed, grey column) after 50 days. The group fed with control diet acts as negative control (white column). Values presented are expressed as means ± SEM of three replicates (n=12 per replicate) and groups denoted by different letters represent a significant difference at P <0.05(ANOVA followed by Fisher's LSD test).

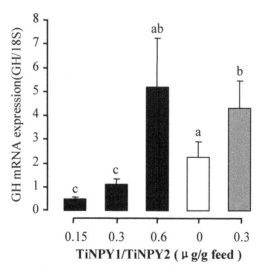

Fig. 15. Growth hormone (GH) mRNA expression of tilapia fed with TiNPY1 (0.15, 0.3 and 0.6µg/g feed, black columns) or TiNPY2 (0.3µg/g feed, grey column) after 50 days. The pituitaries of tilapia were homogenized for RNA extraction and RT-PCR. Then, Real-time PCR was used to detect the expression level of GH. The group fed with control diet acts as negative control (white column). Values presented are expressed as means ± SEM of three replicates (n=12 per replicate) and groups denoted by different letters represent a significant difference at P<0.05(ANOVA followed by Fisher's LSD test).

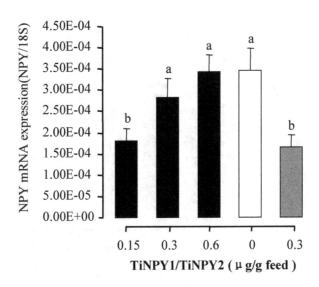

Fig. 16. NPY mRNA expression of tilapia fed with TiNPY1 (0.15, 0.3 and 0.6 µg/g feed, black columns) or TiNPY2 (0.3µg/g feed, grey column) after 50 days. The hypothalamuses of tilapia were homogenized for RNA extraction and RT-PCR. Then, Real-time PCR was used to detect the expression level of NPY. The group fed with control diet acts as negative control (white column). Values presented are expressed as means ± SEM of three replicates (n=12 per replicate) and groups denoted by different letters represent a significant difference at P <0.05(ANOVA followed by Fisher's LSD test).

4. Discussion

Regulation of food intake is very important for the survival and growth of animals. As in mammals, NPY is also the most potent orexigenic peptide in fish (Matsuda, 2009; Volkoff, 2006; Volkoff et al., 2005). GIFT tilapia is a hybrid of Nile tilapia (*Oreochromis niloticus*) and it is a major fish species widely used in aquaculture of China. As the first step to study the functions of recombinant NPY protein in food intake regulation of GIFT tilapia, a cDNA for GIFT tilapia NPY was isolated by molecular cloning. The deduced a.a. sequence of GIFT tilapia NPY revealed that this peptide is the precursor of NPY that comprises the signal peptide, a region coding for the 36 a.a. mature peptide and a C-terminal domain. Sequence alignment of amino acids showed that the NPY mature peptide of GIFT tilapia is the identity of that red tilapia (GenBank: AAV49168) and highly homologous to human NPY with the identity of 86%. This result again clearly proved that NPY is the most highly conserved neuropeptide in vertebrates(Blomqvist et al., 1992).

In the study of protein function, *E. coli* is commonly used to express large quantities of protein. However, there are several obvious deficiencies exists in the *E. coli* expression system. Firstly, the recombinant proteins expressed using this system are intracellular types and are easy to form inclusion bodies of expressions. Secondly, the system lacks post-

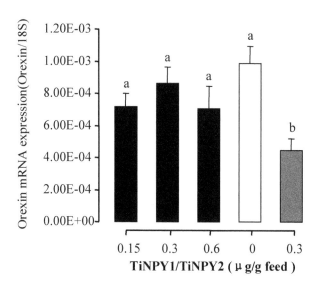

Fig. 17. Orexin mRNA expression of tilapia fed with TiNPY1 (0.15, 0.3 and 0.6 µg/g feed, black columns) or TiNPY2 (0.3µg/g feed, grey column) after 50 days. The hypothalamuses of tilapia were homogenized for RNA extraction and RT-PCR. Then, Real-time PCR was used to detect the expression level of orexin. The group fed with control diet acts as negative control (white column). Values presented are expressed as means ± SEM of three replicates (n=12 per replicate) and groups denoted by different letters represent a significant difference at P<0.05(ANOVA followed by Fisher's LSD test).

translational modification for foreign proteins. Thirdly, the immunogenic sources of *E. coli* such as exotoxin are often mixed with the products during cell fragmentation. Moreover, *E. coli* itself is an important source of water contamination. Therefore, these deficiencies limit its application in protein expression studies. As a eukaryote, yeast *Pichia pastoris*, a useful system for the expression of milligram-to-gram quantities of proteins for both basic laboratory research and industrial manufacture, owns advantages of higher eukaryotic expression systems such as protein processing, protein folding, and posttranslational modification, while being as easy to manipulate as *E. coli* or *Saccharomyces cerevisiae* (Carpio et al., 2009; Cregg et al., 2000).

Expression of target protein in *Pichia pastoris* can be either intracellular or secreted, and secretion requires a signal sequence on the expressed protein to target it to the secretory pathway. Although several different secretion signals have been used successfully, including the native signal peptide of the heterologous proteins, the secretion signal sequence from the *Saccharomyces cerevisiae* α factor prepro-peptide has been used with the most success(Cregg et al., 2000). The major advantage of expressing heterologous proteins as secreted proteins is that *Pichia pastoris* secretes very low levels of native proteins (Cregg et al., 2000), which facilitates the purification and acquisition of a large scale recombinant heterologous proteins. Additionally, it has recently been demonstrated that the culture

supernatant proteins of *P. pastoris* can have beneficial effects on fish larval growth and
innate immunity (Carpio et al., 2009). These characteristics make *P. pastoris* a very useful
heterologous proteins expression system in production of recombinant proteins for
aquaculture purposes. The processing of the α-factor mating signal sequence in pPICZα
occurs in two steps: the preliminary cleavage of the signal sequence by the KEX2 gene
product, with the final Kex2 cleavage occurring between arginine and glutamine in the
sequence Glu-Lys-Arg * Glu-Ala-Glu-Ala, where * is the site of cleavage; and the Glu-Ala
repeats are further cleaved by the STE13 gene product (user manual of EasySelect™ Pichia
Expression Kit, Catalog no. K1740-01).

After obtained the ORF of GIFT tilapia NPY, two recombinant Pichia X-33 stains of
PICZαA-TiNPY1 and pPICZαA-TiNPY2 were established and they can efficiently express
recombinant TiNPY1 and TiNPY2, respectively. The two recombinant proteins were
supposed to be expressed homogenously with no glycosylation, and comprise only one
protein band in Tricine-SDS-PAGE and western blot analysis, respectively. However,
three bands with different molecular weight of each recombinant NPY were observed
after methanol induction for more than 12 hours, and all of them could be isolated and
purified by Ni-NTA His•Bind Column, which means all of them conjugated with 6× His
tag designed in our study. Interestingly, only the upper two bands (with larger molecular
weight) could be recognized by rabbit polyclonal antibody against porcine NPY. Our
hypothesis is that the N-terminal signal peptide from the α factor was not completely cut
off and Glu-Ala repeats were left on the N-terminus of the expressed protein of the first
band (with largest molecular weight), the second band contained mainly recombinant
protein with native N-terminus of tilapia NPY; and the third band, with a smallest
molecular weight and couldn't be recognized by NPY antibody, was the degradation of
recombinant NPY with the degradation of native N-terminus and the preservation of C-
terminus. This speculation was verified by N-terminal a. a. sequence with Edman
stepwise degradation.

Oral delivery of peptide and protein has been proved to be the most suitable route and least
intrusive for delivery to fish in the aquaculture industry (Kiris GA, 2007; Ledger et al., 2002).
As mentioned above, NPY is the most important factor in regulating food intake and energy
metabolism in vertebrates. To test the physiological functions of recombinant TiNPY and
TiNPY2 of GIFT tilapia, yeast culture supernatants with different dosages of the two
proteins were directly sprayed on the surface of ordinary commercial extruded floating feed
and acts as daily diets to feed to the juvenile tilapia. As expected, both TiNPY1 and TiNPY2
could significantly stimulate the food intake of juvenile tilapia. Compared to the control
group, the food intake of tilapia fed with 0.15 or 0.3µgTiNPY1/g feed, or fed with
0.3µgTiNPY2/g feed was increased to 18.03%, 20.80% and 30.22%, respectively. This result
demonstrated again that NPY does not lose its feeding stimulatory effect when passed
through the alimentary canal of fish as was found in the red tilapia (Kiris GA, 2007). Similar
stimulated food intake results were found when Juvenile tilapia received intraperitoneal
injection of recombinant neuropeptide Y expressed by *Escherichia coli* (1 µg/g of body
weight) (Carpio et al., 2006), or i.p. injection (0.6 µg /g of body weight) or orally given (0.25
µg/g of feed) of human NPY (Kiris GA, 2007). And this result is also highly consistent with
those reported in other fish species. For example, injections of mammal NPY or fish NPY
promoted food intake of goldfish (Narnaware et al., 2000; Peng et al., 1993a) and rainbow

trout (Aldegunde and Mancebo, 2006). Moreover, our study also showed that the FCRs of tilapia fed with 0.15 or 0.3µg/g feed of TiNPY1 and fed with 0.3µg/g feed of TiNPY2 were significantly lower than the control group, which perhaps suggests some significance in the aquaculture of tilapia. However, FCR was not altered in tilapia treated with recombinant NPY expressed by *Escherichia coli* (1 µg/g of body weight) (Carpio et al., 2006).

More food intake and low FCR often lead to faster growth. In the present study, the percentage of weight gain in the tilapia fed with 0.15µg/g feed, 0.3µg/g feed or 0.6µg/g feed of recombinant TiNPY1 were 29.65%, 32.11% or 12.60% respectively higher than the control group, which was fed with the control diet. The feed with 0.3µgTiNPY2/g feed made the highest growth speed, with a mean body weight gain of 43.05% higher than the control group. The similar fasted growth results were found in other studies. NPY injection significantly induced energy consumption and body weight of goldfish (Narnaware and Peter, 2001a; Narnaware and Peter, 2001b) and tilapia (Carpio et al., 2006; Kiris GA, 2007); 18 and 30 days after immersion baths with recombinant NPY expressed by *Escherichia coli* three times a week, body weight and body length of catfish were significantly higher than the control (Carpio Y, 2007); Both injection and oral administration with human NPY significantly promoted the growth and body weight of tilapia(Kiris GA, 2007).

The effect of NPY on food intake and growth seems dosage and species specific and too high or too low dosage could not elevate food intake in fish and shrimp (Kiris GA, 2007; Narnaware and Peter, 2001b), The growth and food intake of tilapia *Oreochromis niloticus* were both significantly higher at dosage of 0.25µg/g feed compared to the control, but lower dosage of 0.125 µg/g feed only stimulated food intake(Kiris GA, 2007); Although the group of red tilapia injected with 0.1mg/gbw of recombinant NPY showed a weight increase of 26% when compared to the control group, it is still not statistically significant (Carpio et al., 2006). In our study, weight increase of tilapia fed with a dosage of 0.6µgTiNPY1/g feed was 12.60% higher than control, but with no statistical significance, and significantly lower than fish fed with lower dosages of 0.15 and 0.3 TiNPY1µg/g feed. The tilapia fed with 0.3 µg TiNPY2/g feed obtained the fastest growth rate compared with groups fed with TiNPY1 and the control diet.

Some studies have reported that NPY is involved in the neuroendocrine regulation of growth hormone. For example, NPY stimulates GH secretion in vitro and in vivo in goldfish (Peng et al., 1993b; Peng et al., 1993a) and catfish (Mazumdar et al., 2006). Similar as in mammals, NPY also interacts with a number of appetite factors, e.g. orexin, leptin and CART, to regulate food intake in fish (Volkoff, 2006; Volkoff et al., 2005). In the present study, we also investigated the effects of recombinant proteins of TiNPY1 and TiNPY2 on mRNA expressions of GH in pituitary and NPY as well as orexin in hypothalamus. The results showed that TiNPY2 (0.3µg/g feed) significantly induced GH mRNA expression. In contrast to TiNPY2, low dosages of TiNPY1 (0.15 and 0.3µg/g feed) obviously inhibited GH mRNA expression and high dosage of TiNPY1 (0.6µg/g feed) showed no effect on GH mRNA level. For NPY and orexin, the same dosage of TiNPY2 significantly inhibited mRNA expression of NPY as well as orexin to 50% compared to the control group and only 0.15 µg TiNPY1/g feed has similar inhibitory effect on NPY mRNA level. In contrast, 0.3 and 0.6µgTiNPY1/g feed showed no effect on NPY mRNA expression and all treatments of TiNPY1 haven't any obvious effect on orexin mRNA level. These results, taken together, suggested that long-term feeding of tilapia with recombinant NPY proteins could up-regulate GH mRNA expression and down-regulate the gene expressions of NPY and orexin. Further experiments are needed to test our hypothesis. In the whole experiment, we noticed that the effects of recombinant protein of TiNPY2 are much significant than that induced by TiNPY1. As the two forms of recombinant tilapia NPY expressed by yeast are only different in conjugated tags for identification and purification. The conjugated tag of TiNPY1, which was added a sequence with the molecular weight of 2.2KD to the recombinant protein, contains c-myc, 6× His tag and the amino-acid residues between them. While, the conjugated tag of TiNPY2, which was added to a sequence with the molecular weight of 0.8KDa to the recombinant protein, only contains six amino-acid residues of 6× His. The difference of their effects on the food intake and mRNA expression of GH, NPY and orexin may come from the difference of the conjugated tag attached with them .These results perhaps indicated that a larger conjugated tag of recombinant NPY would interfere its absorption or transportation across the blood-brain barrier. The function of recombinant NPY were also perhaps disturbed by the tags, as lipid content of the white muscle was higher in tilapia fed with TiNPY2 than those feed with TiNPY1 or control diet.

5. Conclusion

We obtained the cDNA encoding the precursor of NPY from GIFT tilapia. The deduced amino acids sequence of the mature peptide of GIFT tilapia is the same as that of red tilapia and it is highly conserved with human NPY. Two Pichia X-33 stains of PICZαA-TiNPY1 and pPICZαA-TiNPY2 were established and they can express the recombinant proteins of TiNPY1 and TiNPY2, respectively. Long-term feeding tilapia with TiNPY1 and TiNPY2 could significantly stimulate the food intake and growth of tilapia and at the same time to reduce the feeding conversion ratio of feed. Moreover, TiNPY2 can induce GH mRNA expression in the pituitary of tilapia and while potently suppressed mRNA expressions of hypothalamic NPY and orexin. For TiNPY1, lower dosages of which could inhibit GH and NPY mRNA expression. All dosages of TiNPY1 used in our experiment showed no effect on orexin mRNA expression. The present study clearly demonstrated that the recombinant protein of NPY expressed from the yeast *Pichia pastoris* has biological activity and oral delivery of NPY is a useful method in the aquaculture industry.

6. Acknowledgment

This work was supported by the National Basic Research Program (2010CB126302), the China Agriculture Research System (CARS-49), the Agriculture Research Special Funds of 3-49, the National High Technology Research Program (2007AA10Z165) and the Fundamental Research Funds for the Central Universities awarded to Professor Wensheng Li.

7. References

Aldegunde, M., Mancebo, M., (2006). Effects of neuropeptide Y on food intake and brain biogenic amines in the rainbow trout (Oncorhynchus mykiss). Peptides. 27, 719-27.

Blomqvist, A. G., et al., (1992). Strong evolutionary conservation of neuropeptide Y: sequences of chicken, goldfish, and Torpedo marmorata DNA clones. Proc Natl Acad Sci U S A. 89, 2350-4.

Carpio, Y., et al., (2006). Cloning, expression and growth promoting action of Red tilapia (Oreochromis sp.) neuropeptide Y. Peptides. 27, 710-8.

Carpio, Y., et al., (2009). Regulation of body mass growth through activin type IIB receptor in teleost fish. Gen Comp Endocrinol. 160, 158-67.

Carpio Y, L. K., Acosta J, Morales R, Estrada MP., (2007). Recombinant tilapia Neuropeptide Y promotes growth and antioxidant defenses in African catfish (Clarias gariepinus) fry. . Aquaculture 272 649-655.

Cerda-Reverter, J. M., Larhammar, D., (2000a). Neuropeptide Y family of peptides: structure, anatomical expression, function, and molecular evolution. Biochem Cell Biol. 78, 371-92.

Cerda-Reverter, J. M., et al., (2000b). Molecular evolution of the neuropeptide Y (NPY) family of peptides: cloning of three NPY-related peptides from the sea bass (Dicentrarchus labrax). Regul Pept. 95, 25-34.

Chavez, M., et al., (1998). Effect of a high-fat diet on food intake and hypothalamic neuropeptide gene expression in streptozotocin diabetes. J Clin Invest. 102, 340-6.

Cregg, J. M., et al., (2000). Recombinant protein expression in Pichia pastoris. Mol Biotechnol. 16, 23-52.

Faber, K. N., et al., (1995). Review: methylotrophic yeasts as factories for the production of foreign proteins. Yeast. 11, 1331-44.

Gelineau, A., Boujard, T., (2001). Oral administration of cholecystokinin receptor antagonists increase feed intake in rainbow trout. J. Fish Biol. . 58, 716–724.

Halford, J. C., et al., (2004). The pharmacology of human appetite expression. Curr Drug Targets. 5, 221-40.

Kalra, S. P., et al., (1999). Interacting appetite-regulating pathways in the hypothalamic regulation of body weight. Endocr Rev. 20, 68-100.

Kehoe, A. S., Volkoff, H., (2007). Cloning and characterization of neuropeptide Y (NPY) and cocaine and amphetamine regulated transcript (CART) in Atlantic cod (Gadus morhua). Comp Biochem Physiol A Mol Integr Physiol. 146, 451-61.

Kiris GA, K. M., Dikel S., (2007). Stimulatory effects of neuropeptide Y on food intake and growth of Oreochromis niloticus. Aquaculture. 264, 383-389.

Ledger, R., et al., (2002). The metabolic barrier of the lower intestinal tract of salmon to the oral delivery of protein and peptide drugs. J Control Release. 85, 91-103.

Lin, S., et al., (2004). NPY and Y receptors: lessons from transgenic and knockout models. Neuropeptides. 38, 189-200.

Lopez-Patino, M. A., et al., (1999). Neuropeptide Y has a stimulatory action on feeding behavior in goldfish (Carassius auratus). Eur J Pharmacol. 377, 147-53.

Matsuda, K., (2009). Recent advances in the regulation of feeding behavior by neuropeptides in fish. Ann N Y Acad Sci. 1163, 241-50.

Mazumdar, M., et al., (2006). Involvement of neuropeptide Y Y1 receptors in the regulation of LH and GH cells in the pituitary of the catfish, Clarias batrachus: an immunocytochemical study. Gen Comp Endocrinol. 149, 190-6.

Narnaware, Y. K., Peter, R. E., (2001a). Effects of food deprivation and refeeding on neuropeptide Y (NPY) mRNA levels in goldfish. Comp Biochem Physiol B Biochem Mol Biol. 129, 633-7.

Narnaware, Y. K., Peter, R. E., (2001b). Neuropeptide Y stimulates food consumption through multiple receptors in goldfish. Physiol Behav. 74, 185-90.

Narnaware, Y. K., Peter, R. E., (2002). Influence of diet composition on food intake and neuropeptide Y (NPY) gene expression in goldfish brain. Regul Pept. 103, 75-83.

Narnaware, Y. K., et al., (2000). Regulation of food intake by neuropeptide Y in goldfish. Am J Physiol Regul Integr Comp Physiol. 279, R1025-34.

Pedrazzini, T., (2004). Importance of NPY Y1 receptor-mediated pathways: assessment using NPY Y1 receptor knockouts. Neuropeptides. 38, 267-75.

Pedrazzini, T., et al., (2003). Neuropeptide Y: the universal soldier. Cell Mol Life Sci. 60, 350-77.

Peng, C., et al., (1993b). Neuropeptide-Y stimulates growth hormone and gonadotropin-II secretion in the goldfish pituitary: involvement of both presynaptic and pituitary cell actions. Endocrinology. 132, 1820-9.

Peng, C., et al., (1993a). Actions of goldfish neuropeptide Y on the secretion of growth hormone and gonadotropin-II in female goldfish. Gen Comp Endocrinol. 90, 306-17.

Romanos, M. A., et al., (1992). Foreign gene expression in yeast: a review. Yeast. 8, 423-88.

Sundstrom, G., et al., (2005). Ray-fin fish tetraploidization gave rise to pufferfish duplicates of NPY and PYY, but zebrafish NPY duplicate was lost. Ann N Y Acad Sci. 1040, 476-8.

Sundstrom, G., et al., (2008). Evolution of the neuropeptide Y family: new genes by chromosome duplications in early vertebrates and in teleost fishes. Gen Comp Endocrinol. 155, 705-16.

Tatemoto, K., et al., (1982). Neuropeptide Y--a novel brain peptide with structural similarities to peptide YY and pancreatic polypeptide. Nature. 296, 659-60.

Valassi, E., et al., (2008). Neuroendocrine control of food intake. Nutr Metab Cardiovasc Dis. 18, 158-68.

Volkoff, H., (2006). The role of neuropeptide Y, orexins, cocaine and amphetamine-related transcript, cholecystokinin, amylin and leptin in the regulation of feeding in fish. Comp Biochem Physiol A Mol Integr Physiol. 144, 325-31.

Volkoff, H., et al., (2005). Neuropeptides and the control of food intake in fish. Gen Comp Endocrinol. 142, 3-19.

Volkoff, H., et al., (2010). Influence of intrinsic signals and environmental cues on the endocrine control of feeding in fish: potential application in aquaculture. Gen Comp Endocrinol. 167, 352-9.

Woods, S. C., et al., (1998). NPY and food intake: discrepancies in the model. Regul Pept. 75-76, 403-8.

6

'Exercise-Eating Linkage' Mediated by Neuro-Endocrine Axis and the Relevance in Regulation of Appetite and Energy Balance for Prevention of Obesity

Takahiro Yoshikawa
Department of Sports Medicine, Osaka City University Graduate School of Medicine,
Osaka,
Japan

1. Introduction

A significant number of modern people of all ages are affected by obesity epidemic in developed and parts of developing world, resulting in immense health and financial burden (Field, 2002; Ogden et al., 2006; Orsi et al., 2011). Obesity is thought to be an independent risk factor for development of various medical conditions, such as type 2 diabetes, hypertension, dyslipidemia, and cardiovascular disease (Daniels, 2009; Fontaine, 2003; Ginsberg, 2000; Kahn & Flier, 2000; National Institutes of health [NIH], 1998), necessitating weight management for prevention and treatment of these serious diseases. Obesity epidemic reflects modern growing trends to promote excess energy intake (EI) and to discourage energy expenditure (EE) (Egger et al., 2001; Food and Agriculture Organization of the United Nations [FAO], 2003; Hill et al., 2003). Thus, it is well recognized that lifestyle intervention, such as changes in behavior by combination of reductions in EI and increases in physical activity, can achieve ideal weight control (Bray, 2008). Nevertheless, it seems impossible for most of people to fight down consciously their impulses of overeating in modern societies where they have easy access to unlimited supply of highly palatable and energy-dense food (Cohen, 2008).

In such circumstance, appetite is receiving extensive attention for one of key factors to adjust or disrupt energy balance (EB). In particular, an important group of the intricate factors for the appetite control are gut hormone family, including ghrelin, peptide YY (PYY), glucagon-like peptide-1 (GLP-1), oxyntomodulin (OXM), and cholecystokinin (CCK) (Huda et al., 2006; Näslund & Hellström, 2007). Recent advances have been made in understanding the structures, sources, releasers, target organs and receptors, and how these gut hormones influence brain systems for the control of appetite and EI. In brief, these gut hormones are secreted from gastrointestinal organs in response to nutrient conditions and give signals to hypothalamic and brainstem nuclei both of which are in close anatomical proximity to a circumventricular organ with an incomplete blood-brain barrier (BBB), such as median eminence and area postrema. Ghrelin is only an orexigenic hormone and secreted shortly before meals, whereas other gut hormones are all anorectic and released into circulation postprandially in proportion to calorie intake.

While these gut hormones have been well-studied for over a decade, numerous studies have so far investigated a possible association of lifestyle habit, such as exercise, with appetite and EI (King, 1999). Interestingly, recent studies, including ours, have revealed inhibitory effects of exercise on the sensation of hunger and satiety and amount of EI associated with the gut hormone release in various population (Broom et al., 2009; Martins et al., 2007; Ueda et al., 2009a, 2009b), suggesting the presence of an 'exercise-eating linkage' mediated by neuro-endocrine axis in human body. The evidence also suggest an intriguing possibility that physical activity has an impact not simply on EE but also on variations in appetite, leading to negative EB.

The present review provides an overview of 1) changes in sensation of hunger and satiety and amount of EI by various types of exercise and next highlights 2) association of exercise with blood kinetics of gut hormones and its relevance in regulation of appetite and EB. Lastly, 3) future perspective of this research field will be discussed.

2. 'Exercise-eating linkage', is it real?

So far, there has been considerable research on changes in subjective appetite parameters and amount of EI by various types of exercise. Exercise is generally assumed to induce a transient energy deficit and subsequent automatic drive in hunger and EI for energy compensation. However, a majority of previous studies failed to show that a single bout of exercise increase hunger or EI. Such discrepancy between EE and EI can be observed in a wide range of population, irrespective of age, gender, body weight, dietary restraint and exercise intensity. For instance, acute high-intensity exercise (about 70% VO_2 max) is unlikely to cause the subsequent increase in EI in unrestraint males with normal body weight, favoring negative EB (Imbeault et al., 1997; Thompson et al., 1988). Similarly, poor compensation was observed in response to energy deficit by a single bout of high-intensity exercise (cycling 50 min, 70% VO_2 max) in restrained young females with normal body weight (Lluch et al., 1998). Although unrestrained female counterparts rated a range of foods to be more palatable after similar type of exercise, it had no significant short-term effect on energy or macronutrient intake (King et al., 1996). Moderate physical activity (a single bout of 20-min brisk walking) suppressed appetite in middle-aged obese women who were not on special diet (i.e. unrestrained eaters) (Tsofliou, 2003). Similar to acute effects of exercise on appetite, a graded increase in EE by 7-day repeated exercise regimens did not show any significant increases in subjective feeling of hunger and food consumption in lean individuals, generating considerable negative EB (Stubbs et al., 2002a, 2002b). Given the evidence above, 'exercise-eating linkage' is, if any, unlikely to benefit the maintenance of EB, at least short term. Rather, 'exercise-eating linkage' might give rise to transient appetite suppression after exercise. However, it is known that various metabolic and behavioral responses i.e. decrease in EE and increase in appetite and EI after exercise, automatically or volitionally, operate in a long-term process of compensation for the exercise-induced energy deficit, minimizing the negative EB and body weight reduction, and the compensatory responses considerably vary among individuals (King et al., 2007, 2008). And it is assumed that such accurate adjustments of EI to an increase in EE seem to take matter of weeks (Whybrow et al., 2008).

In this regard, however, caution should be exercised when interpreting the findings from these studies. Unlike other animals, internal physiological signals for energy repletion and depletion were not sufficient for the control of appetite and eating behavior in humans. It is

'Exercise-Eating Linkage' Mediated by Neuro-Endocrine Axis and the Relevance in Regulation of Appetite and
Energy Balance for Prevention of Obesity
103

well recognized that human eating behavior is a multifactorial process where various external stimuli, including sensory, cognitive, environmental (e.g. social and habitual) variables might play important roles as well as internal signals arising peripherally from gastric distension and energy imbalance (De Castro, 1996). Thus, it is reasonable that eating behavior after exercise can be largely affected by these external factors (British Nutrition Foundation, 1999) and the findings might depend on the background, such as each study setting and subject characteristics. In most previous studies in which association of (short- or long-term) exercise with EI were investigated, test meals were given to subjects *ad libitum*, where the subjects can recognize how much they have eaten, and the subject characteristics (gender, body type and taste) are inconsistent among studies and psychological condition (stress), habitual factors (binge eating) and cognitive factors (reward and preoccupation with food), such as 'food is a reward for exercise' (King, 1999), were often uncontrolled, thus often leading to mixed findings among studies.

3. Exercise and gut hormones: implication for 'exercise-eating linkage'

3.1 Ghrelin
An increasing amount of research has investigated the possibilities that exercise stimulates various gut hormone release into circulation. And, some of recent studies focused on the impact of the exercise-induced gut hormone release on subsequent appetite and EI. In particular, evidence is accumulating for the effect of exercise on the plasma ghrelin levels, but somewhat inconsistent. A single bout of exercise at fasted condition has been shown not to induce significant changes in plasma levels of total ghrelin in normal weight subjects (Kraemer et al., 2004; Zoladz et al., 2005), whereas similar exercise at premeal condition can raise the circulating ghrelin concentrations in moderately overweight postmenopausal women (Borer et al., 2005). Total ghrelin levels were not affected by aerobic exercise intervention for 5 days without body weight reduction (Mackelvie et al., 2007), whereas the plasma levels gradually increased during the 12-weeks aerobic and resistance exercise with significant decreases in body weight and fat (Kim et al., 2008), suggesting that exercise has only a limited impact on the fasting total ghrelin levels unless the body weight of subjects is reduced. Changes in the fasting plasma levels of total ghrelin are likely to depend not on the duration but on the intensity of exercise (Erdmann et al., 2007). Total ghrelin is classified into two categories; orexigenic acylated ghrelin (AG) and anorectic desacyl ghrelin (DG). In contrast to the total ghrelin, orexigenic AG is suppressed by a single bout of exercise at fasted state, resulting in the negative energy balance (Broom et al., 2007). And the postexercise reduction in AG was observed in the lean as well as obese subjects (Marzullo et al., 2008). The effects of long-term exercise training on plasma AG / DG levels seem to be dependent on the duration of exercise. The longer the exercise is performed, the more decrease in AG/DG is observed in favor of body weight reduction (Kim et al., 2008).

3.2 Satiety hormones
Similar to ghrelin, it is only in the last few years that studies have focused on the effects of exercise-induced changes in plasma levels of satiety hormones on appetite regulation and most of these studies have been performed mainly in normal weight individuals. Majority of the early studies focused on plasma PP levels in various setting of exercise preprandially (Hilsted et al., 1980; Sullivan et al., 1984), and postprandially (Greenberg et al., 1986). PP release is likely to be exercise intensity-dependent (Holmqvist et al., 1986). Early studies

measured the circulating PP levels as the index of sympathetic activity rather than its physiological roles for appetite regulation (Holmqvist et al., 1986). Plasma GLP-1 levels have been shown to change by exercise in a small number of studies, most of which investigated the association of high intensity exercise with the fasting plasma levels in athletes (O'Connor et al., 1995, 2006). While a single bout of aerobic exercise at fasted state for 10hrs enhanced a response of plasma PYY levels to a test meal after the exercise, such changes were not shown by resistance exercise (Broom 2009).

In most of these studies, the nutrient stimuli are simply replaced by those of exercise, that is, preprandial exercise. However, because these satiety gut hormones are basically released after nutrient intake, it seems worthwhile to examine whether the postprandial plasma levels of these hormones can be affected by exercise and these hormonal changes could affect the subsequent appetite regulation. Recently, some studies, including ours, have investigated kinetics in postprandial release of gut hormones into circulation by a single bout of exercise (Martins et al., 2007; Ueda et al., 2009a, 2009b). One of these studies has demonstrated the postprandial increase in plasma levels of PYY and GLP-1 during and after 1hr exercise at the intensity of 60% of maximal HR. In particular, the time course changes in plasma PYY concentration seem to be mirror image to those in hunger ratings, suggesting that postprandial release of PYY suppress the hunger feeling during and after exercise (Martins et al., 2007). We also investigated acute effect of a single bout of 1 hr aerobic cycling exercise (50% $\dot{V}O_2$max) on the postprandial plasma levels of gut hormones after standard breakfast in overweight and normal young males and determined the involvement of the hormonal changes in regulation of EB in subjects with normal body weight and overweight (Ueda et al., 2009a, 2009b). We assessed the total release of individual gut hormone during and after the exercise as the area under the curve (AUC) of the time course curve of each hormone. In both body type groups, the aerobic exercise significantly increased subsequent release of PYY and GLP-1 in plasma, while plasma levels of acylated ghrelin were not significantly altered. Of note, exercise-induced suppression of relative EI (absolute EI minus absolute EE) in overweight subjects was significantly larger than in control subjects despite lack of significant difference in PYY and GLP-1 levels between two subject groups. The discrepancy might stem from variability of cognitive and sensory factors between two body type groups. In line with this, when the data were analyzed separately in overweight and normal body type group, a significant linear correlation between the increase in AUC values of plasma PYY and GLP-1 levels by exercise and the concurrent decrease in relative EI was observed within each subject group (unpublished data). Collectively, one could argue that neuro-endocrine axis consisting of satiety gut hormones and brain appetite center could play some important roles in 'exercise-eating linkage' of exercise-induced appetite suppression for a while after a single bout of exercise.

Based on the long-term compensation of exercise-induced energy deficit described above, it seems to be necessary to examine whether sustained exercise training also have an impact on the circulating levels of satiety gut hormone and appetite control through the hormonal axis as well as a single bout exercise. The point is important for planning programs in practice for better appetite and weight control. And a few studies have only recently addressed the issue. A significant rise in fasting plasma levels of PYY was shown in overweight adolescent males and females after 32 weeks of exercise training (60-85% peak VO_2, 45min/day, and 3days/week) (Jones et al., 2009). However, neither effects on ratings of appetite feelings nor those on EB were examined. Another study showed that, while postprandial suppression of plasma AG levels seems to be enhanced, postprandial plasma levels of PYY and GLP-1 also tend to be higher after 12 weeks of exercise intervention (75% maximal heart rate, 500kcal energy deficit/day, and 5days/week) while the subjective feelings of hunger increased paradoxically after a test meal (Martins et al., 2010). Although these findings might suggest the possibility that long-term exercise might modify the profiles of orexigenic and satiety gut hormones in circulation, available data are still scarce, particularly as to whether these hormonal changes could suppress superfluous appetite. Further information will be needed for understanding how these gut hormones could affect the long-term regulation of appetite and EI.

4. Future perspectives

As described above, findings of recent studies to date indicate the presence of 'exercise-eating linkage' via neuro-endocrinal axis. Now the following important questions remain unanswered.

Does the responsiveness vary among different intensity and style of exercise or among different body weight types? Does the responsiveness of hypothalamus to the gut hormones fluctuate during exercise? Interestingly, a single bout of 6hr exercise improves the responsiveness of hypothalamus to leptin and appetite control in male rats (Flores et al., 2006; Ropelle et al., 2008). Another study demonstrated that habitual exercise influence appetite and EI in response to covert preload energy manipulation (Long et al., 2002; van Walleghen et al., 2007). In particular, Long SJ *et al.* raised the possibility that exercise may enhance the accuracy of appetite control by the exercise-induced improvement in insulin sensitivity (Aldred et al., 1995; Haber et al., 1977; Holt et al., 1992; Poehlman et al., 2000). Insulin exerts appetite-inhibiting effects via hypothalamus activation (Schwartz 2000). It is still unknown whether the response to satiety gut hormones also can be altered by exercise. Based on previous studies in which these peptides are dosed peripherally, obesity *per se* does not seem to affect the responsiveness to some satiety gut hormones, such as PYY (Batterham et al., 2003).

Does the change in gut hormone levels with exercise have significant effects on other physiological systems as well as appetite regulation? Interestingly, PYY administration decreases respiratory quotient (RQ) and reduces adiposity in diet-induced obese mice (Adams et al., 2006). In human study, high fasting and postprandial peak PYY was observed in subjects with low resting metabolic rate (RMR) (daily EE) and low RQ (Guo et al., 2006). The findings raise an intriguing possibility that exercise might induce PYY secretion and regulate not only the appetite but also EE and fuel partitioning in favour of fat oxidation, providing the additional evidence of advantage of exercise intervention for weight and body fat reduction.

Possible association of the fluctuating gut hormone levels with subsequent appetite and EB are intriguing. However, more important question is how much effect we can expect such intrinsic signal of exercise-induced hormonal changes to modulate the overall appetite system in which other diverse extrinsic factors are largely involved. Hypothalamus is one of pivotal entry points of the peripheral internal signals into central pathways mediating brain appetite regulation along with nucleus tractus solitarius (NTS) in brainstem. There are reciprocal connections between these two entry points and these areas communicate with higher centers such as brain reward centers (e.g. ventrotegmental area, nucleus accumbens, ventral pallidum, and orbitofrontal cortex) which play a role in integration of various sensory information and hedonic signals (Wynne et al., 2005). One of recent neurophysiological studies revealed that the sensory inputs produced by sight, smell, taste and texture of food converge at specific brain regions, such as orbitofrontal cortex, and interact with peripheral hunger/satiety signals at hypothalamus, including autonomic nerve activation and gut hormones, and finally determine eating behavior (Rolls, 2005, 2006). In addition, taste information is also sent to the reward system, which mediates the motivation of eating of palatable food, and finally transfers the signals to the hypothalamus (Yamamoto, 2008). While human intrinsic appetite control systems remain unchanged in recent few decades, the excess food stimuli override appetite suppressive responses, such as humoral and neural satiety signals arising from gastrointestinal organs, resulting in overeating and subsequent obesity. Exercise might partly correct the disparity between the primitive appetite control systems and the current expanding food consumption by upregulating the peripheral satiety signals. Interestingly, a recent human study using brain functional MRI demonstrated that, after intravenous infusion of PYY at physiological plasma concentrations, mimicking the fed state, hypothalamic neural activity was not correlated with caloric intake, while the changes in neural signals within higher center, the orbitofrontal cortex, correlated with caloric intake, suggesting that brain activity predicting caloric intake appeared to switch from hypothalamus to higher center, orbitofrontal cortex in the presence of PYY (Batterham et al., 2007). Based on this observation, the exercise-induced increase in the plasma PYY levels might cause some possible effects on the neural

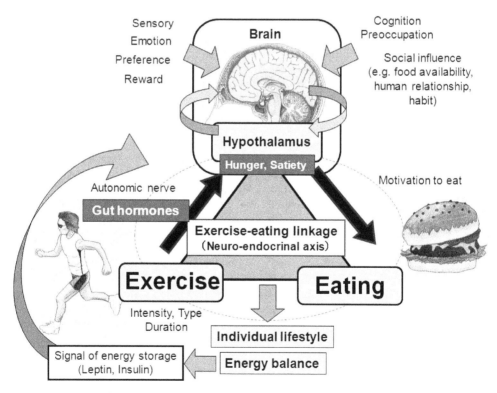

Fig. 1. Overview of exercise-eating linkage via neuro-endocrinal axis

'Exercise-Eating Linkage' Mediated by Neuro-Endocrine Axis and the Relevance in Regulation of Appetite and
Energy Balance for Prevention of Obesity

107

activity in higher centers for appetite control. In addition to the changes in gut hormones, exercise also influences brain dopaminergic, GABAergic, noradrenergic and serotonergic systems (Meeusen & De Meirleir, 1995). In rat models, changes in synthesis and metabolism of these neurotransmitters and receptors during exercise were observed in distinct brain regions including hypothalamus (Kramer et al., 2000). Although it is beyond the scope of this review to include these neurophysiological findings, we should keep in mind the large general picture of these control systems before we consider the implication for the association of exercise with appetite, EB and gut hormones. Future studies will be needed to investigate the effects of (acute or long-term) exercise on the overall appetite regulatory systems (exercise-eating linkage) based on the crosstalk interactions between peripheral endocrine system and central appetite centers (neuro-endocrinal axis) (Figure). Furthermore, the understanding might give us clues to reveal the reasons why there is inter-individual variability in ratings of hunger and amount of food ingested after exercise (King et al., 2007), leading to tailored strategies of preventive programs and treatment for overeating and obesity.

In conclusion, The evidence of exercise-induced changes in satiety gut hormones with suppression of hunger feeling and subsequent relative EI provides considerable support for the value of exercise not only in a measure of expenditure but also in preventing from overeating and obesity. Understanding of this area in endocrinology combined with neurophysiology of eating behaviour in higher brain centers might facilitate the development of promising approach to maintain better dietary life with appropriate exercise and healthy body weight.

5. References

Adams SH, Lei C, Jodka CM, Nikoulina SE, Hoyt JA, Gedulin B, Mack CM, Kendall ES. PYY[3-36] administration decreases the respiratory quotient and reduces adiposity in diet-induced obese mice. *J Nutr.* 2006;136:195-201.

Aldred HE, Hardman AE, Taylor S. Influence of 12 weeks of training by brisk walking on postprandial lipemia and insulinemia in sedentary middle-aged women. *Metabolism.* 1995;44:390-7.

Batterham RL, Cohen MA, Ellis SM, Le Roux CW, Withers DJ, Frost GS, Ghatei MA, Bloom SR. Inhibition of food intake in obese subjects by peptide YY3-36. *N Engl J Med.* 2003;349:941-8.

Batterham RL, ffytche DH, Rosenthal JM, Zelaya FO, Barker GJ, Withers DJ, Williams SC. PYY modulation of cortical and hypothalamic brain areas predicts feeding behaviour in humans. *Nature.* 2007;450:106-9.

Borer KT, Wuorinen E, Chao C, Burant C. Exercise energy expenditure is not consciously detected due to oro-gastric, not metabolic, basis of hunger sensation. *Appetite.* 2005;45:177-81.

Bray GA. Lifestyle and pharmacological approaches to weight loss: efficacy and safety. *J Clin Endocrinol Metab.* 2008;93(11 Suppl 1):S81-8.

British Nutrition Foundation. *Obesity.* Blackwell Science: Oxford, 1999.

Broom DR, Stensel DJ, Bishop NC, Burns SF, Miyashita M. Exercise-induced suppression of acylated ghrelin in humans. *J Appl Physiol.* 2007;102:2165-71.

Broom DR, Batterham RL, King JA, Stensel DJ. Influence of resistance and aerobic exercise on hunger, circulating levels of acylated ghrelin, and peptide YY in healthy males. *Am J Physiol Regul Integr Comp Physiol.* 2009;296:R29-35.

Cohen DA. Neurophysiological pathways to obesity: below awareness and beyond individual control. *Diabetes*. 2008;57:1768-73.

Daniels SR. Complications of obesity in children and adolescents. *Int J Obes (Lond)*. 2009;33:S60-5.

De Castro JM. How can eating behavior be regulated in complex environments of free-living humans? *Neurosci Biobehav Rev*. 1996;20:119-31.

Egger GJ, Vogels N, Westerterp KR. Estimating historical changes in physical activity levels Med J Aust. 2001;175(11-12):635-6.

Erdmann J, Tahbaz R, Lippl F, Wagenpfeil S, Schusdziarra V. Plasma ghrelin levels during exercise - effects of intensity and duration. *Regul Pept*. 2007;143:127-35.

Field AE, Epidemiology and health and economic consequences of obesity. In: Wadden TA, Stunkard AJ, editors. Handbook of obesity treatment. New York: Guilford Press; 2002. p3-18.

Flores MB, Fernandes MF, Ropelle ER, Faria MC, Ueno M, Velloso LA, Saad MJ, Carvalheira JB. Exercise improves insulin and leptin sensitivity in hypothalamus of Wistar rats. *Diabetes*. 2006;55:2554-61.

Fontaine KR, Years of life lost due to obesity. JAMA. 2003;289:187-193.

Food and Agriculture Organization of the United Nations (FAO). Global and regional food consumption pattern and trends; http://www.fao.org/DOCREP/005/AC911E/ac911e05.htm

Ginsberg HN. Insulin resistance and cardiovascular disease. *J Clin Invest*. 2000;106:453-8.

Greenberg GR, Marliss EB, Zinman B. Effect of exercise on the pancreatic polypeptide response to food in man. *Horm Metab Res*. 1986;18:194-6.

Guo Y, Ma L, Enriori PJ, Koska J, Franks PW, Brookshire T, Cowley MA, Salbe AD, Delparigi A, Tataranni PA. Physiological evidence for the involvement of peptide YY in the regulation of energy homeostasis in humans. *Obesity (Silver Spring)*. 2006;14:1562-70.

Haber GB, Heaton KW, Murphy D, Burroughs LF. Depletion and disruption of dietary fibre. Effects on satiety, plasma-glucose, and serum-insulin. *Lancet*. 1977;2:679-82.

Hill JO, Wyatt HR, Reed GW, Peters JC. Obesity and the environment: where do we go from here? *Science*. 2003;299:853-5.

Hilsted J, Galbo H, Sonne B, Schwartz T, Fahrenkrug J, de Muckadell OB, Lauritsen KB, Tronier B. Gastroenteropancreatic hormonal changes during exercise. *Am J Physiol*. 1980;239:G136-40.

Holmqvist N, Secher NH, Sander-Jensen K, Knigge U, Warberg J, Schwartz TW. Sympathoadrenal and parasympathetic responses to exercise. *J Sports Sci*.1986;4:123-8.

Holt S, Brand J, Soveny C, Hansky J. Relationship of satiety to postprandial glycaemic, insulin and cholecystokinin responses. *Appetite*. 1992;18:129-41.

Huda MS, Wilding JP, Pinkney JH. Gut peptides and the regulation of appetite. *Obes Rev*. 2006;7:163-82.

Imbeault P, Saint-Pierre S, Alméras N, Tremblay A. Acute effects of exercise on energy intake and feeding behaviour. *Br J Nutr*. 1997;77:511-21.

Jones TE, Basilio JL, Brophy PM, McCammon MR, Hickner RC. Long-term exercise training in overweight adolescents improves plasma peptide YY and resistin. *Obesity (Silver Spring)*. 2009;17:1189-95 .

Kahn BB, Flier JS. Obesity and insulin resistance. J Clin Invest. 2000;106:473-481.

Kim HJ, Lee S, Kim TW, Kim HH, Jeon TY, Yoon YS, Oh SW, Kwak H, Lee JG. Effects of exercise-induced weight loss on acylated and unacylated ghrelin in overweight children. *Clin Endocrinol (Oxf)*. 2008;68:416-22.

King NA, Snell L, Smith RD, Blundell JE. Effects of short-term exercise on appetite responses in unrestrained females. *Eur J Clin Nutr*. 1996;50:663-7.

King NA. What processes are involved in the appetite response to moderate increases in exercise-induced energy expenditure? *Proc Nutr Soc*. 1999;58:107-13.

King NA, Caudwell P, Hopkins M, Byrne NM, Colley R, Hills AP, Stubbs JR, Blundell JE. Metabolic and behavioral compensatory responses to exercise interventions: barriers to weight loss. *Obesity (Silver Spring)*. 2007;15:1373-83.

King NA, Hopkins M, Caudwell P, Stubbs RJ, Blundell JE. Individual variability following 12 weeks of supervised exercise: identification and characterization of compensation for exercise-induced weight loss. *Int J Obes (Lond)*. 2008;32:177-84.

Kraemer RR, Durand RJ, Acevedo EO, Johnson LG, Kraemer GR, Hebert EP, Castracane VD. Rigorous running increases growth hormone and insulin-like growth factor-I without altering ghrelin. *Exp Biol Med*. 2004;229:240-6.

Kramer JM, Plowey ED, Beatty JA, Little HR, Waldrop TG. Hypothalamus, hypertension, and exercise. *Brain Res Bull*. 2000;53:77-85.

Lluch A, King NA, Blundell JE. Exercise in dietary restrained women: no effect on energy intake but change in hedonic ratings. *Eur J Clin Nutr*. 1998;52:300-7.

Long SJ, Hart K, Morgan LM. The ability of habitual exercise to influence appetite and food intake in response to high- and low-energy preloads in man. *Br J Nutr*. 2002;87:517-23.

Mackelvie KJ, Meneilly GS, Elahi D, Wong AC, Barr SI, Chanoine JP. Regulation of appetite in lean and obese adolescents after exercise: role of acylated and desacyl ghrelin. *J Clin Endocrinol Metab*. 2007;92:648-54.

Martins C, Morgan LM, Bloom SR, Robertson MD. Effects of exercise on gut peptides, energy intake and appetite. *J Endocrinol*. 2007;193:251-8.

Martins C, Kulseng B, King NA, Holst JJ, Blundell JE. The effects of exercise-induced weight loss on appetite-related peptides and motivation to eat. *J Clin Endocrinol Metab*. 2010;95:1609-16.

Marzullo P, Salvadori A, Brunani A, Verti B, Walker GE, Fanari P, Tovaglieri I, De Medici C, Savia G, Liuzzi A. Acylated ghrelin decreases during acute exercise in the lean and obese state. *Clin Endocrinol (Oxf)*. 2008;69:970-1.

Meeusen R, De Meirleir K. Exercise and brain neurotransmission. *Sports Med*. 1995;20:160-88.

National Institutes of health (NIH). Clinical guidelines on the identification, evaluation, and treatment of overweight and obesity in adults: the evidence report. *Obes Res*. 1998;6:51S-210S.

Näslund E, Hellström PM. Appetite signaling: from gut peptides and enteric nerves to brain. *Physiol Behav*. 2007;92:256-62.

O'Connor AM, Johnston CF, Buchanan KD, Boreham C, Trinick TR, Riddoch CJ. Circulating gastrointestinal hormone changes in marathon running. *Int J Sports Med*. 1995;16:283-7.

O'Connor AM, Pola S, Ward BM, Fillmore D, Buchanan KD, Kirwan JP. The gastroenteroinsular response to glucose ingestion during postexercise recovery. *Am J Physiol Endocrinol Metab*. 2006;290:E1155-61.

Ogden CL, Carroll MD, Curtin LR, McDowell MA, Tabak CJ, Flegal KM. Prevalence of overweight and obesity in the United States, 1999-2004. *JAMA*. 2006;295:1549-55.

Orsi CM, Hale DE, Lynch JL. Pediatric obesity epidemiology. *Curr Opin Endocrinol Diabetes Obes*. 2011;18:14-22.

Poehlman ET, Dvorak RV, DeNino WF, Brochu M, Ades PA. Effects of resistance training and endurance training on insulin sensitivity in nonobese, young women: a controlled randomized trial. *J Clin Endocrinol Metab.* 2000;85:2463-8.

Rolls ET. Taste, olfactory, and food texture processing in the brain, and the control of food intake. *Physiol Behav.* 2005;85:45-56.

Rolls ET. Brain mechanisms underlying flavour and appetite. *Philos Trans R Soc Lond B.* 2006;361:1123-36.

Ropelle ER, Fernandes MF, Flores MB, Ueno M, Rocco S, Marin R, Cintra DE, Velloso LA, Franchini KG, Saad MJ, Carvalheira JB. Central exercise action increases the AMPK and mTOR response to leptin. *PLoS One.* 2008;3:e3856.

Schwartz MW, Woods SC, Porte D Jr, Seeley RJ, Baskin DG. Central nervous system control of food intake. *Nature.* 2000;404:661-71.

Stubbs RJ, Sepp A, Hughes DA, Johnstone AM, Horgan GW, King N, Blundell J. The effect of graded levels of exercise on energy intake and balance in free-living men, consuming their normal diet. *Eur J Clin Nutr.* 2002a;56:129-40.

Stubbs RJ, Sepp A, Hughes DA, Johnstone AM, King N, Horgan G, Blundell JE. The effect of graded levels of exercise on energy intake and balance in free-living women. *Int J Obes Relat Metab Disord.* 2002b;26:866-9.

Sullivan SN, Champion MC, Christofides ND, Adrian TE, and Bloom SR. Gastrointestinal regulatory peptide responses in long-distance runners. *Phys Sports Med.* 1984;12:77-82.

Thompson DA, Wolfe LA, Eikelboom R. Acute effects of exercise intensity on appetite in young men. *Med Sci Sports Exerc.* 1988;20:222-7.

Tsofliou F, Pitsiladis YP, Malkova D, Wallace AM, Lean ME. Moderate physical activity permits acute coupling between serum leptin and appetite-satiety measures in obese women. *Int J Obes Relat Metab Disord.* 2003;27:1332-9.

Ueda SY, Yoshikawa T, Katsura Y, Usui T, Nakao H, Fujimoto S. Changes in gut hormone levels and negative energy balance during aerobic exercise in obese young males. *J Endocrinol.* 2009a;201:151-9.

Ueda SY, Yoshikawa T, Katsura Y, Usui T, Fujimoto S. Comparable effects of moderate intensity exercise on changes in anorectic gut hormone levels and energy intake to high intensity exercise. *J Endocrinol.* 2009b;203:357-64.

van Walleghen EL, Orr JS, Gentile CL, Davy KP, Davy BM. Habitual physical activity differentially affects acute and short-term energy intake regulation in young and older adults. *Int J Obes (Lond).* 2007;31:1277-85.

Whybrow S, Hughes DA, Ritz P, Johnstone AM, Horgan GW, King N, Blundell JE, Stubbs RJ. The effect of an incremental increase in exercise on appetite, eating behaviour and energy balance in lean men and women feeding ad libitum. *Br J Nutr.* 2008;100:1109-15.

Wynne K, Stanley S, McGowan B, Bloom S. Appetite control. *J Endocrinol.* 2005;184:291-318.

Yamamoto T. Central mechanisms of roles of taste in reward and eating. *Acta Physiol Hung.* 2008;95:165-86.

Zoladz JA, Konturek SJ, Duda K, Majerczak J, Sliwowski Z, Grandys M, Bielanski W. Effect of moderate incremental exercise, performed in fed and fasted state on cardio-respiratory variables and leptin and ghrelin concentrations in young healthy men. *J Physiol Pharmacol.* 2005;56:63-85.

7

Attenuin: What It Is, How It Works and What It Does

Ana Gordon, José C. Garrido-Gracia, Rafaela Aguilar, Carmina Bellido,
Juana Martín de las Mulas and José E. Sánchez-Criado
University of Córdoba
Spain

1. Introduction

The reproductive function in female mammals, unlike that of males, is cyclical in nature. Whilst testosterone exerts a wholly negative control, regulation of the ovarian cycle is effected through a complex series of positive and negative feedback mechanisms involving the ovary, the pituitary and the hypothalamus. Although the role of these feedback mechanisms has been known for many years, our knowledge of the detailed workings involved continues to expand. Reproductive-axis hormones have proved to be similar in all the mammalian species studied to date. The female cycle can generally be divided into the follicular, periovulatory (preovulatory and ovulatory) and luteal phases. The pituitary hormones – the gonadotropins luteinizing hormone (LH) and follicle-stimulating hormone (FSH) – remain at basal levels throughout most of the reproductive cycle, due to negative regulation by ovarian hormones (mainly estradiol and progesterone; see fig. 1 for additional details). The physiological capacity of steroids to control gonadotropin secretion is evident in a marked increase in plasma LH and FSH levels after the menopause or following ovariectomy. During the preovulatory phase, the estradiol negative feedback switches to positive. Major positive actions by estrogens include: a 20- to 50-fold increase in pituitary sensitivity to gonadotropin-releasing hormone (GnRH) (Speight et al., 1981); an increase in pituitary GnRH receptors, in concert with GnRH (Clayton et al., 1980); an increase in progesterone receptors (PR) in both pituitary and hypothalamus (Conneely et al., 1989); stimulation of GnRH synthesis and release, resulting in preovulatory GnRH secretion (Sarkar et al., 1976); and a drop in GnRH metabolism by pituitary cells (Danforth et al., 1990). These positive actions of estradiol lead to the appearance of GnRH self-priming. GnRH self-priming is an event with a twofold effect: it prompts an exponential increase in pituitary responsiveness to GnRH, and it coordinates increased responsiveness with enhanced GnRH release, ensuring that both occur at the same time and thus guaranteeing preovulatory LH secretion (Fink, 1995). In rats, this self-priming effect has been found to be more effective when GnRH pulses occur at hourly intervals (Fink, 1995), a frequency also reported to be optimal in monkeys with hypothalamic lesions (Knobil, 1980) and in women with idiopathic hypogonadotropic hypogonadism (Crowley et al., 1985). How does GnRH come to possess this unique property? Probably because the preovulatory LH surge is indispensable for species reproduction, and the fact that a very small amount of GnRH induces a disproportionate release of LH makes the process both economic and efficient

(Fink, 1995). In conclusion, although the cyclical nature of reproduction has been recognized in both humans and animals for centuries, the sequence of events involved has only recently become clear, and a number of questions remain unanswered (Schwartz, 2000).

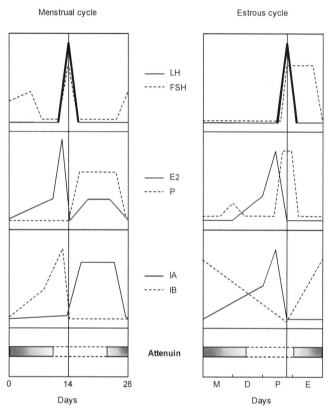

Fig. 1. **Diagram showing pituitary and ovarian hormone fluctuation during menstrual (woman) and estrous (rat) cycles.** LH: luteinizing hormone; FSH: follicle-stimulating hormone; E2: estradiol; P: progesterone; IA: inhibin A; IB: inhibin B; M: metestrus; D: diestrus; P: proestrus; E: estrus. Days of cycle are synchronized with the LH surge (day 14 in women and proestrous afternoon in rats). During the menstrual cycle, and shortly after functional luteolysis (drop in E2, P and IA) the secretion of FSH increased, stimulating the ovaries and inducing follicular recruitment. In the rat, secondary FSH secretion during early estrus stimulated the ovaries, similarly inducing follicular recruitment. In both cases, increased FSH secretion augmented attenuin bioactivity by stimulating the ovaries (lower panels). Attenuin bioactivity prevented premature occurrence of the LH surge (see text for additional details).

One crucial and still-unresolved question is how the negative feedback exerted by estradiol suddenly switches to positive, resulting in the preovulatory LH surge. Though this issue has been argued back and forth, no agreement has yet been reached. The positive effects of estradiol do not all occur at the same time, nor are they present only during preovulatory secretion. For example, the increased steroid-induced pituitary response to GnRH is directly linked to steroid levels during the follicular phase (Yen et al., 1972). Moreover, GnRH self-priming can be observed experimentally long before the LH surge is due (Waring & Turgeon, 1980). All this would suggest that steroids have to reach a critical threshold before generating any LH surge (de Koning, 1995), or alternatively that some factor is exerting a "braking" effect on the estradiol positive feedback (Whitehead, 1990). Studies of *in vitro* fertilization (IVF) methods argue against the idea of a critical level of estradiol (200 pg/ml during 36-48 h): reports indicate that in FSH-treated women with multiple follicles able to produce supraphysiological levels of estradiol from the beginning of the follicular phase, preovulatory LH secretion does not occur prematurely, and when it does appear it is diminished (Ferraretti et al., 1983; Glasier et al., 1988; Messinis et al., 1986). High levels of steroids are unlikely to inhibit the preovulatory LH surge, and high exogenous doses of estradiol are unable to suppress LH secretion in normal menstrual cycles (Messinis & Templeton, 1987). There is thus no evidence to support the hypothesis that abnormal estradiol levels inhibit preovulatory LH secretion in stimulated cycles; indeed, the evidence so far points to the existence of some non-steroidal factor, produced by stimulated ovaries and able to suppress steroidal positive feedback. Over recent decades, the search for putative new substances secreted by the ovaries has provided new insights into the role of the ovaries in gonadotropin secretion. This chapter focuses on the factor known as attenuin (Messinis & Templeton, 1989; Sopelak & Hodgen, 1984).

1.1 Evidence for the existence of attenuin

The development of IVF methods for addressing infertility in the 1970s and 1980s also shed new light on the role of FSH. In addition to its classic functions (stimulation of aromatase activity and estradiol secretion in granulosa cells, and participation in follicular selection mechanisms), FSH was found to stimulate the production of an ovarian factor with a special ability to reduce preovulatory LH secretion in women. The first evidence for an ovarian factor that attenuated GnRH-induced LH secretion appeared in the late 70s, when de Jong et al. (1979), using bovine follicular fluid (bFF), observed a drop in the responsiveness of rat pituitary cells to GnRH. Over the following decade, a number of studies pointed to the existence of a non-steroidal ovarian factor that reduced preovulatory LH release when FSH was administered during the follicular phase in women (Ferraretti et al., 1983; Messinis & Templeton, 1986), monkeys (Littman & Hodgen, 1984; Schenken et al., 1984) and rats (Busbridge et al., 1988; Geiger et al., 1980). This factor was called gonadotropin surge-attenuating factor (GnSAF), gonadotropin surge-inhibiting factor (GnSIF) or simply attenuin. In 1984, Schenken et al. demonstrated for the first time a direct effect of FSH on gonadotropin secretion, involving one or more ovarian factor(s). Ovarian venous serum (OVS) was collected from FSH-treated monkeys before and after aspiration of the right ovarian follicle; the left ovarian follicle remained intact. Serum from right ovaries before aspirated and from intact left ovaries inhibited GnRH responsiveness in rat pituitary cultures, suggesting that exogenous FSH increased OVS concentrations of a non-steroidal ovarian factor with gonadotropin-inhibiting activity. The ovarian origin of attenuin was confirmed when Fowler et al. (2002), culturing theca, stroma and granulosa cells from cyclic women, showed that attenuin bioactivity was present only in granulosa-cell-conditioned medium. Use of a superovulated protocol as a model for increased attenuin bioactivity posed a number of problems, including elevated peripheral estradiol and inhibin levels during gonadotropin administration (de Jong, 1988; Messinis & Templeton, 1988;

Muttukrishna et al., 1994), which raised doubts as to the origin of this bioactivity. With regard to estradiol, studies carried out in women have proved that effects on LH secretion are not due to negative feedback: Messinis et al. (1991, 1993) demonstrated that a single FSH injection had dose-dependent suppressive effects on pituitary responsiveness to exogenous GnRH pulses. This effect was seen as early as 8 h after FSH administration, although circulating estradiol did not increase significantly until at least 24 h after gonadotropin administration. Subsequently, this group also concluded that attenuin bioactivity in FSH-treated women could not be due to an increase in circulating total α-inhibin (Messinis et al., 1991, 1993, 1994, 1996).

Attenuin bioactivity has so far been found in serum, FF and ovarian extracts from superovulated (Fowler et al., 1994a) and cyclic women (Fowler et al., 1995a), in bFF (Van Dieten et al., 1999), in porcine FF (pFF; Danforth et al., 1987; Kita et al., 1994), in rat ovarian extracts (de Koning et al., 1989) and in rat testicular extracts (Tio et al., 1994). It should be stressed that attenuin bioactivity has been observed in human FF (hFF) from women during an untreated spontaneous cycle, suggesting that it plays a physiological role as a central regulator (Busbridge et al., 1990; Byrne et al., 1993).

1.2 Current status of attenuin characterization

In 1987 Danforth et al., using pFF, showed that attenuin bioactivity displayed certain characteristics: it was resistant to moderate heating (60 °C for 60 min), fully recoverable from an acetone precipitation, and not bound by a heparin/sepharose affinity matrix of the sort widely used to isolate inhibin. To date, attempts to characterize attenuin have proved relatively unsuccessful. Purification strategies have obtained very small amounts of bioactive material and an abundance of different proteins. The fact that the protein is present at very low concentrations makes it difficult to use Edman sequencing, leading to a whole range of different results. Tio et al. (1994) isolated inhibin and attenuin by high performance liquid chromatography from 32 liters of rat Sertoli cell-conditioned medium. Both peptides were separated on polyacrylamide gel; however the partial N-terminal sequence of the 37 kDa protein with attenuin bioactivity did not match gene and protein databases (Genbank and PIR). Subsequently, employing an elegant sequential series of purification techniques, Danforth & Cheng (1995) found a 69 kDa monomeric polypeptide in pFF that inhibited GnRH-stimulated LH secretion, but partial N-terminal analysis showed no homology with other reproductive hormones. Mroueh et al. (1996) also found a protein with attenuin bioactivity in hFF, similar to that reported in pFF (63 kDa). However, Pappa et al. (1999), starting from the same source (hFF) treated with multiple and complex purification techniques, described a protein with a molecular mass of 12.5 kDa. This protein was identified by mass spectrometry as a truncated part of the C-terminus of human serum albumin (HSA). The next published purification procedure side-stepped serum albumin contamination problems by using a serum- and BSA-free granulosa-luteal cell culture system (Fowler et al., 2002). The isolated attenuin-bioactivity protein had a molecular weight of 60-70 kDa and an isoelectric point (pI) of 5.7-5.8 pH. The internal and N-terminal amino acid sequences did not display significant homology with other accessions in the protein-sequence database. Attenuin is therefore thought to be a peptide, different from inhibin, with a postulated molecular weight which varies from less than 37 kDa (Tio et al., 1994) to 64-69 kDa (Danforth & Cheng, 1995; Fowler et al., 2002). These differences may reflect the presence either of small active subunits or of larger aggregates with or without carrier proteins, and may also reflect species differences. Ingeniously, using the expression-secretion system of a yeast (*Pichia Pastoris* GS115), it has proved feasible to produce recombinant polypeptides of HSA. Various polypeptides thus obtained were added to rat pituitary cultures and only those corresponding to subdomain IIIB (specifically residues 490-585) presented attenuin bioactivity, while the whole molecule and even the whole subdomain IIIB were inactive (Tavoulari et al., 2004). More recently, Karligiotou et al. (2006) used the retrotranscriptase-polymerase chain reaction (RT-PCR) technique and appropriate primers to amplify different transcripts from HSA gene in granulosa cells. Results showed that while all HSA fragments were expressed in the nucleus, only two fragments (the promoter and a C-terminal fragment) were expressed in granulosa cell cytoplasm, indicating a differential expression of the HSA gene, probably leading to attenuin synthesis. Finally, the current attenuin purification strategy involves the use of phage display techniques to produce antibodies against partially-purified human-granulosa-luteal cell-conditioned medium. Three of these antibodies were found to block human attenuin bioactivity on GnRH-induced LH secretion from rat pituitary cell cultures. Subsequently, these antibodies were used to immunopurify attenuin; the antigen-antibody complexes obtained were separated by electrophoresis. Candidate attenuin spots (around 66 kDa and pI 5.5-6.0) were excised for peptide mass mapping. The main molecules identified were HSA precursor and variants. All these data suggest that attenuin may be a post-translationally modified form of serum albumin, or else may be very tightly bound to, and transported by, serum albumin (Sorsa-Leslie et al., 2005).

1.3 Synthesis and secretion pattern of attenuin

In women, the production of attenuin in the ovarian follicle is clearly related to follicular size in both spontaneous and stimulated cycles. FF from follicles smaller than 11 mm (stimulated cycles, Fowler et al., 1994b) or 6-8 mm (spontaneous cycles, Fowler et al., 2001) has been found to contain the greatest amount of attenuin. In women receiving fertility treatment, there is an increase both in the number of follicles and in serum attenuin bioactivity with respect to spontaneous cycles (Byrne et al., 1993). Similarly, small follicles in pig ovaries contain the highest attenuin concentrations, while bioactivity falls sharply in preovulatory follicles (Kita et al., 1994). Thus, medium from granulosa cell cultures showed more attenuin bioactivity when these cells were obtained from aspiration of small follicles (Seo & Danforth, 1994). All these findings suggest that small and growing follicles are the major producers of attenuin. In summary, attenuin levels are highest during the early part of the menstrual cycle (days 1 to 8), falling thereafter as follicular size increases, and disappearing at the appropriate preovulatory time (Fowler et al., 2003). The corpus luteum does not appear to produce attenuin in women, but small developing follicles may produce attenuin during the luteal phase (Messinis et al., 1996; fig. 1 lower panel).

2. Methods of study

2.1 In vivo

In the absence of purified bioactive molecule, for the reasons indicated above, the effect of attenuin on the LH surge in rats is currently studied using both *in vivo* and *in vitro* procedures. The *in vivo* approach consists in administration of exogenous FSH during the diestrous phase in cycling rats as a tool to increase the biological activity of endogenous attenuin (Geiger et al., 1980; Gordon et al., 2008). In addition to attenuin, FSH also stimulates the synthesis and secretion by granulosa cells of a number of steroidal and non-steroidal factors (mainly estradiol and inhibin) that affect pituitary gonadotropin secretion (Arai et al., 1996; Watanabe et al., 1990). However, this treatment attenuates the magnitude of the proestrous afternoon LH surge despite the presence of high circulating levels of estradiol (Geiger et al., 1980; Gordon et al., 2008, de Koning et al., 1987; see fig. 2A for additional details).

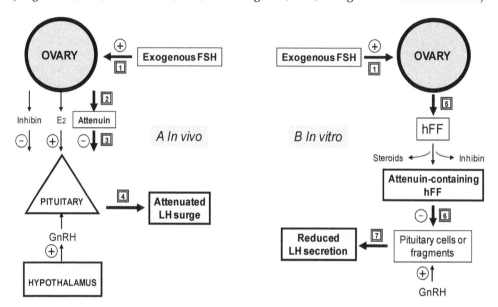

Fig. 2. **Schematic representation of current approaches to the study of attenuin effects on luteinizing hormone (LH) secretion.** GnRH: gonadotropin releasing hormone; E2: 17β-estradiol; FSH: follicle-stimulating hormone; hFF: human follicular fluid. A: *in vivo*. [1] Administration of FSH stimulates the synthesis/secretion of ovarian hormones (E2, inhibin and attenuin) [2]. Whereas in proestrus inhibin suppresses FSH secretion (Gordon et al., 2010a, 2010c) and E2 acts on LH secretion in its positive feedback mode [2], attenuin acting on gonadotrope membrane receptor [3] results in a reduction of the magnitude of the LH surge [4]. B: *in vitro*. Administration of FSH stimulates follicular growth and recruitment [1]. Pooled hFF from women undergoing IVF treatments [5] is submitted to steroid charcoal-extraction and inhibin immunoprecipitation (Gordon et al., 2010c). Attenuin-containing hFF is then added to cultured pituitary cells or fragments [6]. This results in a reduction of GnRH-stimulated LH secretion [7].

At the same time, the bioactivity of attenuin can be promoted and/or prolonged by removing endogenous inhibin and consequently increasing endogenous FSH. One option is the neutralization of inhibin's biological activity by injection of an anti-inhibin serum on metestrus that increases FSH serum levels during diestrus and proestrus, induces superovulation and again reduces the magnitude of the proestrous afternoon LH surge (Ishigame et al., 2004).

2.2 In vitro
However, it is difficult to delineate, *in vivo*, the precise bioactivity of attenuin in the rat pituitary using exogenous FSH. Alternatively, attenuin bioactivity can be studied by *in vitro*

procedures, using cultured anterior pituitary cells or pituitary fragments treated with murine FF (Busbridge et al., 1990; Fowler & Spears, 2004), pFF (Danforth & Cheng, 1995) or hFF from women undergoing IVF treatments (Byrne et al., 1995a, 1996; Fowler & Templeton 1996) as a source of exogenous attenuin, following steroid and inhibin depletion (see fig. 2B for additional details).

3. Mechanism of attenuin action

3.1 Background

Despite considerable research and the availability of improved molecular techniques, little is known about how attenuin acts. This section outlines the key findings reported to date. *In vitro* experiments have highlighted the potentiating effects of increased intracellular calcium, stimulation of both intracellular GnRH signalling pathways (calcium- and cAMP-dependent protein kinases, PKC and PKA respectively), as well as progesterone treatment on GnRH-induced LH secretion (Kile & Nett, 1994; Sánchez-Criado et al., 2006). A further clue regarding the mechanism by which attenuin acts was discovered when, in rat pituitary monolayers, GnRH was co-incubated with either estradiol, progesterone, PMA (phorbol 12-myristate 13-acetate, a stimulator of PKC) or calcium ionophore. All treatments potentiated the effects of GnRH on LH synthesis and release, but administration of hFF counteracted the enhancing effects of all these compounds, with one exception: the augmentative effect of progesterone on GnRH-induced LH synthesis (Cowking et al., 1995). Shortly afterwards, the authors found that while progesterone augmented GnRH self-priming in rat pituitary monolayers, this secretion was blocked when hFF and the antiprogestagen RU486 were added to the medium (Byrne et al., 1995b). All these findings suggest that the mechanism of action of attenuin on preovulatory LH secretion might involve the pituitary PR. There is considerable evidence, both *in vivo* and *in vitro*, to suggest that attenuin has a suppressant effect on GnRH self-priming (Byrne et al., 1996; Koppenaal et al., 1992, 1993). This action has been shown to be linked to a blockade of GnRH second messenger pathways rather than to competition between attenuin and GnRH for GnRH receptors (Fowler et al., 1994c; Tijssen et al., 1997). A study by Helder et al. (1997) reported that the unknown attenuin receptor located in the gonadotrope membrane might act through the cAMP pathway. It might thus be hypothesized that the inhibiting effect of attenuin on LH secretion is exerted through this GnRH second pathway. Both hypotheses, i.e. attenuin acting through a GnRH second pathway or through the PR, are feasible, since it has been shown that GnRH can activate the PR in a ligand-independent manner through the PKA and/or PKC pathways (Garrido-Gracia et al., 2006; Turgeon & Waring, 1994).

3.2 The relationship between attenuin and LH release

A number of published studies report a reduction of the preovulatory LH surge *in vivo* in rats treated with FSH during metestrus and diestrus (Culler, 1992; Geiger et al., 1980; Gordon et al., 2008; de Koning et al., 1987; Shuiling et al., 1999). Additionally, this FSH treatment *in vivo* causes an *in vitro* suppression of GnRH-stimulated LH secretion, GnRH self-priming and progesterone-potentiating effect on GnRH-stimulated LH secretion, without affecting basal LH levels (Byrne et al., 1996; Gordon et al., 2008; Koppenaal et al., 1992, 1993). *Pace* Geiger et al. (1980), the possibility that these effects are produced by an increase in estradiol levels can be ruled out, since animals treated with estradiol benzoate display greater LH secretion both *in vivo* and *in vitro*; more important, FSH plus estradiol-injected ovariectomized rats do not display any suppressant effect on LH secretion (Gordon et al., 2008). All this proves conclusively that FSH treatment stimulates the production of some ovarian factor(s) other than estradiol, that reduces the preovulatory LH surge but not basal LH secretion. Subsequent *in vitro* research has shown that attenuin produces this inhibiting effect on pituitary sensitivity to GnRH in a dose-dependent manner: administration of different doses of FSH (0.1, 1 and 10 I.U.) caused variable inhibition of LH secretion, partially reversed by simultaneous administration of estradiol (Gordon et al., 2009a). Attenuin would thus appear to bind to its gonadotrope membrane receptor and activate a secondary pathway in order to inhibit preovulatory LH secretion (Fowler & Templeton, 1996). The potentiating effects of progesterone, 8-bromo cAMP and PMA on GnRH-stimulated LH secretion are antagonized in rat hemipituitaries incubated with steroid-free bFF (bFF) or with FF from women undergoing a superovulation protocol (Cowking et al., 1995; Tijssen et al., 1997). All this suggests that attenuin may exert a suppressant effect on the GnRH secondary pathway. Subsequent research has shown that neither progesterone, nor GnRH, nor activation of PKA and PKC has any effect on GnRH-stimulated LH secretion in FSH-treated cyclic rats (Gordon et al., 2008; 2009b), indicating that this effect is probably produced downstream of PKA, PKC and progesterone. Given these findings, and the fact that attenuin decreases all PR-dependent parameters of LH secretion, it may be postulated that this action is exerted through a modification of PR expression and/or action (Garrido-Gracia et al., 2007).

3.3 The relationship between attenuin, PR and LH release

With regard to the effect of FSH-treatment on PR gene expression in rats, RT-PCR analysis has revealed a partial decrease in PR mRNA (Gordon et al., 2008). Nevertheless, immunohistochemical examination revealed no difference in the number of PR-positive pituitary cells in FSH injected rats (Gordon et al., 2008, 2009b) or rats in which inhibin was immunoneutralized; the latter group, however, did not display a similar partial decrease in PR mRNA (Gordon et al., 2010a). These differences may be due to different FSH and/or attenuin levels between experimental groups. In most species and tissues, PR is expressed by a single gene but transcribed into separate mRNAs as two distinct molecular forms, PR-A and PR-B. The B (stimulatory) form contains an additional N-terminal sequence and is the main transcription factor, while the A form is modulatory of B in nature (Vegeto et al., 1993; Wen et al., 1994). For this reason, the present authors decided to analyze two inhibiting possibilities: an increase in PR-A and a decrease in PR-B protein levels. While passive immunization against inhibin with an anti-inhibin serum attenuated preovulatory LH secretion in cyclic rats, pituitary protein levels of both PR isoforms were unaffected by the absence of inhibin. This was the first time the two PR isoform protein levels had been demonstrated using the western blot technique in rat pituitaries (Gordon et al., 2010a). Although attenuin could exert its negative action on LH secretion by several mechanisms, the results pointed to a possible involvement of attenuin in post-translational modifications of PR, leading to its inactivation. Phosphorylation at serine residues is the most frequent post-translational processing event in PR modification (Beck et al., 1992; Takimoto & Horwitz, 1993) and is involved in PR-regulated gene transcription (Denner et al., 1990; Faus & Haendler, 2006). To explore this question, two studies were carried out: the first sought to measure PR phosphorylation levels, while the second aimed to determine the effect of phosphatases on pituitary sensitivity to GnRH.

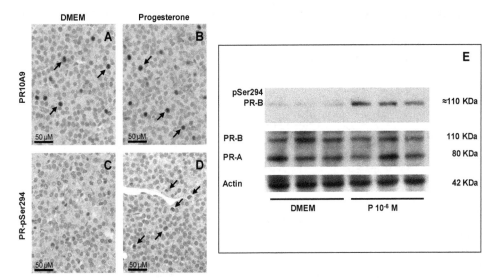

Fig. 3. **Methods of studying progesterone receptor (PR) phosphorylation in rat gonadotropes.** Left panel: Immunoreactive products to PR10A9 antibody in the nulei of gonadotropes, the only rat pituitary cell expressing PR (Garrido-Gracia et al., 2008). Pituitaries were incubated with medium alone (A, DMEM) or progesterone (B). No differences were found between the number of PR positive gonadotropes. Immunohistochemical expression of phosphorylated PR gonadotropes (C, D) in anterior pituitaries from proestrous rats (Gordon et al., 2009b). Immunoreactive products to pSer294 antibody are observed only in gonadotropes of pituitaries incubated with progesterone (D). The relative expression of pSer294-positive gonadotropes and PR109A9-positive gonadotropes provides an approximation of the PR phosphorylation rate. Right panel: PR A and B isoforms and phosphorylated PR-B content in pituitaries from proestrous rats incubated either with medium alone (DMEM) or with progesterone (P 10^{-6} M). Only PR-B phosphorylated product is seen in pituitaries incubated with progesterone (Gordon et al., 2011).

In the first study, the PR phosphorylation protocol in pituitaries was optimized by adding progesterone to the incubation medium. Subsequently, pituitaries from rats treated with FSH or with anti-inhibin serum were immunostained with an antibody that recognizes the immunogen corresponding to amino acid residues 288–300 from human PR-B, Ser294 being phosphorylated (Clemm et al. 2000). All the experimental groups in which attenuin was increased and preovulatory secretion diminished showed a significant drop in the number of cells expressing pSer294 (Gordon et al., 2009b, 2010a; fig. 3, left panel).

The following study analyzed the *in vitro* effect of calyculin, a potent inhibitor of intracellular phosphatases (Condrescu et al. 1999), on GnRH-stimulated LH secretion and GnRH self-priming in FSH-treated rats. The results showed that this drug was able, albeit partially, to reverse GnRH-stimulated LH secretion in a dose-dependent manner (Gordon et al., 2009b). Altogether, these results suggest that the ovarian-dependent inhibitory effect of FSH injection on the preovulatory LH secretion in the rat may involve an imbalance between the activities of protein kinases and phosphatases, resulting in a dephosphorylation of pituitary PR (see fig. 4 for additional details). In the light of previous immunohistochemical data (Gordon et al., 2009b, 2010a; fig. 3, left panel), the preliminary results obtained using the western blot technique (Gordon et al., 2011; fig. 3 right panel) supported the hypothesis that attenuin produces an inhibiting effect on LH secretion by dephosphorylation of pituitary PR.

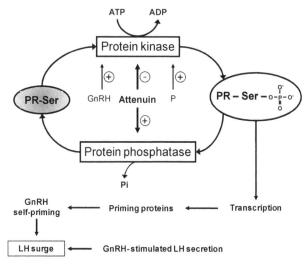

Fig. 4. **Proposed effects of attenuin on the LH surge**. GnRH: gonadotropin releasing hormone; PR-Ser: gonadotrope unphosphorylated progesterone receptor (PR); PR-Ser-PO$_4$$^{2-}$: gonadotrope phosphorylated PR. PR can be activated/phosphorylated in a ligand-dependent (progesterone) or independent (GnRH second pathways) manner. Attenuin reduces phosphorylation of Ser (serine) of the immunogen MAPGRS(p)PLATTV located in the N-terminal domain of PR-B. Activated PR-B transcribes "priming proteins" resulting in GnRH self-priming. This unique property of gonadotropes, together with estradiol sensitization of gonadotropes to GnRH, results first in GnRH-stimulated LH secretion and finally in the LH surge.

3.4 The relationship between attenuin and LH synthesis

The preovulatory secretion of LH is the result not only of increased LH synthesis (Tse et al., 1993) but also of increased LH secretion by gonadotropes (Ramey et al., 1987). While the effects of attenuin on LH secretion have been exhaustively studied, it is not known whether attenuin has any effect on LH synthesis. Fowler et al. (1995b), using rat pituitary cultures, studied the effects of steroid-free and inhibin-depleted hFF on GnRH- augmented LH synthesis and secretion in rat pituitary cultures. Results showed a decrease in both parameters, suggesting that this factor reduces pituitary responsiveness to GnRH by suppressing both the *de novo* synthesis and the acute and long term release of LH. However, there is no evidence to show how attenuin might effect this suppression. The present authors found that the addition of ionomycin (a calcium ionophore) to the incubation medium did not result, as expected, in a massive release of LH in pituitaries from FSH-treated rats. Moreover, no differences were found in LH secretion between calyculin plus GnRH and ionomycin, indicating a possible failure in LH synthesis (Gordon et al., 2009b). LH pituitary content and LHβ mRNA expression were therefore evaluated; results showed that FSH treatment decreased pituitary LH content in intact, but not in ovariectomized, rats injected with estradiol benzoate, without affecting LHβ mRNA levels. Altogether, these results suggest lower LH synthesis caused by attenuin, potentiating its inhibiting effects on LH secretion (Gordon et al., 2009a).

3.5 The relationship between attenuin, PR and LH synthesis

To determine whether pituitary PR was involved in LH synthesis inhibition by attenuin, cyclic rats were injected with different doses of FSH and progesterone. Results showed that while progesterone by itself had no effect (control groups), saturation of PR with the cognate ligand reversed the inhibitory effect of attenuin on LH protein levels, although not on LH secretion (Gordon et al., 2010b). Apart from these results showing that attenuin probably inhibits LH synthesis at post-transcriptional level, little is known about the mechanism involved in that inhibition – probably by increasing LH degradation (Kitahara et al., 1990) and/or decreasing GnRH-induced LH polypeptide glycosylation (Ramey et al., 1987) – except that, as indicated earlier, the inhibitory pathway in LH synthesis involves the gonadotrope PR. However, the detailed mechanism underlying the PR-mediated attenuin-induced inhibition of LH protein levels requires further detailed investigation. Even so, the available evidence supports the view of PR as a keystone in the neuroendocrine integrator at both hypothalamic and pituitary levels (Levine et al., 2001). In conclusion, it is postulated that, just as inhibin controls FSH synthesis and release (Attardi et al., 1991; Scott & Burger 1981), attenuin reduces proestrous GnRH-dependent LH secretion through a dual mechanism of action: inhibition of both LH synthesis and LH release.

4. The possible physiological role of attenuin

4.1 Humans

Menstrual cyclicity in women is highly dependent on positive and negative ovarian feedback mechanisms. During the follicular phase of the cycle, estradiol plays a key role in the control of both gonadotropins. Together with this steroid, low concentrations of circulating progesterone and inhibin B also contribute to the control of LH and FSH secretion, respectively. During the luteal phase, both estradiol and progesterone regulate secretion of the two gonadotropins, while inhibin A plays a role in FSH secretion. The transition from follicular to luteal phase involves a preovulatory secretion of both LH and FSH, helped by the estradiol positive mode (fig. 1, left panel). However, the change from negative to positive estradiol feedback at some threshold cannot entirely account for the change from pituitary insensitivity to the maelstrom of events leading to the LH surge. Although the question remains unresolved, there is evidence that estradiol and attenuin interact on the pituitary in the context of the positive feedback mechanism. It may be assumed that estradiol sensitizes the pituitary to GnRH, while attenuin antagonizes that sensitizing effect. Based on existing knowledge regarding attenuin action and its secretion pattern, it has been suggested that attenuin activity is greater during the early and midfollicular phases and lower both in the late follicular phase and at midcycle. Therefore, the pituitary LH response to GnRH is low during the early and midfollicular phase and is markedly enhanced during the late follicular phase, triggering the full expression of the preovulatory LH surge. According to this hypothesis, the role of attenuin in humans is to control the amplitude and not the onset of the LH surge (Messinis et al., 2006). It should be highlighted the possible role of attenuin in the polycystic ovary syndrome (PCOS). In PCOS, the mechanism responsible for abnormal gonadotropin secretion (elevated serum LH) has not been completely elucidated. One possible etiopathology mechanism is an increased of pituitary responsiveness to GnRH, caused by a decreased in attenuin production (Ruiz et al., 1996). This would offer an explanation for the most common endocrine disease that affects ovulation and fertility. At the same time, and once attenuin had been isolated, this peptide could be used as a GnRH antagonist and as a physiological contraceptive agent.

4.2 Rats

Administration of FSH during the diestrous phase prompts a reduction in proestrous LH secretion in the rat. It is worth noting that the effects of attenuin on proestrus can only be observed with this treatment (Culler, 1992; Geiger et al., 1980; Koppenaal et al., 1991). However, it is difficult to determine with any precision the role of attenuin in physiological conditions using this experimental model. Previous findings by the present authors (Gordon et al., 2010c) give grounds for speculation regarding the possible physiological role of attenuin. The incubation protocol for pituitary glands from intact cycling rats on each of the 4 days of the estrous cycle demonstrated the existence of GnRH self-priming in diestrous and proestrous phases. Subsequently, steroid-free inhibin-depeleted hFF was added to the medium. Results reported by Fowler et al. (Fowler et al., 1994b, 2001, 2003) suggest a reduction in attenuin synthesis and/or secretion when the ovarian follicle is close to preovulatory size. For this reason, we used hFF from follicles of two sizes: small (<15 mm in diameter) and large (>15 mm in diameter). Surprisingly, results in terms of secretion levels showed that only diestrous GnRH self-priming, but not proestrous self-priming as expected from the effects of injected FSH, was susceptible to the inhibiting action of attenuin contained in hFF. It should be noted that hFF from both large and small follicles had the same effects on all the LH and FSH secretion parameters so far studied. Nevertheless, the possibility that a different inhibitory bioactivity of hFF may be found using hFF from smaller follicles cannot be ruled out (Fowler et al., 2003; Fowler & Spears, 2004). Overall, these facts were interpreted as signifying that, during the normal estrous cycle, ovarian attenuin inhibited pituitary PR-dependent GnRH self-priming in diestrus only. Later on, in proestrus, pituitaries become either desensitized to the inhibitory bioactivity of attenuin and/or sensitized to the stimulatory activity of GnRH (fig. 1, right panel). By contrast, Tijssen et al. (1997) showed that attenuin was able to suppress both diestrous and proestrous GnRH self-priming. These discrepancies may be due to the different origins of FF (human vs. bovine), to the experimental model used (static vs. dynamic incubation) and to the absence or presence of inhibin. Previous results published by this research group (Tébar et al., 1996, 1998) support the hypothesis that the pituitary loses sensitivity to attenuin when follicles reach the preovulatory size, which would account for estradiol suddenly exerting a positive feedback. This intriguing mechanism, by which pituitaries become insensitive to attenuin and/or sensitive to the stimulatory action of GnRH, may provide an extra clue for understanding estrous cycle length regulation. This factor would limit the physiological timing (proestrous afternoon) as well as the magnitude (preovulatory secretion) of pituitary responsiveness to GnRH. This research thus shows how a decrease in endogenous FSH levels during diestrus, with a consequent reduction in attenuin production but no significant effect on estradiol levels, gives rise to a 1- or 2-day advancement of blunted preovulatory LH surges in 4- (Tébar et al., 1996, 1998) and 5-day (Sánchez-Criado et al., 1996) cyclic rats, respectively. This suggests that, in physiological circumstances, submaximal FSH-dependent ovarian attenuin bioactivity prevents the premature LH surge in diestrus by antagonizing the secretory effect of GnRH (Koppenaal et al., 1991; Tébar et al., 1998) and/or the sensitizing effect of estradiol on the pituitary (Schuiling et al., 1999). On the whole, all these findings, together with the existence of pituitary PR on diestrus, would suggest that PR-dependent GnRH self-priming in the diestrous phase in the 4-day cyclic rat is blocked by attenuin bioactivity.

5. Conclusions

Our work over the last few years suggests that attenuin is a FSH-dependent ovarian factor different from inhibin, which decreases preovulatory LH secretion in rats by activating gonadotrope membrane receptors, resulting in PR dephosphorylation. The reduction in PR activity is associated with a decrease in both LH secretion and LH synthesis.

The bioactivity of attenuin appears to play a major role in synchronizing physiological pituitary and ovarian events, so that preovulatory LH secretion is limited to proestrus, when the ovarian follicle and the oocyte are in optimal conditions to respond to the LH surge and to be fertilized, respectively.

However, all these findings must be viewed as speculative until experiments can be repeated using purified attenuin.

6. Acknowledgments

This review has been subsidized by grants BFU2008-00480 from DGICYT and P07-CVI2559 from CICE-Junta de Andalucia (Spain).

7. References

Arai K, Watanabe C, Taya K & Sasamoto S 1996 Roles of inhibin and estradiol in the regulation of follicle-stimulating hormone and luteinizing hormone secretion during the estrous cycle of the rat. Biology of Reproduction 55: 127–133.

Attardi B, Keeping HS, Winters SJ, Kotsuji F & Troen P 1991 Comparison of the effects of cycloheximide and inhibin on the gonadotropin subunit messenger ribonucleic acids. Endocrinology 128: 119–125.

Beck CA, Weigel NL & Edwards DP 1992 Effects of hormone and cellular modulators of protein phosphorylation on transcriptional activity, DNA binding, and phosphorylation of human progesterone receptor. Molecular Endocrinology 6: 607–620.

Busbridge NJ, Buckley DM, Cornish M & Whitehead SA 1988 Effects of ovarian hyperstimulation and isolated preovulatory follicles on LH responses to GnRH in rats. Journal of Reproduction and Fertility 82: 329–336.

Busbridge NJ, Chamberlain GV, Griffiths A & Whitehead SA 1990 Non-steroidal follicular factors attenuate the self-priming action of gonadotropin-releasing hormone on the pituitary gonadotroph. Neuroendocrinology 51: 493–499.

Byrne B, Fowler PA, Messinis IE & Templeton A 1993 Gonadotrophin surge-attenuating factor secretion varies during the follicular phase of the menstrual cycle of spontaneously cycling women. Journal of Endocrinology 139 (Suppl. p53).

Byrne B, Fowler PA, Fraser M, Culler MD & Templeton A 1995a Gonadotropin surge-attenuating factor bioactivity in serum from superovulated women is not blocked by inhibin antibody. Biology of Reproduction 52: 88-95.

Byrne B, Fowler PA & Templeton A 1995b GnSAF suppresses progesterone augmented GnRH self-priming. Journal of Reproduction and Fertility; Abstract Series 16: 3.

Byrne B, Fowler PA & Templeton A 1996 Role of progesterone and nonsteroidal ovarian factors in regulating gonadotropin-releasing hormone self-priming in vitro. Journal of Clinical Endocrinology and Metabolism 81: 1454–1459

Clayton RN, Solano AR, Garcia-Vela A, Dufau ML & Catt KJ 1980 Regulation of pituitary receptors for GnRH during the rat estrous cycle. Endocrinology 107: 699–706.

Clemm DL, Sherman L, Boonyaratanakornkit V, Schrader WT, Weigel NL & Edwards DP 2000 Differential hormone-dependent phosphorylation of progesterone receptor A and B forms revealed by a phosphoserine site-specific monoclonal antibody. Molecular Endocrinology 14: 52-65.

Condrescu M, Hantash BM, Fang Y & Reeves JP 1999 Mode-specific inhibition of sodium-calcium exchange during protein phosphatase blockade. Journal of Biological Chemistry. 274: 33279-33286.

Conneely OM, Kettelberger DM, Tsai MJ, Schrader WT & O'Malley BW 1989 The chicken progesterone receptor A and B isoforms are products of an alternate translation initiation event. Biological Chemistry 264: 14062-14064.

Cowking L, Fowler PA & Templeton A 1995 Acute exposure to ovarian steroids and a PKC activator do not overcome GnSAF bioactivity in vitro. Journal of Reproduction and Fertility; Abstract Series 15: 56-50.

Crowley WF Jr, Filicori M, Spratt DI & Santoro NF 1985 The physiology of gonadotropin-releasing hormone (GnRH) secretion in men and women. Recent Progress in Hormone Research 41: 473-531.

Culler MD 1992 In vivo evidence that inhibin is a gonadotropin surge-inhibiting/attenuating factor. Endocrinology 131: 1556-1558.

Danforth DR, Sinosich MJ, Anderson TL, Cheng CY, Bardin CW & Hodgen GD 1987 Identification of gonadotropin surge-inhibiting factor (GnSIF) in follicular fluid and its differentiation from inhibin. Biology of Reproduction 5: 1075-1082.

Danforth DR, Elkind-Hirsch K & Hodgen GD 1990 In vivo and in vitro modulation of gonadotropin-releasing hormone metabolism by estradiol and progesterone. Endocrinology 127: 319-324.

Danforth DR & Cheng CY 1995 Purification of a candidate gonadotropin surge inhibiting factor from porcine follicular fluid. Endocrinology 136: 1658-1665.

Denner LA, Weigel NL, Maxwell BL, Schrader WT & O'Malley BW 1990 Regulation of progesterone receptor-mediated transcription by phosphorylation. Science 250: 1740-1743.

van Dieten JA, Helder MN, van den Oever C & de Koning J 1999 Non-steroidal factors in bovine follicular fluid inhibit or facilitate the action of pulsatile administration of GnRH on LH release in the female rat. Journal of Endocrinology 161: 237-243.

Faus H & Haendler B 2006 Post-translational modifications of steroid receptors. Biomedicine and Pharmacotherapy 60: 520-528.

Ferraretti AP, Garcia JE, Acosta AA & Jones GS 1983 Serum luteinizing hormone during ovulation induction with human menopausal gonadotropin for in vitro fertilization in normally menstruating women. Fertility and Sterility 40: 742-747.

Fink G 1995 The self-priming effect of LHRH: a unique servomechanism and possible cellular model for memory. Frontiers in Neuroendocrinology 16: 183-190.

Fowler PA, Cunningham P, Fraser M, McGregor F, Byrne B, Pappa A, Messinis IE & Templeton A 1994a Circulating gonadotrophin surge-attenuating factor from superovulated women suppresses in vitro gonadotrophin releasing-hormone self-priming. Journal of Endocrinology 143: 45–54.

Fowler PA, Fraser M, Cunningham P, Knight PG, Byrne B, McLaughlin E, Wardle PG, Hull MGR & Templeton A 1994b Higher gonadotrophin surge-attenuating factor (GnSAF) bioactivity is found in small follicles from superovulated women. Journal of Endocrinology 143: 33–44.

Fowler PA, Bramley TA, MacGregor F & Templeton A 1994c Does GnSAF act through the pituitary protein kinase C pathway? Journal of Reproduction and Fertility; Abstract Series 13: 40.

Fowler PA, Fahy U, Culler MD, Knight PG, Wardle PG, McLaughlin EA, Cunningham P, Fraser M, Hull MG, Templeton A 1995a Gonadotrophin surge-attenuating factor bioactivity is present in follicular fluid from naturally cycling women. Human Reproduction 10: 68-74.

Fowler PA, Fraser M, Cunningham P & Templeton A 1995b GnSAF suppresses both the synthesis and release of LH induced by GnRH. Journal of Reproduction and Fertility; Abstract Series 15: 55-50.

Fowler PA & Templeton A 1996 The nature and function of putative gonadotropin surge-attenuating/inhibiting factor (GnSAF/IF). Endocrine Reviews 17: 103-120.

Fowler PA, Sorsa T, Harris WJ, Knight PG & Mason HD 2001 Relationship between follicle size and gonadotrophin surge attenuating factor (GnSAF) bioactivity during spontaneous cycles in women. Human Reproduction 16: 1353-1358.

Fowler PA, Sorsa-Leslie T, Cash P, Dunbar B, Melvin W, Wilson Y, Mason HD & Harris W 2002 A 60-66 kDa protein with gonadotrophin surge attenuating factor bioactivity is produced by human ovarian granulosa cells. Molecular Human Reproduction 8: 823-832.

Fowler PA, Sorsa-Leslie T, Harris W & Mason HD 2003 Ovarian gonadotrophin surge-attenuating factor (GnSAF): where are we after 20 years of research? Reproduction 126: 689-699.

Fowler PA & Spears N 2004 The cultured rodent follicle as a model for investigations of gonadotrophin surge-attenuating factor GnSAF production. Reproduction 127: 679-688.

Garrido-Gracia JC, Bellido C, Aguilar R & Sánchez-Criado JE 2006 Protein kinase C cross-talk with gonadotrope progesterone receptor is involved in GnRH-induced LH secretion. Journal of Physiology and Biochemistry 62: 35-42.

Garrido-Gracia JC, Gordon A, Bellido C, Aguilar R, Barranco I, Millán Y, Martín de las Mulas J & Sánchez-Criado JE 2007 The integrated action of oestrogen receptor isoforms and sites with progesterone receptor in the gonadotrope modulate LH secretion: evidence from tamoxifen-treated ovariectomized rats. Journal of Endocrinology 193: 107-119.

Garrido-Gracia JC, Gordon A, Aguilar R, Monterde JG, Blanco A, Martín de Las Mulas J & Sánchez-Criado JE 2008 Morphological effects of oestradiol-17beta, and selective oestrogen receptor alpha and beta agonists on luteinising hormone-secreting cells in tamoxifen-treated ovariectomised rats. Histology and Histopathology 23: 1453-1463.

Geiger JM, Plas-Roser S & Aron Cl 1980 Mechanisms of ovulation in female rats treated with FSH at the beginning of the estrous cycle: changes in pituitary responsiveness to luteinizing hormone releasing hormone (LHRH). Biology of Reproduction 22: 837-845.

Glasier A, Thatcher SS, Wickings EJ, Hillier SG & Baird DT 1988 Superovulation with exogenous gonadotropins does not inhibit the luteinizing hormone surge. Fertility and Sterility 49: 81-85.

Gordon A, Garrido-Gracia JC, Aguilar R, Bellido C, Velasco JA, Millan Y, Tena-Sempere M, Martín de Las Mulas J & Sánchez-Criado JE 2008 The ovary-mediated FSH attenuation of the LH surge in the rat involves a decreased gonadotroph progesterone receptor (PR) action but not PR expression. Journal of Endocrinology 196: 583-592.

Gordon A, Garrido-Gracia JC, Aguilar R & Sánchez-Criado JE 2009a Ovarian stimulation with FSH in the rat reduces proestrous GnRH-dependent LH secretion through a dual mechanism: inhibition of LH synthesis and release. Neuroscience Letters 460: 219-222.

Gordon A, Garrido-Gracia JC, Aguilar R, Guil-Luna S, Millán Y, de Las Mulas JM & Sánchez-Criado JE 2009b Ovarian stimulation with FSH reduces phosphorylation of gonadotrope progesterone receptor and LH secretion in the rat. Reproduction 137: 151-159.

Gordon A, Aguilar R, Garrido-Gracia JC, Guil-Luna S, Sánchez Cespedes R, Millán Y, Watanabe G, Taya K, Martín de Las Mulas J & Sánchez-Criado JE 2010a Immunoneutralization of Inhibin in Cycling Rats Increases Follicle-Stimulating Hormone Secretion, Stimulates the Ovary and Attenuates Progesterone Receptor-Dependent Preovulatory Luteinizing Hormone Secretion. Neuroendocrinology 91: 291-301.

Gordon A, Garrido-Gracia JC, Sánchez-Criado JE & Aguilar R 2010b Involvement of rat gonadotrope progesterone receptor in the ovary-mediated inhibitory action of FSH on LH synthesis. Journal of Physiology and Biochemistry In press.

Gordon A, Aguilar R, Garrido-Gracia JC, Bellido C, Millán Y, Guil-Luna S, García-Velasco JA, Bellido-Muñoz E, Martín de Las Mulas J & Sánchez-Criado JE 2010c Human follicular fluid (hFF) from superovulated women inhibits progesterone receptor (PR)-dependent GnRH selfpriming in an estrous cycle-dependent manner in the rat. Journal of Endocrinological Investigation 33: 564-570.

Gordon A, Garrido-Gracia JC, Aguilar R & Sánchez-Criado JE 2011 La atenuina (GnSI/AF) ovárica reduce la secreción preovulatoria de LH en la rata por desfosforilación de la isoforma B del receptor de progesterona. 53° Congress of Spanisn Society of Endocrinology and Nutrition, Santiago de Compostela, Spain.

Helder MN, van Eersel SE, van Heurn JW & de Koning J 1997 Gonadotrophin surge-inhibiting factor inhibits GnRH-stimulated mitogen-activated protein kinase activation. Human Reproduction 1: 67-68.

Ishigame H, Medan MS, Watanabe G, Shi Z, Kishi H, Aray KY & Taya K 2004 A new alternative method for superovulation using passive immunization agaist inhibin in adult rats. Biology of Reproduction 71: 236-243.

de Jong FH, Welschen R, Hermans WP, Smith SD & van der Molen HJ 1979 Effects of factors from ovarian follicular fluid and Sertoli cell culture medium on in-vivo and in-vitro release of pituitary gonadotrophins in the rat: an evaluation of systems for the assay of inhibin. Journal of Reproduction and Fertility (Suppl.) 26: 47-59.

de Jong FH 1988 Inhibin. Physiological Reviews 68: 555-607.

Karligiotou E, Kollia P, Kallitsaris A & Messinis IE 2006 Expression of human serum albumin (HSA) mRNA in human granulosa cells: potential correlation of the 95 amino acid long carboxyl terminal of HSA to gonadotrophin surge-attenuating factor. Human Reproduction 21: 645-650.

Kile JP & Nett TM 1994 Differential secretion of follicle-stimulating hormone and luteinizing hormone from ovine pituitary cells following activation of protein kinase A, protein kinase C, or increased intracellular calcium. Biology of Reproduction 50: 49-54.

Kita M, Taii S, Kataoka N, Shimatsu A, Nakao K & Mori T 1994 Changes of gonadotrophin surge inhibiting/attenuating factor activity in pig follicular fluid in relation to follicle size. Journal of Reproduction and Fertility 101: 59-66.

Kitahara S, Winters SJ, Attardi B, Oshima H & Troen P 1990 Effects of castration on luteinizing hormone and follicle-stimulating hormone secretion by pituitary cells from male rats. Endocrinology 126: 2642-2649.

Knobil E 1980 The neuroendocrine control of the menstrual cycle. Recent Progress in Hormone Research 36: 53-88.

de Koning J, Tijssen AM & van Rees GP 1987 The involvement of ovarian factors in maintaining the pituitary glands of female rats in a state of low LH responsiveness to LHRH. Journal of Endocrinology 112: 265-273.

de Koning J, Tijssen AM & van Rees GP 1989 The self-priming action of LHRH increases the low pituitary LH and FSH response caused by ovarian factors: observations in vitro. Journal of Endocrinology 120: 439-447.

de Koning J 1995 Gonadotrophin surge-inhibiting/attenuating factor governs luteinizing hormone secretion during the ovarian cycle: physiology and pathology. Human Reproduction 10: 2854-2861.

Koppenaal DW, Tijssen AM, van Dieten JA & de Koning J 1991 The self-priming action of LHRH is under negative FSH control through a factor released by the ovary: Observations in female rats in vivo. Journal of Endocrinology 129: 205-211.

Koppenaal DW, Tijssen AM & de Koning J 1992 The effect of gonadotrophin surge-inhibiting factor on the self-priming action of gonadotrophin-releasing hormone in female rats in vitro. Journal of Endocrinology 134: 427-436.

Koppenaal DW, van Dieten JA, Tijssen AM & de Koning J 1993 Induction of the gonadotrophin surge-inhibiting factor by FSH and its elimination: a sex difference in the efficacy of the priming effect of gonadotrophin-releasing hormone on the rat pituitary gland. Journal of Endocrinology 138: 191-201.

Levine JE, Chappell PE, Schneider JS, Sleiter NC & Szabo M 2001 Progesterone receptors as neuroendocrine integrators. Frontiers in Neuroendocrinology 22: 69-106.

Littman BA & Hodgen GD 1984 Human menopausal gonadotropin stimulation in monkeys: blockade of the luteinizing hormone surge by a highly transient ovarian factor. Fertility and Sterility 41: 440-447.

Messinis IE & Templeton A 1986 The effect of pulsatile follicle stimulating hormone on the endogenous luteinizing hormone surge in women. Clinical Endocrinology 25: 633-640.

Messinis IE, Templeton A & Baird DT 1986 Relationships between the characteristics of endogenous luteinizing hormone surge and the degree of ovarian hyperstimulation during superovulation induction in women. Clinical Endocrinology 25: 393-400.

Messinis IE & Templeton A 1987 Effect of high dose exogenous oestrogen on midcycle luteinizing hormone surge in human spontaneous cycles. Clinical Endocrinology 27: 453-459.

Messinis IE & Templeton A 1988 The endocrine consequences of multiple folliculogenesis. Journal of Reproduction and Fertility (Suppl.) 36: 27-37.

Messinis IE & Templeton A 1989 Pituitary response to exogenous LHRH in superovulated women. Journal of Reproduction and Fertility 87: 633-639.

Messinis IE, Hirsch P & Templeton A 1991 Follicle stimulating hormone stimulates the production of gonadotrophin surge attenuating factor (GnSAF) in vivo. Clinical Endocrinology 35: 403-407.

Messinis IE, Lolis D, Papadopoulos L, Tsahalina T, Papanikolaou N, Seferiadis K & Templeton A 1993 Effect of varying concentrations of follicle stimulating hormone on the production of gonadotrophin surge attenuating factor (GnSAF) in women. Clinical Endocrinology 39: 45-50.

Messinis IE, Lolis D, Zikopoulos K, Tsahalina E, Seferiadis K & Templeton AA. 1994 Effect of an increase in FSH on the production of gonadotrophin-surge-attenuating factor in women. Journal of Reproduction and Fertility 101: 689-95.

Messinis IE, Lolis D, Zikopoulos K, Milingos S, Kollios G, Seferiadis K & Templeton A 1996 Effect of follicle stimulating hormone or human chorionic gonadotrophin treatment on the production of gonadotrophin surge attenuating factor (GnSAF) during the luteal phase of the human menstrual cycle. Clinical Endocrinology 44: 169-175.

Messinis IE 2006 Ovarian feedback, mechanism of action and possible clinical implications. Human Reproduction Update 12: 557-571.

Mroueh JM, Arbogast LK, Fowler P, Templeton AA, Friedman CI & Danforth DR 1996 Identification of gonadotrophin surge-inhibiting factor (GnSIF)/attenuin in human follicular fluid. Human Reproduction 11: 490-496.

Muttukrishna S, Fowler PA, Groome NP, Mitchell GG, Robertson WR & Knight PG 1994 Serum concentrations of dimeric inhibin during the spontaneous human menstrual cycle and after treatment with exogenous gonadotrophin. Human Reproduction 9: 1634-1642.

Pappa A, Seferiadis K, Fotsis T, Shevchenko A, Marselos M, Tsolas O & Messinis IE 1999 Purification of a candidate gonadotrophin surge attenuating factor from human follicular fluid. Human Reproduction 14: 1449-1456.

Ramey JW, Highsmith RF, Wilfinger WW & Baldwin DM 1987 The effects of gonadotropin-releasing hormone and estradiol on luteinizing hormone biosynthesis in cultured rat anterior pituitary cells. Endocrinology 120: 1503-1513.

Ruiz A, Aguilar R, Tébar M, Gaytán F & Sánchez-Criado JE 1996 RU486-treated rats show endocrine and morphological responses to therapies analogous to responses of women with polycystic ovary syndrome treated with similar therapies. Biology of Reproduction 55: 1284-1291.

Sanchez-Criado JE, Ruiz A, Tebar M & Mattheij JA 1996 Follicular and luteal progesterone synergize to maintain 5-day cyclicity in rats. Revista Española de Fisiología 52: 223-229.

Sánchez-Criado JE, Garrido-Gracia JC, Bellido C, Aguilar R, Guelmes P, Abreu P, Alonso R, Barranco I, Millán Y & de Las Mulas JM 2006 Oestradiol-17beta inhibits tamoxifen-induced LHRH self-priming blocking hormone-dependent and ligand-independent activation of the gonadotrope progesterone receptor in the rat. Journal of Endocrinology 190: 73-84.

Sarkar D, Chiappa SA, Fink G & Sherwood NM 1976 Gonadotropin-releasing hormone surge in pro-oestrous rats. Nature 264: 461-463.

Schenken RS, Anderson WH & Hodgen GD 1984 Follicle-stimulating hormone increases ovarian vein nonsteroidal factors with gonadotropin-inhibiting activity. Fertility and Sterility 42: 785-790.

Schwartz NB 2000 Neuroendocrine regulation of reproductive cyclicity. En Neuroendocrinology in Physiology and Medicine, pp 135-145. Eds PMConn & ME Freeman. Totowa, NJ: Humana Press Inc.

Schuiling GA, Valkhof N & Koiter TR 1999 FSH inhibits the augmentation by oestradiol of the pituitary responsiveness to GnRH in the female rat. Human Reproduction 14: 21-26.

Scott RS & Burger HG 1981 Mechanism of action of inhibin. Biology of Reproduction 24: 541-550.

Seo SH & Danforth DR 1994 Porcine granulosa cells produce gonadotropin surge inhibiting factor (GnSIF) activity in vitro. Serono Symposia Xth Ovarian Workshop. Raven Press, New York, p 62.

Sopelak VM & Hodgen GD 1984 Blockade of the estrogen-induced luteinizing hormone surge in monkeys: a nonsteroidal, antigenic factor in porcine follicular fluid. Fertility and Sterility 41: 108-113.

Sorsa-Leslie T, Mason HD, Harris WJ & Fowler PA 2005 Selection of gonadotrophin surge attenuating factor phage antibodies by bioassay. Reproductive Biology and Endocrinology 3: 49.

Speight A, Popkin R, Watts AG & Fink G 1981 Oestradiol-17 beta increases pituitary responsiveness by a mechanism that involves the release and the priming effect of luteinizing hormone releasing factor. Journal of Endocrinology 88: 301-308.

Takimoto GS & Horwitz KB 1993 Progesterone receptor phosphorylation: Complexities in defining a functional role. Trends in Endocrinology and Metabolism 4: 1-7.

Tavoulari S, Frillingos S, Karatza P, Messinis IE & Seferiadis K 2004 The recombinant subdomain IIIB of human serum albumin displays activity of gonadotrophin surge-attenuating factor. Human Reproduction 19: 849-858.

Tebar M, Ruiz A, Bellido C & Sanchez-Criado JE 1996 Ovary mediates the effects of RU486 given during proestrus on the diestrous secretion of luteinizing hormone in the rat. Biology of Reproduction 54: 1266-1270.

Tebar M, Ruiz A & Sanchez-Criado JE 1998 Involvement of estrogen and follicle-stimulating hormone on basal and luteinizing hormone (LH)-releasing hormone-stimulated LH secretion in RU-486-induced 3-day estrous cycle in the rat. Biology of Reproduction 58: 615-619.

Tijssen AM, Helder MN, Chu ZW & de Koning J 1997 Intracellular antagonistic interaction between GnRH and gonadotrophin surge-inhibiting/attenuating factor bioactivity downstream of second messengers involved in the self-priming process. Journal of Reproduction and Fertility 111: 235-242.

Tio S, Koppenaal D, Bardin CW & Cheng CY 1994 Purification of gonadotropin surge-inhibiting factor from Sertoli cell-enriched culture medium. Biochemical and Biophysical Research Communications 199: 1229-1236.

Tse A, Tse FW, Almers W & Hille B 1993 Rhythmic exocytosis stimulated by GnRH-induced calcium oscillations in rat gonadotropes. Science 260: 82-84.

Turgeon JL & Waring DW 1994 Activation of the progesterone receptor by the gonadotropin-releasing hormone self-priming signaling pathway. Molecular Endocrinology 8: 860-869.

Vegeto E, Shahbaz MM, Wen DX, Goldman ME, O'Malley BW & McDonnell DP 1993 Human progesterone receptor A form is a cell- and promoter-specific repressor of human progesterone receptor B function. Molecular Endocrinology 7: 1244-55.

Waring DW & Turgeon JL 1980 Luteinizing hormone-releasing hormone-induced luteinizing hormone secretion in vitro: cyclic changes in responsiveness and self-priming. Endocrinology 106: 1430-1436.

Watanabe G, Taya K & Sasamoto S 1990 Dynamics of ovarian inhibin secretion during the oestrous cycle of the rat. Journal of Endocrinology 126: 151-157.

Wen DX, Xu YF, Mais DE, Goldman ME & McDonnell DP 1994 The A and B isoforms of the human progesterone receptor operate through distinct signaling pathways within target cells. Molecular and Cellular Biology 14: 8356-8364.

Whitehead SA 1990 A gonadotrophin surge attenuating factor? Journal of Endocrinology 126: 1-4.

Yen SS, Tsai CC, Vandenberg G & Rebar R 1972 Gonadotropin dynamics in patients with gonadal dysgenesis: a model for the study of gonadotropin regulation. Journal of Clinical Endocrinology and Metabolism 35: 897-904.

8

Hormones and Metabolism in Poultry

Colin G. Scanes
University of Wisconsin Milwaukee,
USA

1. Introduction

Poultry are domesticated species of birds. Birds were domesticated for eggs (chickens, ducks and geese), meat (chickens, ducks, geese, turkeys, ostriches, emus, pigeons and game birds) or other uses including feathers (ostriches, ducks and geese), leather (ostriches), specific oils (ostriches, emus), cock-fighting (chickens) and homing (pigeons). Table 1 summarizes the approximate time when and the location where the species were domesticated.

Poultry by global production	Domestication			Production in 2009	
	Species	When	Location(s)	Meat million metric tons	Eggs million metric tons
Chickens	Gallus gallus	5000 Before Common Era (BCE)	North East China	79.6	62.4
Turkeys	Meleagris gallopavo	200-2500 BCE	Meso-America	5.3	< 1.0
Ducks	Anas platyrinchos	3000 BCE	Fertile Crescent and East Asia/China	3.8	5.0[b]
Geese	Anser anser/Anser cynoides	3000 BCE	Fertile Crescent and East Asia/China	2.4[a]	
Pigeons	Columbia livia	3000 BCE	Fertile Crescent	< 1.0	< 1.0
Ostriches	Struthio camelus	1857	South Africa	< 1.0	< 1.0
Emus	Dromaius novaehollandiae	within last 100 years	Australia	< 1.0	< 1.0

[a] Goose and guinea fowl combined; [b] Eggs other than chicken – predominantly duck and goose

Table 1. Poultry – Their Domestication and Production (based on Scanes, 2011 and data from the Food and Agricultural Organization)

Investigations of the hormonal control of growth and/or metabolism in poultry have predominantly been performed using chickens (reviewed Scanes, 2009). Not only have such studies focused on the chicken as an important agricultural animal but also the chick embryo has long been a model for developmental biology. Moreover, the chicken is the model species for birds. There are numerically many fewer studies in turkeys, ducks and ostriches together with a substantial body of research in Japanese quail as another avian model species.

Research approaches have included ablation and replacement studies, assay of circulating hormone concentrations or gene expression in response to physiological perturbations, genetic models associated with a singe gene such a dwarf or obese chickens and genetic models produced by multi-generation selection for specific phenotypes such as fast or slow growth. There have been limited transgenic studies on the hormonal control of growth or metabolism. There is presently not a robust knock-out model in poultry.

2. Glucose homeostasis

Steady state or basal circulating concentrations of glucose are much higher in poultry than in mammals. Indeed the circulating concentrations of glucose reported in poultry species would be considered grossly hyperglycemic or symptomatic of diabetes mellitus in mammals. For instance, circulating concentrations of glucose were reported in chickens as being between 190 to 220 mg/dL (reviewed by Hazelwood, 1986) or more recently based on 15 studies as 234 ± 11.8 (SEM) mg/dL [13 ± 0.7 mM](Scanes, 2008).

Physiological state	Change in circulating concentration of glucose mM	Reference
Fasting (24hours)	No change or - 1.2	Belo et al., 1976; Harvey et al., 1976; Hazelwood & Lorenz, 1959
Insulin Administration	- 6 mM	Harvey et al., 1976;
Glucagon administration	+ 12 mM	Harvey et al., 1976;

Table 2. Changes in circulating concentrations of glucose in chickens with physiological state or perturbation

Despite the difference in set point, circulating concentrations are maintained within tight limits by a series of homeostatic mechanisms (see table 2). The physiological mechanisms are discussed below. Table 3 summarizes changes in various metabolites during fasting in chickens.

3. Hormones controlling circulating concentrations of glucose and metabolism

Circulating concentrations are maintained within tight limits by a series of physiological mechanisms. Synthesis of fatty acid and triglycerides in poultry are anatomically separated in poultry. Lipogenesis occurs predominantly in the liver of poultry while adipose tissue is the site of triglyceride synthesis and breakdown or lipolysis. These processes are under the

Physiological state	Change in circulating concentration of glucose	Reference
Glucose	No change or -4mM or -1.2 mM	Belo et al., 1976; Harvey et al., 1976; Hazelwood & Lorenz, 1959
Beta Hydroxy butyrate	+1.2 µM	Belo et al., 1976
Alanine	+110 µM	Belo et al., 1976
Serine	+250 µM	Belo et al., 1976
Glycine	-150 µM	Belo et al., 1976
Heart Glycogen	- 8.3 µmoles per g	Hazelwood & Lorenz, 1959
Liver Glycogen	- 85 µmoles per g	Hazelwood & Lorenz, 1959

Table 3. Changes in circulating concentrations of glucose, other metabolites and tissue glycogen in chickens when fasted

control of metabolic hormones with pancreatic glucagon, arguably, the most important. The role of glucagon and glucagons-like peptides of intestinal origin has received less attention. When circulating concentrations of glucose are elevated, there is a rapid increase in the rate of secretion of insulin from the pancreatic islet beta (β) cells and a concomitant rise in the circulating concentrations of insulin. The effects of insulin include the following:

• Increase in glucose uptake by muscle, liver and adipose tissue with glucose accumulating as glycogen together with increases in triglyceride in adipose tissue
• Increase in lipogenesis

When circulating concentrations of glucose are depressed, there is rapid increases secretion of glucagon from the pancreatic islet alpha (α) or A cells and a concomitant rise in the circulating concentrations of glucagon. The effects of glucagon include the following:

• Increased lipolysis in adipose tissue
• Decreased muscle and liver glycogen
• Decreased glucose utilization
• Increased gluconeogenesis
• Decrease in lipogenesis.

Other important hormones controlling metabolism in poultry include the avian adrenal glucocorticoid, corticosterone, and the thyroid hormone, triiodothyronine (T_3).

3.1 Insulin

The structure of chicken pro-insulin is long established (Perler et al., 1980). The amino-acid sequence for ostrich and chicken insulin are identical (Evans et al., 1988). The structure of insulin is identical in Pekin ducks, Muscovy ducks and domestic geese (Chevalier et al., 1996). Duck insulin has a lower potency and binding affinity to the mammalian insulin receptor compared to chicken insulin (Constans et al., 1991).

Insulin is released at times of surplus glucose, for instance following post prandial absorption of nutrients from the small intestine (DeBeer et al., 2009). The factors controlling insulin secretion are summarized in table 4. Insulin secretion from chicken pancreas *in situ* is increased by elevated glucose concentrations; this being potentiated by glucagon (King & Hazelwood, 1976). Similarly, elevated glucose concentrations increase insulin from chicken B islets *in vitro* (Datar et al., 2006). The stimulatory effect of glucagon is unlikely to be physiological as circulating concentrations of glucagon are very low when high insulin secretion is evident as, for instance, is seen following feeding (DeBeer et al., 2008). Circulating concentrations of insulin increased by the glucocorticoid, dexamethasone (Song et al., 2011). Similarly in ducks, insulin secretion is increased by glucose or arginine or oleic acid or glucagon (Foltzer & Miahle, 1980).

Stimulus	Insulin	Glucagon	Reference
Glucose	↑↑↑	↓↓	Chicken: Lanslow et al., 1970; King & Hazelwood, 1976; Honey et al., 1980 Duck: Foltzer & Miahle, 1980
Arginine	↑	↑	Chicken: King & Hazelwood, 1976; Honey et al., 1980 Duck: Foltzer & Miahle, 1980
Oleic Acid	↑	?	Chicken: Lanslow et al., 1970; King & Hazelwood, 1976; Duck: Foltzer & Miahle, 1980
Insulin	Not applicable	--	Chicken: Honey & Weir, 1979 Duck: Sitbon & Mialhe, 1978.
Glucagon	↑ in the presence of high glucose	Not applicable	Chicken: King & Hazelwood, 1976; Duck: Foltzer & Miahle, 1980
Somatostatin	↓	↑	Duck: Strosser et al., 1980
Corticosterone	↑↑	?	Chicken: Song et al., 2011
Epinephrine	↓	?	Chicken: Lanslow et al., 1970;

Table 4. Control of insulin and glucagon secretion in chickens and ducks

Despite the very high ambient circulating concentrations of glucose in poultry, insulin still plays an important role in the control of carbohydrate and to some extent also lipid metabolism. Insulin acts to increase energy storage as glycogen (liver and muscles) and triglyceride in adipose tissue (see figure 1). The physiological role of insulin in poultry is supported by the elevated circulating concentrations of glucose observed after fed chickens receive antisera against insulin (Simon et al., 2000).

3.1.1 Carbohydrate metabolism

Insulin evokes a movement of glucose from the blood. For instance, when administered to chickens insulin will induce a decline in circulating concentrations of glucose, albeit to levels that would be considered hyperglycemic in mammals (Hazelwood & Lorenz, 1959).

Chickens respond to insulin with a depression in circulating concentrations of glucose (Hazelwood & Lorenz, 1959) but are relatively insensitive to insulin (Vasilatos-Younken, 1986; Edwards et al., 1999). Insulin increases glucose uptake by skeletal muscle (M. fibularis longus) *in vitro* as indicated 2 deoxy--D-[1,2-3H]-glucose uptake (Zhao et al., 2009). In ducks, insulin increase in glucose uptake by skeletal muscle sarcolemmal vesicles while also inducing translocation of GLUT-4 like proteins from intracellular pools to the sarcolemma (Thomas-Delloye et al., 1999).

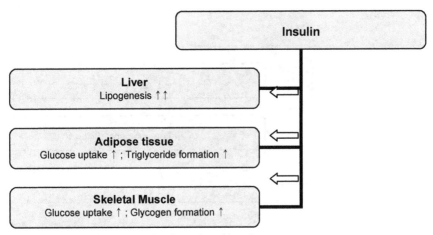

Fig. 1. Schema of physiological role of insulin in poultry

3.1.2 Lipid metabolism
Insulin can influence lipid metabolism but the physiological significant of these effects is uncertain. Fatty acid synthesis occurs predominantly in the liver of poultry and is under the control of metabolic hormones. Lipogenesis is increased *in vitro* in the presence of insulin together with T_3 (Goodridge, 1973; Wilson et al., 1986). Insulin also stimulates free fatty acid uptake by duck hepatocytes (Gross and Mialhe, 1984). However, insulin does not suppress the lipolytic effects of glucagon on chicken adipose tissue (Langslow & Hales, 1969).

3.2 Glucagon
In poultry, the major role of glucagon is to modulate carbohydrate and lipid metabolism to provide readily utilizable energy, at times of nutritional restriction. Ostrich glucagon is identical to duck glucagon (Ferreira et al., 1991).

Glucagon effects the mobilization of glucose and fatty acids from storage into the circulation together with decreasing glucose utilization (see figure 2). As might be expected, in the absence of feeding, as in regimens where chickens are fed on alternative days, there are large increases in the circulating concentrations of glucagons between meals (DeBeer et al., 2009). Surprisingly in view of its release during fasting, glucagon decreases food intake when administered centrally to chicks (Honda et al., 2007). The factors controlling glucagon secretion are summarized in table 4. Broadly, glucagon secretion is inhibited by glucose but stimulated by amino-acids. For instance, in ducks, glucagon secretion is increased by the amino-acid, arginine (Foltzer & Miahle, 1980).

3.2.1 Carbohydrate metabolism
Glucagon administration increases the circulating concentration of glucose (see table 2)(chicken: Harvey et al. 1978; turkey: McMurtry et al., 1996; ducks: Foltzer & Miahle, 1980). This is due to increases in hepatic glycogenolysis and gluconeogenesis together with decreased glucose utilization, for instance for fatty acid synthesis (Wilson et al., 1986). Glucagon has been found to stimulate gluconeogenesis, for instance, in the perfused chicken liver (Sugano et al., 1982).

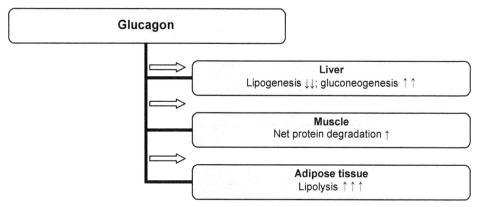

Fig. 2. Schema of physiological role of glucagon in poultry

3.2.2 Lipid metabolism
Glucagon suppresses lipogenesis in chicken hepatocytes in vitro (Wilson et al., 1986). Glucagon is the major lipolytic hormone in birds (Langslow & Hales, 1969) with its effect decreased in the presence of GH (e.g. Campbell & Scanes, 1987).

3.3 Protein metabolism
Glucagon increases gluconeogenesis and presumably net protein degradation in stores such as muscle. In ducks, glucagon increases both circulating concentrations of amino-acids (Foltzer & Miahle, 1980).

3.4 Thyroid hormones
As in mammals, the thyroid glands produce thyroxine (T_4). This is converted to the active Form, T_3. There is further deiodination and inactivation of T_3 by the T_3-degrading type III deiodinase. This enzyme is decreased in the presence of growth hormone (GH) (Darras et al., 1993). Metabolic effects of T_3 chickens include the following:

- T_3 increases heat production. Exposure of chickens to cool environmental temperatures has been reported to increase circulating concentrations of T_3, heat production and expression of uncoupling proteins (UCPs) (Collin et al., 2003). Thyroid hormones increase thermogenesis by a mechanism involving UCPs. Expression of UCPs in chickens is related to circulating concentrations of thyroid hormones, particularly T_3 (Collin et al., 2005).
- The amount of adipose tissue in chickens is related to thyroid status with increased adipose tissue in hypothyroid chickens treated with methimazole and reduced adipose

tissue in hyperthyroid chickens, receiving T_3 administration chronically (Decuypere et al., 1987)

- T_3, together with insulin, elevates the rate of lipogenesis in chicken hepatocytes *in vitro* (Wilson et al., 1986)
- Thyroid hormones influence metabolism in the small intestine with T_4 *in vitro* for 72 hours increasing glucose active transport in the duodenum of chick embryos (Black, 1988)
- T_3 decreasing the expression of genes related to obesity including brain-derived neurotrophic factor (BDNF), leptin receptor (LEPR), pro-opiomelanocortin (POMC), thyrotropin releasing hormone (TRH), and agouti-related protein (AGRP) in chicken hypothalamic neurons in vitro (Byerly et al., 2009).

3.5 Corticosterone

Corticosterone is the major glucocorticoid in birds. It has marked effects on carbohydrate, lipid and protein metabolism. Production of corticosterone is stimulated by ACTH and other hormones including calcitonin (e.g. Nakagawa-Mizuyachi et al., 2009). The glucocorticoid receptor (GR) is expressed in multiple tissues in the chicken including the liver and anterior pituitary gland (Porter at al., 2007). The activation of receptor and its translocation into the nucleus is stimulated by corticosterone and this is blocked by the specific glucocorticoid antagonist, ZK98299, when the chicken GR is expressed in Cos-7 cells (Proszkowiec-Weglarz & Porter, 2010). Hepatic expression of the glucocorticoid receptor in chickens is reported to be inversely correlated with circulating concentrations of corticosterone (Marelli et al., 2010) suggesting the corticosterone down regulates expression of its own receptor..

3.5.1 Carbohydrate metabolism

Effects of corticosterone on carbohydrate metabolism include the following:

- Increasing circulating concentrations of glucose (Lin et al., 2007; Jiang et al., 2008; Yuan et al., 2008; Zhao et al., 2009) although depressed circulating concentrations of glucose have also been reported (Gao et al., 2008)
- Increasing circulating concentrations of insulin (Jiang et al., 2008; Yuan et al., 2008; Zhao et al., 2009)
- Increasing glucose uptake as indicated 2 deoxy--D-[1,2-3H]-glucose uptake by fibularis longus muscle *in vitro* (Zhao et al., 2009)
- Decreasing glucose uptake response to either insulin or nitric oxide as indicated 2 deoxy--D-[1,2-3H]-glucose uptake by fibularis longus muscle in vitro (Zhao et al., 2009)
- Decreasing circulating concentrations of nitric oxide (Zhao et al., 2009)
- Increased breast muscle glycogen (Lin et al., 2007) but lower levels have also been reported (Gao et al., 2008).

Despite the marked effects on glucose metabolism, circulating concentrations of lactate are unchanged in chickens receiving glucocorticoid administration (Lin et al., 2007).

There is a growing viewpoint that corticosterone acts via induction of insulin resistance. Evidence for corticosterone inducing insulin resistance comes from the consistent increasing in circulating concentrations of both glucose and insulin (see above e.g. Yuan et al., 2008) and the decreased glucose uptake evoked by insulin as indicated 2 deoxy--D-[1,2-3H]-glucose uptake by fibularis longus muscle in vitro (Zhao et al., 2009)

3.5.2 Protein metabolism
The effects on corticosterone on protein metabolism include the following effects reported in chickens:
*   Depressing body weight, and particularly breast muscle weight, following chronic administration of corticosterone (Lin et al., 2006)
*   Increasing net breakdown of muscle protein due to both decreased synthesis and increased degradation (discussed in more detail under corticosterone and growth)
*   Decreasing circulating concentrations of total amino-acids (Gao et al., 2008) and increased concentrations of urate (Lin et al., 2007). These are indicative of both increases in deamidation of amino-acids and consequently of gluconeogenesis (Lin et al., 2007)
*   Increasing gluconeogenesis by perfused liver (Kobayashi et al., 1989)
*   Reductions in super-oxide dismutase activity (Lin et al., 2009).

3.5.3 Lipid metabolism
Corticosterone has marked effects on lipid metabolism including:
*   Increased liver weight (Jiang et al., 2008)
*   Increased hepatic lipogenesis (Lin et al., 2006; Yuan et al., 2008)
*   Increased abdominal and subcutaneous adipose weight (Bartov, 1982; Buyse et al., 1987; Jiang et al., 2008; Yuan et al., 2008)
*   Increased circulating concentrations of non-esterified fatty acids (NEFA) (Jiang et al., 2008; Yuan et al., 2008)
*   Increased circulating concentrations of triglyceride and very low density lipoprotein (VLDL) (Jiang et al., 2008)
*   Increased adipose lipo-protein lipase (LPL) (Jiang et al., 2008; Yuan et al., 2008).

3.5.4 Immune effects of corticosterone
Administration of corticosterone to chicken results in reductions in the weights (and weights as a percentage of body weight) of the bursa Fabricius and spleen (Shini et al., 2008) Other effects include an initial transitory improvement of the antibody response to infectious bronchitis virus (IBV) vaccination followed by a marked impairment of the response to IBV (Shini et al., 2008)/ Other effects including increasing the heterophil to lymphocyte (H/L) ratio in the circulation (Shini et al., 2009). Corticosterone increases expression interleukins -1beta, IL-6, IL-10, IL-12alpha and IL-18 while decreasing that of chemokine C-C motif ligand (CCL)16 and transforming growth factor-beta4 in heterophils in the circulation of chickens (Shini et al., 2010).

3.5.5 Other metabolic effects of corticosterone
Other metabolic effects of corticosterone in chickens include the following:
*   Increasing expression sodium and glucose co-transporter 1 (SGLT-1 vitamin D-dependent calcium-binding protein-28,000 molecular weight (CaBP-D28k), and peptide transporter 1 (PepT-1) mRNA in the duodenum (Hu et al., 2010)
*   Increasing expression of genes related to obesity in the chicken hypothalamus including brain-derived neurotrophic factor (BDNF), neuropeptide Y and agouti-related protein (AGRP) (Byerly et al., 2009)
*   Depressing adenosine deaminase activity in all regions of the chicken gastro-intestinal tract except the proventriculus (Bhattacharjee et al., 2009).

3.6 Other hormones and metabolism
3.6.1 Estrogen and metabolism

Estrogen has some effects on metabolism. Estrogen increases adiposity in poultry. For instance, synthetic estrogens increase adipose tissue in chickens (Carew & Hill, 1967; Snapir et al., 1983). Moreover, the anti-estrogen, tamoxifen, decreases adiposity in female chickens (Rozenboim et al., 1989; 1990). In addition, estrogens are responsible for the dramatic increase in the hepatic synthesis of the yolk lipo-proteins (Reviewed: Scanes et al., 2004).

3.6.2 Ghrelin and metabolism

Lipogenesis in the chicken liver is increased by ghrelin as indicated by expression of fatty acid synthase (Buyse et al., 2009). Moreover, ghrelin reduces the respiratory quotient in young chickens (Geelissen et al., 2006).

3.6.3 Growth Hormone (GH) and metabolism

Both native and biosynthetic growth hormone (GH) *per se* can stimulate lipolysis *in vitro* (Campbell & Scanes, 1985). Moreover, GH inhibits glucagon stimulated lipolysis (Campbell & Scanes, 1986).

3.6.4 Somatostatin and metabolism

The major gastro-intestinal hormone, somatostatin is reported to be a potent inhibitor of glucagon stimulated lipolysis with chicken adipose tissue (Di Scala et al., 1985).

4. Hormonal control of growth

In poultry, the two major hormones required for the full expression of growth are GH and T_3. Both require the anterior pituitary gland. GH is directly synthesized by somatotrophs in the caudal lobe of the anterior pituitary gland in poultry. T_3 is produced by monodeiodination of the thyroid hormones, thyroxine (T_4). In turn, secretion of T_4 is stimulated by the anterior pituitary hormone, thyrotropin (thyroid stimulating hormone TSH). Moreover, the circulating concentrations of T_3 are maintained by GH reducing deactivation by T3-degrading type III deiodinase (Darras et al., 1993).

Evidence for the importance of anterior pituitary hormones in the growth of poultry (see figure 3) comes from ablation and replacement therapy studies. In young chickens, hypophysectomy depressed growth (body weight or skeletal growth) with growth rate being partially restored with either GH or T_3 replacement therapy (King & Scanes, 1986; Scanes et al., 1986). Similarly in young turkeys, hypophysectomy reduced growth rate but no effects of GH are observed (Proudman et al., 1994).

4.1 Growth Hormone (GH) and Growth

Dwarf chickens exhibit markedly reduced growth (Scanes et al., 1983) due to lack of GH receptors (Burnside et al., 1991; Agarwal et al., 1994) and the reduced circulating concentrations of T_3 (Scanes et al., 1983). While GH may be essential for growth, additional exogenous GH have either no (chickens: Cogburn et al. 1989, Cravener et al., 1989; Rosebrough et al., 1991; turkeys: Bacon et al., 1995) or only a small positive effect on poultry growth (Leung et al., 1986; Vasilatos-Younken et al., 1988; Scanes et al., 1990) with the latter potentially transitory. Instead, it may be hypothesized that the set points for GH/IGF-I

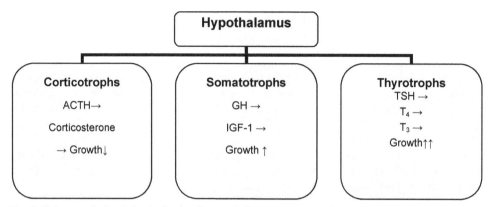

Fig. 3. Schema of physiological role of growth hormone in poultry

mediated growth are tightly controlled to insure optimal growth. It is argued that excess weight/size would be selected heavily against birds because of the energy requirements for flight.

GH acts specifically on the growth of immune tissues in birds. In birds, there is special separation between T and B cells during development in respectively the thymus and bursa Fabricius. In young chickens, hypophysectomy depresses thymus growth with GH partially overcoming this effect (King and Scanes, 1986; Johnson et al., 1993).

4.1.1 Control of GH synthesis and release

Release of GH from somatotrophs in the chicken pituitary is controlled by the following:

- The number of somatotrophs;
- The amount of GH available to be released, which is in turn dependant on GH gene expression and translation (GH synthesis);
- Stimulatory control by hypothalamic peptides such as GH releasing hormone (GHRH), thyrotropin releasing hormone (TRH), ghrelin and pituitary adenylate cyclase-activating peptide (PACAP) together with possibly leptin;
- Inhibitory control by the hypothalamic and peripheral somatostatin, together with negative feedback by hormones whose release/synthesis are increased by GH, namely insulin-like growth factor 1 (IGF-1) and triiodothyronine (T_3);
- The stimulatory and inhibitory effects depend upon both the concentrations of the stimulator or inhibitor and the responsiveness of somatotrophs to them. Not all chicken somatotrophs respond to all secretagogues; some respond to both GHRH and PACAP (85%), or to GHRH and TRH (73%) or to GHRH and leptin (51%) or to GHRH and ghrelin (21%) (Scanes et al., 2007).

Expression of the GH gene is inhibited by T_3 or IGF-1 in chickens (Radecki et al., 1994; Scanes et al., 1999).

4.2 Thyroid hormones and growth

In poultry, normal growth rate requires critical or optimal concentrations of T_3 and perhaps T_4 also. Administration of T_3 to dwarf chicks to restore normal circulating concentrations of T_3 produces some increase in growth rate (Marsh et al., 1984; Bowen et al., 1987). However, T_3 administration to chickens with circulating concentrations within the normal range

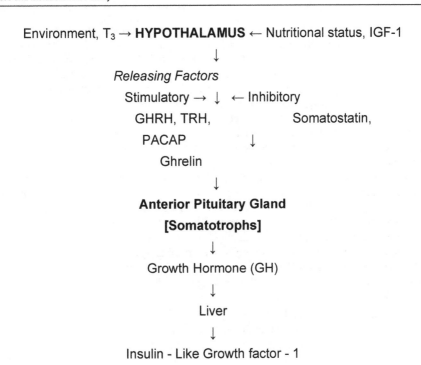

Fig. 4. The hypothalamic growth hormone – insulin-like growth factor 1 – growth axis in poultry

depresses growth rate (Marsh et al., 1984; Bowen et al., 1987). Thyroid ablation by the goitrogen methimazole results in markedly lower growth rates (Chaisson et al., 1979; Decuypere et al., 1987) and circulating concentrations of IGF-1(Decuypere et al., 1987; Rosebrough et al., 2003). Growth rates of chickens are depressed by T3 administration and to a less extent T4 (Decuypere et al., 1987). This would support the concept that normal growth rate in poultry depends on a physiological "set- point".
Other growth related effects of thyroid hormones include the following:

- T$_3$ increases the growth rate of young hypophysectomised chickens (Scanes et al., 1986);
- Thyroid hormones induce development of the small intestine with thyroxine *in vitro* for 72 hours increasing microvillar growth and the rate of mitosis in the epithelia in chick embryo duodena (Black, 1978) and glucose active transport in the duodenum of chick embryos (Black, 1988);
- T3 decreases GH secretion by effects at both the levels of the anterior pituitary and the hypothalamus. For instance, T3 increases the expression of both type 2 and 5 somatostatin receptor sub-types (De Groef et al., 2007) and reduces the expression of thyrotropin releasing hormone (TRH) both in vivo and in vitro in chicken hypothalamic neurons (Byerly et al., 2009).

4.3 Insulin like growth factor-1 and growth
There is strong evidence that the effects of GH and thyroid hormones are mediated by hepatic production of insulin-like growth factor-1 (IGF-1). Circulating concentrations of IGF-

1are markedly decreased in hypophysectomized young chickens with GH partially reversing this effect (Huybrechts et al., 1985; Lazarus and Scanes, 1988). GH also elevates plasma IGF-1 in intact adult chickens (Scanes et al., 1999). Moreover, IGF-I release from chicken hepatocytes *in vitro* is elevated in the presence of GH and synergistically with GH and insulin (Houston & O'Neill, 1991). Circulating concentrations of IGF-1 are reduced by chronic methimazole administration with concentrations partially restored by T3 administration (Rosebrough and McMurtry, 2003). Chicks treated with the goitrogens, propylthiouracil, have depressed growth rate, circulating concentrations of IGF-I and hepatic expression of IGF-I (Tsukada et al., 1998) and T_4 administration partially restoring these parameters (Tsukada et al., 1998).

There is a report that the administration of IGF-I stimulate growth rate in chickens (Tomas et al., 1998). Moreover, there are increases in skeletal muscle mass and elevated rates of protein synthesis (Conlon & Kita, 2002) and depressed rates of degradation (Tomas et al., 1998). The effect of IGF-1 on chick growth has not been observed in other studies (McGuinness & Cogburn, 1991; Huybrechts et al., 1992; Tixier-Boichard et al., 1992). One mechanism by which, glucocorticoid hormones depress growth is by depressing IGF-1; circulating concentrations of IGF-1 have recently been observed to be decreased by the glucocorticoid, dexamethasone, in chickens (Song et al., 2011).

4.4 Other hormones and growth

Other hormones such as the adrenal cortical hormone, corticosterone, estradiol and testosterone can have marked effects on growth.

4.4.1 Corticosterone and growth

Glucocorticoids including the endogenous avian steroid, corticosterone, and the synthetic dexamethasone depress growth in chickens (Li et al., 2009; Hu et al., 2010; Song et al., 2011).

- Decreased skeletal muscle weight (Yuan et al., 2008; Song et al., 2011)
- Increased protein degradation as indicated by increases in the concentrations of 3-methyl histidine in both pectoralis and femoris muscles (Dong et al., 2007)
- Increases muscle proteolysis (Gao et al., 2008)
- Reduced skeletal protein synthesis as indicated by the RNA:protein ratio (Dong et al., 2007) Decreasing the growth of the small intestine in chickens although the effect is of a small magnitude than that with overall growth as weight of the small intestine relative to body weight is increased (Hu et al., 2010)
- Increases expression of myostatin (Song et al., 2011).
- Depressing duodenal and jejunal villus height and crypt depth (Hu et al., 2010)

Corticosterone plays the pivotal role in inducing functioning somatotropes during late embryonic development (Dean and Porter, 1999; Porter et al., 2001).

4.4.2 Estrogen and growth

Estrogen has effects on the growth of specific organs being responsible for the massive growth of the oviduct during sexual maturation (reviewed: Scanes et al., 2004). Estrogens play an important role in the formation of the calcium storing tissue, medullary bone, at the time of sexual maturation. Formation of medullary bone matrix is stimulated by estradiol and testosterone in immature male quail chicks with mineralization requiring vitamin D3 (Takahashi et al., 1983). Estradiol, in combination with testosterone, is has found to stimulate proliferation of chicken medullary osteoblasts and inhibit their apoptosis (Chen et al., 2010). Moreover, medullary bone formation is suppressed when aromatase, critical for estradiol synthesis, is inhibited (Deng et al., 2010).

4.4.3 Glucagon-like peptide 2 (GLP-2) and growth
Glucagon-like peptide 2 increases growth in chickens (Hu et al., 2010).

4.4.4 Testosterone and growth
The major circulating androgen in birds is testosterone. Testosterone acting via conversion to 5α Dehydro-testosterone (DHT) depresses growth in chickens (Fennell & Scanes, 1992a) while stimulating that of turkeys (Fennell & Scanes, 1992b).Androgens in combination with estrogens induce the formation of medullary bone at the time of sexual maturation (e.g. Chen et al., 2010).

5. References

Agarwal, S.K., Cogburn, L.A. & Burnside, J. (1994). Dysfunctional growth hormone receptor in a strain of sex-linked dwarf chickens: evidence for a mutation in the intra-cellular domain. *Journal of Endocrinology*, Vol.142, No.3, pp. 427-434, ISSN 0022-0795

Bacon, W.L., Long, D.W. & Vasilatos-Younken, R. (1995). Responses to exogenous pulsatile turkey growth hormone by growing 8-week-old female turkeys. *Comparative Biochemistry and Physiology A Molecular Biology*, Vol.111, No.3, pp. 471-482, ISSN 1095-6433.

Bartov, I. (1982). Corticosterone and fat deposition in broiler chicks: effect of injection time, breed, sex and age. *British Poultry Science*, Vol. 23, No. 2, pp.161-170, ISSN 0007-1668.

Belo, P. S., Romsos, D. R. & Leveille, G. A. (1976). Blood metabolites and glucose metabolism in the fed and fasted chicken. *Journal of Nutrition*, Vol. 106, No.8, pp. 1135–1143, ISSN 0022-3166.

Bhattacharjee, P. & Sharma, R. (2009). Antithetical effects of corticosterone and dibutyryl cAMP on adenosine deaminase in the gastrointestinal tract of chicken during postnatal development. *Molecular and Cellular Biochemistry*, Vol. 327, No. 1-2, 79-86, ISSN 0300-8177.

Black, B.L. (1978) Morphological development of the epithelium of the embryonic chick intestine in culture: influence of thyroxine and hydrocortisone. *American Journal of Anatomy*, Vol.153, No. 4, pp. 573-599, ISSN 1097-0177.

Black, B.L. (1988) Development of glucose active transport in embryonic chick intestine. Influence of thyroxine and hydrocortisone. *Comparative Biochemistry and Physiology A Comparative Physiology*, Vol. 90, No. 3, pp.379-386, ISSN 1095-6433.

Bowen, S.J., Huybrechts, L.M., Marsh, J.A. & Scanes, C.G. (1987). Influence of triiodothyronine and growth hormone on growth of dwarf and normal chickens: interactions of hormones and genotype. *Comparative Biochemistry and Physiology A Comparative Physiology*, Vol. 86, No. 1, pp. 137-142, ISSN 1095-6433.

Burnside, J., Liou, S.S. & Cogburn, L.A. (1991). Molecular cloning of the chicken growth hormone receptor complementary deoxyribonucleic acid: mutation of the gene in sex-linked dwarf chickens. *Endocrinology*, Vol. 128, No. 6, pp. 3183-3192, ISSN 0013-7227.

Buyse, J., Decuypere, E., Sharp, P.J., Huybrechts, L.M., Kühn, E.R. & Whitehead, C. (1987). Effect of corticosterone on circulating concentrations of corticosterone, prolactin, thyroid hormones and somatomedin C and on fattening in broilers selected for high or low fat content. *Journal of Endocrinology*, Vol. 112, No. 2, pp. 229-237, ISSN 0022-0795.

Buyse, J., Janssen, S., Geelissen, S., Swennen, Q., Kaiya, H., Darras, V.M. & Dridi, S. (2009). Ghrelin modulates fatty acid synthase and related transcription factor mRNA levels in a tissue-specific manner in neonatal broiler chicks. *Peptides*, Vol. 30, No. 7, pp.1342-1347, ISSN 0196-9785.

Byerly, M.S., Simon, J., Lebihan-Duval, E., Duclos, M.J., Cogburn, L.A. & Porter, T.E. (2009). Effects of BDNF, T3, and corticosterone on expression of the hypothalamic obesity gene network in vivo and in vitro. *American Journal of Physiology Regulatory Integrative Comparative Physiology*, Vol. 296, No. 4, pp. R1180-1189, ISSN 0363-6143.

Campbell, R.M. & Scanes, C.G. (1985). Lipolytic activity of purified pituitary and bacterially derived growth hormone on chicken adipose tissue *in vitro*. *Proceedings of the Society of Experimental Biology and Medicine*, Vol. 180, No. 3, pp. 513-517, ISSN 0037-9727.

Campbell, R.M. & Scanes, C.G. (1987). Growth hormone inhibition of glucagon and cAMP-induced lipolysis by chicken adipose tissue *in vitro*. *Proceedings of the Society of Experimental Biology and Medicine* Vol.184, No. 4, pp. 456-460, ISSN 0037-9727.

Carew, L.B. & Hill, F.W. (1967). Effect of diethylstilbestrol on energy and protein utilization by chicks fed a diet high in fat content. *Journal of Nutrition*, Vol. 92, No. 3, pp. 393-398, ISSN 0022-3166.

Chaisson, R.B., Sharp, P.J., Klandorf, H., Scanes, C.G. & Harvey, S. (1979). The effect of rapeseed meal and methimazole on levels of plasma hormones in growing broiler cockerels. *Poultry Science*, Vol. 58, No. 3, pp. 1575-1583, ISSN 1537-0437.

Chen, X., Deng, Y., Zhou, Z., Tao, Q., Zhu, J., Li, X., Chen, J. & Hou, J. (2010). 17beta-estradiol combined with testosterone promotes chicken osteoblast proliferation and differentiation by accelerating the cell cycle and inhibiting apoptosis in vitro. *Veterinary Research Communications*, Vol. 34, No. 2, pp. 143-152, ISSN 0165-7380.

Chevalier, B., Anglade, P., Derouet, M., Mollé, D. & Simon, J. (1996). Isolation and characterization of Muscovy (Cairna moschata) duck insulin. *Comparative Biochemistry and Physiology A Comparative Physiology, B Molecular Biology*, Vol. 114, No. 1, pp.19-26, ISSN 1095-6433.

Cogburn, L.A., Liou, S.S., Rand, A.L. & McMurtry, J.P. (1989). Growth, metabolic and endocrine responses of broiler cockerels given a daily subcutaneous injection of natural or biosynthetic chicken growth hormone. *Journal of Nutrition*, Vol. 119, No. 8, pp. 1213-1222, ISSN 0022-3166.

Collin A, Buyse J, van As P, Darras VM, Malheiros RD, Moraes, V.M., Reyns, G.E., Taouis, M. & Decuypere, E. (2003). Cold-induced enhancement of avian uncoupling protein expression, heat production, and triiodothyronine concentrations in broiler chicks. *General and Comparative Endocrinology*, Vol. 130, No. 1, pp. 70-77, ISSN 0016-6480.

Collin A, Cassy, S., Buyse, J., Decuypere, E. & Damon, M. (2005). Potential involvement of mammalian and avian uncoupling proteins in the thermogenic effect of thyroid hormones. *Domestic Animal Endocrinology*, Vol. 29, No.1, pp. 78-87, 0739-7240.

Conlon, M.A. & Kita, K. (2002). Muscle protein synthesis rate is altered in response to a single injection of insulin-like growth factor-I in seven-day-old Leghorn chicks. *Poultry Science*, Vol. 81, No. 10, pp. 1543-1547, ISSN 1537-0437.

Constans, T., Chevalier, B., Derouet, M., Simon, J. (1991). Insulin sensitivity and liver insulin receptor structure in ducks from two genera. A *American Journal of Physiology*, Vol. 261, No. 4, pp. R882-R890, ISSN 0363-6143.

Cravener, T.L., Vasilatos-Younken, R. & Wellenreiter, R.H. (1989). Effect of subcutaneous infusion of pituitary-derived chicken growth hormone on growth performance of broiler pullets. *Poultry Science*, Vol. 68, No. 8, pp. 1133-1140, ISSN 1537-0437.

Darras, V.M., Rudas, P., Visser, T.J., Hall, T.R., Huybrechts, L.M., Vanderpooten, A., Berghman, L.R., Decuypere, E. & Kühn, E.R. (1993). Endogenous growth hormone controls high plasma levels of 3,3',5-triiodothyronine (T3) in growing chickens by decreasing the T3-degrading type III deiodinase activity. *Domestic Animal Endocrinology*, Vol. 10, No. 1, pp. 55-65, ISSN 0739-7240.

Dean, C.E. & Porter, T.E. (1999). Regulation of somatotroph differentiation and growth hormone (GH) secretion by corticosterone and GH-releasing hormone during embryonic development. *Endocrinology*, Vol. 140, No. 3, pp. 1104-1110, ISSN 0013-7227.

De Beer, M., McMurtry, J.P., Brocht, D.M. & Coon, C.N. (2008). An examination of the role of feeding regimens in regulating metabolism during the broiler breeder grower period. 2. Plasma hormones and metabolites. *Poultry Science*, Vol. 87, No. 2, pp. 264-275, ISSN 1537-0437.

Decuypere, E., Buyse, J., Scanes, C.G., Huybrechts, I. & Kuhn, E.R. (1987). Effects of hyper- or hypothyroid status on growth, adiposity and levels of growth hormone, somatomedin C and thyroid metabolism in broiler chickens. *Reproduction Nutrition Développement*, Vol. 27, No.2B, pp. 555-565, ISSN 0926-5287.

De Groef, B., Grommen, S.V. & Darras, V.M. (2007). Feedback control of thyrotropin secretion in the chicken: thyroid hormones increase the expression of hypophyseal somatostatin receptor types 2 and 5. *General and Comparative Endocrinology*, Vol. 152, No. 2-3, pp.178-182, ISSN 0016-6480.

Deng, Y.F., Chen, X.X., Zhou, Z.L. & Hou, J.F. (2010). Letrozole inhibits the osteogenesis of medullary bone in prelay pullets. *Poultry Science*, Vol. 89, No. 5, pp. 917-023, ISSN 1537-0437.

Di Scala-Guenot, D., Strosser, M.T. & Mialhe, P. (1985). The biological activity of duck 'big' somatostatin on chicken adipose tissue. *Biochimica et Biophysica Acta*, Vol. 845, No. 2, pp. 261-264, ISSN 0005-2736.

Dong, H., Lin, H., Jiao, H.C., Song, Z.G., Zhao, J.P. & Jiang, K.J. (2007). Altered development and protein metabolism in skeletal muscles of broiler chickens (Gallus gallus domesticus) by corticosterone. *Comparative Biochemistry and Physiology A Molecular and Integrative Physiology*, Vol. 147, No. 1, pp.189-195, ISSN 1095-6433.

Edwards, M.R., McMurtry, J.P. & Vasilatos-Younken, R. (1999). Relative insensitivity of avian skeletal muscle glycogen to nutritive status. *Domestic Animal Endocrinology*, Vol. 16, No. 4, pp. 239-247, ISSN 0739-7240.

Evans, T.K., Litthauer, D. & Oelofsen, W. (1988). Purification and primary structure of ostrich insulin. *International Journal of Peptide and Protein Research*, Vol. 31, No. 5, pp. 454-462, *ISSN* 0367-8377.

Farhat, A. & Chavez, E.R. (2000). Comparative performance, blood chemistry, and carcass composition of two lines of Pekin ducks reared mixed or separated by sex. *Poultry Science*, Vol. 79, No. 4, pp. 460-465, ISSN 1537-0437.

Fennell, M.J. & Scanes, C.G. (1992a). Inhibition of growth in chickens by testosterone, 5a-dihydrotestosterone, and 19-nortestosterone. *Poultry Science*, Vol. 71, No. 2,pp. 357-366, ISSN 1537-0437.

Fennell, M.J. & Scanes, C.G. (1992b). Effects of androgen (testosterone, 5a-dihydrotestosterone, and 19-nortestosterone in turkeys. *Poultry Science*, Vol. 71, No. 3, pp. 539-549, ISSN 1537-0437.

Ferreira, A., Litthauer, D., Saayman, H., Oelofsen, W., Crabb, J. and Lazure, C. 1991. Purification and primary structure of glucagon from ostrich pancreas splenic lobes. *International Journal of Peptide and Protein Research*, Vol. 38, No. 4, pp. 90-95, *ISSN* 0367-8377.

Foltzer, C. & Mialhe, P. (1980). Pituitary and adrenal control of pancreatic endocrine function in the duck. III. Effects of glucose, oleic acid, arginine, insulin and glucagon infusions in hypophysectomized or normal ducks. *Diabetes & Metabolism*, Vol. 6, No. 4, pp. 257-63, ISSN 1262-3636.

Food and Agricultural Organization Agricultural Statistics. http://faostat.fao.org/site/569/default.aspx#ancor Accessed March 13, 2011

Gao, J., Lin, H., Song, Z.G. & Jiao, H.C. (2008). Corticosterone alters meat quality by changing pre-and postslaughter muscle metabolism. *Poultry Science*, Vol. 87, No. 8, pp. 1609-1617, ISSN 1537-0437.

Geelissen, S.M., Swennen, Q., Geyten, S.V., Kühn, E.R., Kaiya, H., Kangawa, K., Decuypere, E., Buyse, J. & Darras, V.M. (2006). Peripheral ghrelin reduces food intake and respiratory quotient in chicken. *Domestic Animal Endocrinology*, Vol. 30, No. 2, pp. 108-116, ISSN 0739-7240.

Goodridge, A.G. (1973). Regulation of fatty acid synthesis in isolated hepatocytes preparaed from livers of neonatal chicks. *Journal of Biological Chemistry*, Vol. 248, No. 6, pp. 1924-1931, ISSN 0021-9258.

Gross, R. & Mialhe, P. (1987). Glucose, beta adrenergic effects, and pancreatic endocrine function in the isolated perfused duck pancreas. *Acta endocrinologica*, Vol. 115, No. 1, pp. 105-111. ISSN:0001-5598

Gross, R. and Mialhe, P. 1984. Effect of insulin on free fatty acid uptake by hepatocytes in the duck. *Journal of Endocrinology*, Vol. 102, No. 3, pp. 381-386, ISSN 0022-0795.

Harvey, S., Scanes, C.G., Chadwick, A. & Bolton, N.J. (1978). Influence of fasting, glucose and insulin on the levels of growth hormone and prolactin in the plasma of the domestic fowl (Gallus domesticus). *Journal of Endocrinology*. Vol. 76, No. 3, pp. 501-506, ISSN 0022-0795.

Hazelwood, R.L. & Lorenz, F.W. (1959). Effects of fasting and insulin on carbohydrate metabolism of the domestic fowl. *American Journal of Physiology*, Vol. 197, Vol. 1, pp. 47-51, ISSN 0363-6143.

Hazelwood, R.L. (1986). Carbohydrate metabolism. In: *Avian Physiology* (Ed. P. D. Sturkie) pp.303-325. ISBN-13: 9780387961958, Springer Verlag, New York,

Honda, K., Kamisoyama, H., Saito, N., Kurose., Y., Sugahara, K. & Hasegawa, S. (2007). Central administration of glucagon suppresses food intake in chicks. *Neuroscience Letters*, Vol. 416, No. 2, pp. 198-201.*ISSN: 0304-3940*.

Honey, R.N. & Weir, G.C. (1979). Insulin stimulates somatostatin and inhibits glucagon secretion from the perfused chicken pancreas-duodenum. *Life Science*, Vol. 24, No. 19, pp. 1747-1750, ISSN 0024-3205.

Honey, R.N., Schwartz, J.A., Malhe, J. & Weir, G.C. (1980). Insulin, glucagons and somatostatin secretion from isolated perfused rat and chicken pancreas-duodenum. *American Journal of Physiology*, Vol. 238, No.2, pp. E150-E156, ISSN 0363-6143.

Houston, B. & O'Neill, I.E. (1991). Insulin and growth hormone act synergistically to stimulate insulin-like growth factor-I production by cultured chicken hepatocytes. *Journal of Endocrinology*, Vol. 128, No. 3, pp. 389-393, ISSN 0022-0795.

Hu, X.F. , Guo, Y.M. , Huang, B.Y. , Bun, S. , Zhang, L.B. , Li, J.H. , Liu, D. , Long, F.Y. , Yang, X. & Jiao, P. (2010). The effect of glucagon-like peptide 2 injection on performance, small intestinal morphology, and nutrient transporter expression of stressed broiler chickens. *Poultry Science*, Vol. 89, No. 9, pp. 1967-1974, ISSN 1537-0437.

Huybrechts, L.M., King, D.B., Lauterio, T.J., Marsh, J. & Scanes, C.G. (1985). Plasma concentrations of somatomedin-C in hypophysectomized, dwarf and intact growing domestic fowl as determined by heterologous radioimmunoassay. *Journal of Endocrinology*, Vol. 104, No. 2, pp. 233-239, ISSN 0022-0795.

Huybrechts, L.M., Decuypere, E., Buyse, J., Kühn, E.R. & Tixier-Boichard, M. (1992). Effect of recombinant human insulin-like growth factor-I on weight gain, fat content, and hormonal parameters in broiler chickens. *Poultry Science*, Vol. 71, No. 1, pp. 181-187, ISSN 1537-0437.

Jiang, K.J., Jiao, H.C., Song, Z.G., Yuan, L., Zhao, J.P. & Lin, H. (2008). Corticosterone administration and dietary glucose supplementation enhance fat accumulation in broiler chickens. *British Poultry Science*, Vol. 49, No. 5, pp. 625-631, ISSN 0007-0437.

Johnson, B.E., Scanes, C.G., King, D.B. & Marsh, J.A. (1993). Effect of hypophysectomy and growth hormone on immune development in the domestic fowl. Developmental and Comparative Immunology, Vol. 17, No. 4, pp. 331-339, ISSN 0145-305X.

King, D.B. & Scanes, C.G. (1986). Effects of mammalian growth hormone and prolactin on the growth of hypophysectomized chickens. *Proceedings of the Society of Experimental Biology and Medicine*, Vol. 182, No. 2, pp. 201-207, ISSN 0037-9727.

King, D.L. and Hazelwood, R.L. 1976. Regulation of avian insulin secretion by isolated perfused chicken pancreas. *American Journal of Physiology*, Vol. 231, No. 6, pp. 1830-1839, ISSN 0363-6143.

Kobayashi, T., Iwai, H., Uchimoto, R., Ohta, M., Shiota, M. & Sugano, T. (1989). Gluconeogenesis in perfused livers from dexamethasone-treated chickens. *American Journal of Physiology*, Vol. 256, No. 4, pp. R907-R914, ISSN 0363-6143.

Langslow, D.R. & Hales, C.N. (1969). Lipolysis in chicken adipose tissue *in vitro*. *Journal of Endocrinology*, Vol. 43, No. 2, pp. 243-260, ISSN 0022-0795.

Langslow, D.R., Butler, E.J., Hales, C.N. & Pearson, A.W. (1970). The response of plasma insulin, glucose and non-esterified fatty acids to various hormones, nutrients and drugs in the domestic fowl. *Journal of Endocrinology*, Vol. 46, No. 2, pp. 243-260, ISSN 0022-0795.

Lazarus, D.D. & Scanes, C.G. (1988). Acute effects of hypophysectomy and administration of pancreatic and thyroid hormones on circulating concentrations of somatomedin-C in young chickens: relationship between growth hormone and somatomedin C. *Domestic Animal Endocrinology*, Vol. 5, No. 4, pp. 283-289, ISSN 0739-7240.

Leung, F.C. & Taylor, J.E. (1983). In vivo and in vitro stimulation of growth hormone release in chickens by synthetic human pancreatic growth hormone releasing factor (hpGRFs). *Endocrinology*, Vol. 113, No. 5, pp. 1913-1915, ISSN 0013-7227.

Lin, H., Sui, S.J., Jiao, H.C., Buyse, J. & Decuypere, E. (2006). Impaired development of broiler chickens by stress mimicked by corticosterone exposure. *Comparative Biochemistry and Physiology A Molecular and Integrative Physiology*, Vol. 143, No. 3, pp. 400-405, ISSN 1095-6433.

Lin, H., Sui, S.J., Jiao, H.C., Jiang, K.J.., Zhao, J.P. & Dong, H . (2007). Effects of diet and stress mimicked by corticosterone administration on early postmortem muscle metabolism of broiler chickens. *Poultry Science*, Vol. 86, No. 3, pp. 545-554, ISSN 1537-0437.

Lin, H., Gao, J., Song, Z.G. & Jiao, H.C. (2009). Corticosterone administration induces oxidative injury in skeletal muscle of broiler chickens. *Poultry Science*, Vol. 88, No. 5, pp. 1044-1051, ISSN 1537-0437.

Marelli, S.P., Terova, G., Cozzi, M.C., Lasagna, E., Sarti, F.M. & Cavalchini, L.G . (2010). Gene expression of hepatic glucocorticoid receptor NR3C1 and correlation with plasmatic corticosterone in Italian chickens. *Animal Biotechnology*, Vol. 21, No. 2, pp. 140-148, ISSN: 1049-5398.

Marsh, J.A., Lauterio, T.J. & Scanes, C.G. (1984). Effects of triiodothyronine treatments on body and organ growth and development of immune function in dwarf chickens. *Proceedings of the Society of Experimental Biology and Medicine*, Vol. 117, No.1, pp. 82-91, ISSN 0037-9727.

McGuinness, M.C. & Cogburn, L.A. (1991). Response of young broiler chickens to chronic injection of recombinant-derived human insulin-like growth factor-I. *Domestic Animal Endocrinology*, Vol. 8, No. 4, pp. 611-620, ISSN 0739-7240.

McMurtry, J.P., Tsark, W., Cognurn, L., Rosebrough, R. & Brocht, D. (1996). Metabolic responses of the turkey hen (Meleagris gallopavo) to an intravenous injection of chicken or porcine glucagon. *Comparative Biochemistry and Physiology C Pharmacology, Toxicology and Endocrinology*, Vol. 114, No. 2, pp. 159-163, ISSN 1095-6433.

Nakagawa-Mizuyachi, K., Takahashi, T. & Kawashima, M. (2009). Calcitonin directly increases adrenocorticotropic hormone-stimulated corticosterone production in the hen adrenal gland. *Poultry Science*, Vol. 88, No. 10, pp. 2199-2205, ISSN 1537-0437.

Perler F., Efstratiadis A., Lomedico P., Gilbert W., Kolodner R. & Dodgson J.B. (1980). The evolution of genes: the chicken preproinsulin gene. *Cell*, Vol. 20, No.2, pp. 555-566, ISSN: 0092-8674.

Porter, T.E., Dean, C.E., Piper, M.M., Medvedev, K.L., Ghavam, S. & Sandor, J. (2001). Somatotroph recruitment by glucocorticoids involves induction of growth hormone gene expression and secretagogue responsiveness. *Journal of Endocrinology*, Vol. 169, No. 3, pp. 499-509, ISSN 0022-0795.

Porter, T.E., Ghavam, S., Muchow, M., Bossis, I. & Ellestad, L. (2007). Cloning of partial cDNAs for the chicken glucocorticoid and mineralocorticoid receptors and characterization of mRNA levels in the anterior pituitary gland during chick embryonic development. *Domestic Animal Endocrinology*, Vol. 33, No. 2, pp. 226-239, ISSN 0739-7240.

Proszkowiec-Weglarz, M. & Porter, T.E. (2010). Functional characterization of chicken glucocorticoid and mineralocorticoid receptors. *American Journal of Physiology Regulatory Integrative Comparative Physiology*, Vol. 298, No. 5, pp. R1257-1268, ISSN 0363-6143.

Proudman, J.A., McGuinness, M.C., Krishnan, K.A. & Cogburn, L.A. (1994). Endocrine and metabolic responses of intact and hypophysectomized turkey poults given a daily injection of chicken growth hormone. *Comparative Biochemistry and Physiology C Pharmacology, Toxicology and Endocrinology*, Vol. 109, No. 1, pp. 47-56, ISSN 1095-6433.

Radecki, S.V., Deaver D.R. & Scanes, C.G. (1994). Triiodothyronine reduces growth hormone secretion and pituitary growth hormone mRNA in the chicken, *in vivo* and *in vitro*. *Proceedings of the Society of Experimental Biology and Medicine*, Vol. 205, No. 4, pp. 340-346, ISSN 0037-9727.

Rosebrough, R.W. & McMurtry, J.P. (2003). Methimazole and thyroid hormone replacement in broilers. *Domestic Animal Endocrinology*, Vol. 24, No. 3, pp. 231-242, ISSN 0739-7240.

Rosebrough, R.W., McMurtry, J.P. & Vasilatos-Younken, R. (1991). Effect of pulsatile or continuous administration of pituitary-derived chicken growth hormone (p-cGH) on lipid metabolism in broiler pullets. *Comparative Biochemistry and Physiology A Comparative Physiology*, Vol. 99, No. 1-2, pp. 207-214, ISSN 1095-6433.

Rozenboim, I., Robinzon, B., Arnon, E. & Snapir, N. (1989). Effect of embryonic and neonatal administration of tamoxifen on adiposity in the broiler chicken. *British Poultry Science*, Vol. 30, No. 3, pp. 607-612, ISSN 0007-1668.

Rozenboim, I., Robinzon, B., Ron, B., Arnon, E. & Snapir, N. (1990) The response of broilers' adiposity to testosterone after embryonic exposure to androgen and tamoxifen. *British Poultry Science*, Vol. 31, No. 3, pp. 645-650, ISSN 0007-1668.

Scanes, C. G. (2008). Perspectives on Analytical Techniques and Standardization. *Poultry Science*, Vol. 87, No. 11, pp. 2175-2177, ISSN 1537-0437.

Scanes, C.G. (2009) Perspectives on the endocrinology of poultry growth and metabolism. *General and Comparative Endocrinology*, Vol. 163, No. 1-2, pp. 24-32, ISSN 0016-6480.

Scanes, C.G. (2011). *Fundamentals of Animal Science*. Delmar Cengage, ISBN-10: 1428361278, Clifton Park, NY.

Scanes, C.G., Marsh, J., Decuypere, E. & Rudas, P. (1983). Abnormalities in the plasma concentration of thyroxine, triiodothyronine and growth hormone in sex-linked dwarf and autosomal dwarf white leghorn domestic fowl (*Gallus domesticus*). *Journal of Endocrinology*, Vol. 97, No. 1, pp. 127-135, ISSN 0022-0795.

Scanes, C.G., Duyka, D.R., Lauterio, T.J., Bowen, S.J., Huybrechts, L.M., Bacon, W.L. & King, D.B. (1986). Effect of chicken growth hormone, triiodothyronine and hypophysectomy in growing domestic fowl. *Growth*, Vol. 50, No. 1, 12-31, ISSN 1440-169X.

Scanes, C.G., Proudman, J.A. & Radecki, S.V. (1999). Influence of Continuous Growth Hormone or Insulin-Like Growth Factor I Administration in Adult Female Chickens. *General and Comparative Endocrinology*, Vol. 114, No. 3, pp. 315-323, ISSN 0016-6480.

Scanes, C.G., Brant, G. & Ensminger, M.E. (2004). *Poultry Science*. ISBN 0-13-113375-6. Pearson Prentice, Upper Saddle River, NJ.

Scanes, C. G., Glavaski-Joksimovic, A., Johannsen, S. A., Jeftinija, S. & Anderson, L.L. (2007). Subpopulations of Somatotropes with Differing Intracellular Calcium Concentration Responses to Secretagogues. *Neuroendocrinology*, Vol. 85, No. 4, pp. 221-231, ISSN 0028-3835

Snapir, N., Robinzon, B. & Shalita, B. (1983). The involvement of gonads and gonadal steroids in the regulation of food intake, body weight and adiposity in the white Leghorn cock. Pharmacology Biochemistry and Behavior, Vol. 19, No. 4, pp. 617-624, ISSN: 0091-3057.

Shini, S., Kaiser, P., Shini, A. & Bryden, W.L. (2008). Biological response of chickens (Gallus gallus domesticus) induced by corticosterone and a bacterial endotoxin. *Comparative Biochemistry and Physiology B Biochemistry and Molecular Biology*, Vol.149, No. 2, pp. 324-333, ISSN 1095-6433.

Shini, S., Shini, A. & Huff, G.R. (2009). Effects of chronic and repeated corticosterone administration in rearing chickens on physiology, the onset of lay and egg production of hens. Physiology & Behavior, Vol. 98, No. 1-2, pp. 73-77, ISSN: 0031-9384.

Shini, S., Shini, A. & Kaiser, P. (2010). Cytokine and chemokine gene expression profiles in heterophils from chickens treated with corticosterone. *Stress*, Vol. 13, No. 3, pp. 185-194, ISSN 1025-3890.

Simon, J., Derouet, M. & Gespach, C. (2000). An anti-insulin serum, but not a glucagon antagonist, alters glycemia in fed chickens. Hormone and metabolic research, Vol. 32, No. 4, pp. 139-141,ISSN:0018-5043.

Sitbon, G. & Mialhe, P. (1978). Pancreatic hormones and plasma glucose: regulation mechanism in the goose under physiological conditions; 3. Inhibitory effects of insulin on glucagons secretion. *Hormones and Metabolic Research*, Vol. 10, No. 6, pp. 473-477, *ISSN* 0018-5043.

Song, Z., Zhang, X., Zhu, L., Jiao, H. & Lin, H. (2011). Dexamethasone Alters the Expression of Genes Related to the Growth of Skeletal Muscle in Chickens (Gallus gallus domesticus). *Journal of Molecular Endocrinology* Feb 16. [Epub ahead of print]

Strosser, M., Chen, T.L., Harvey, S. & Mialhe, P. (1980). Somatostatin stimulates glucagons secretion in ducks. *Diabetologia*, Vol. 18, No. 4, pp. 319-322. *ISSN* 0012-186X.

Sugano, T., Shiota, M., Khono, H. & Shimada, M. (1982). Stimulation of gluconeogenesis by glucagon and norepinephrine in the perfused chicken liver. Journal of Biochemestry, Vol. 92, No. 1, pp. 111-120, ISSN 0021-924X.

Takahashi, N., Shinki, T., Abe, E., Horiuchi, N., Yamaguchi, A., Yoshiki, S. & Suda, T. (1983). The role of vitamin D in the medullary bone formation in egg-laying Japanese quail and in immature male chicks treated with sex hormones. Calcified Tissue International, Vol. 35, No. 4-5, pp. 465-471, ISSN: 0171-967X

Tixier-Boichard, M., Huybrechts, L.M., Decuypere, E., Kühn, E.R., Monvoisin, J.L., Coquerelle, G., Charrier, J. & Simon, J. (1992). Effects of insulin-like growth factor-I (IGF-I) infusion and dietary tri-iodothyronine (T3) supplementation on growth, body composition and plasma hormone levels in sex-linked dwarf mutant and normal chickens. *Journal of Endocrinology,* Vol.133, No. 1, pp. 101-110, ISSN 0022-0795.

Thomas-Delloye, V., Marmonier, F., Duchamp, C., Pichon-Georges, B., Lachuer, J., Barré, H. and Crouzoulon, G. 1999. Biochemical and functional evidences for a GLUT-4 homologous protein in avian skeletal muscle. *Journal of Physiology,* Vol. 277, No. 6, pp. R1733-R1740, ISSN 0363-6143.

Tomas, F.M., Pym, R.A., McMurtry, J.P. & Francis, G.L. (1998). Insulin-like growth factor (IGF)-I but not IGF-II promotes lean growth and feed efficiency in broiler chickens. *General and Comparative Endocrinology,* Vol. 110, No. 3, pp. 262-275, ISSN 0016-6480.

Tsukada, A., Ohkubo, T., Sakaguchi, K., Tanaka, M., Nakashima, K., Hayashida, Y., Wakita, M. & Hoshino, S. (1998). Thyroid hormones are involved in insulin-like growth factor-I (IGF-I) production by stimulating hepatic growth hormone receptor (GHR) gene expression in the chicken. Growth Hormone & IGF Research, Vol. 8, No. 3, pp. 235-242, ISSN: 1096-6374.

Vasilatos-Younken, R., Cravener, T.L., Cogburn, L.A., Mast, M.G. & Wellenreiter, R.H. (1988). Effect of pattern of administration on the response to exogenous pituitary-derived chicken growth hormone by broiler-strain pullets. *General and Comparative Endocrinology,* Vol. 71, No. 2, pp. 268-283, ISSN 0016-6480.

Vasilatos-Younken, R. (1986). Age-related changes in tissue metabolic rates and sensitivity to insulin in the chicken. *Poultry Science,* Vol. 65, No. 7, pp.1391-1399, ISSN 0016-6480.

Wilson, S.B., Back, D.W., Morris, S.M., Swierczynski, J. & Goodridge, A.G. (1986). Hormonal regulation of lipogenic enzymes in chick embryo hepatocytes in culture. Expression of the fatty acid synthase gene is regulated at both translational and pretranslational steps. Journal of Biological Chemistry, Vol. 261, No. 32, pp. 15179-15182, ISSN 0021-9258.

Yuan, L., Lin, H., Jiang, K.J., Jiao, H.C. & Song, Z.G. (2008). Corticosterone administration and high-energy feed results in enhanced fat accumulation and insulin resistance in broiler chickens. *British Poultry Science*, Vol. 49, No. 4, pp. 487-495, ISSN 0007-1668.

Zhao, J.P., Lin, H., Jiao, H.C. & Song, Z.G. (2009). Corticosterone suppresses insulin- and NO-stimulated muscle glucose uptake in broiler chickens (*Gallus gallus domesticus*). *Comparative Biochemistry and Physiology C Pharmacology, Toxicology and Endocrinology*, Vol. 149, No. 3, pp. 448-454, ISSN 1095-6433.

9

Generation of Insulin Producing Cells for the Treatment of Diabetes

Guo Cai Huang and Min Zhao
Department of Diabetes and Endocrinology,
King's College London School of Medicine, London
Great Britain

1. Introduction

The are approx. 177 million people suffering from diabetes worldwide and this number will be doubled by 2030. Patients with type 1 diabetes require multiple injections of insulin daily with doses careful adjusted on carbohydrate intake, level of activity and stress. Often there is a mismatch between insulin requirements and the calculated dose, resulting in hyper or hypo-glycaemia. Between 20-30% of patients however suffer from recurrent hypoglycaemia, which may require third party help (Geddes et al. 2008). Islet transplantation has been a promising therapy since the "Edmonton protocol" was published in 2000 (Shapiro et al. 2000). However, numbers of transplants remain low for a variety of reasons (Shapiro et al. 2006). One major hurdle to more widespread provision of this treatment remains a shortage of supply of donor organs, with only 25-30% of isolations resulting in islets of sufficient quantity and quality to be used in clinical transplantation, indicating a huge waste of valuable resources (Nano et al. 2005). Studies using animal models have found the evidences of neogenisis of beta cells under non-physiological condition as well the limited proliferation capacity of beta cells. Unfortunately, human beings cannot be manipulated to generate insulin-producing cells. There are increasing evidence suggested that glucose response insulin-producing cells could be generated in large quantity for human use. The following are a few possible aspects that can be explored for this purpose.

1.1 Beta cell replication and regeneration

There are substantial evidences suggesting that the adult pancreas can generate new β-cells in response to pancreatic damage or increased demand for insulin (Wang et al., 1995; Bonner-Weir et al., 1993; Guz et al., 2001). The source of new β-cells is thought to be the replication of existing β-cells under normal growth condition (Dor et al., 2004). However, the capacity of mature β-cells to proliferation and then re-differentiate back into β-cells has not been demonstrated *in vitro* and it still remains a challenge. In addition to the replication, there are mounting evidences indicated that regeneration of beta cells also contribute significantly to the new beta cells when pancreas is under non-physiological conditions such as partial pancreas duct ligation (Wang et al., 1995) or partial pancreatectomy (Finegood et al., 1999). However, such mechanisms are believed to have little implication to diabetes patients, as it is not possible to mimic the situations in animals to humans. Furthermore, even though there is regeneration of beta cells; the patients need immunosuppressive drugs to control the self-destruction of beta cells by autoimmune mechanisms. In addition to the beta cell proliferation, whether there are other cell sources for the beta cell neogenesis is not clear. It has been shown that human adult pancreases contain cells expressing Oct4 and Sox2 proteins (Zhao et al., 2007). The expression of Oct4 and Sox2 is thought to be related to the stemness of stem cells in human pancreas. The location of these cells in the small ducts is interesting (Fig 1) as it reflects the development of pancreas. Whether these cells are a part of the undifferentiated stem cells retained in ducts during the formation of pancreas and are the sources of new beta cells in adulthood remains unknown to us. The question is whether these cells are truly functional adult stem cells? If they are, how these cells contribute to the balance of beta cell number warrants further investigations. Insulin positive cells were indeed observed in the pancreas ducts (Bonner-Weir et al., 1993; Dudek et al., 1991; Pour 1994; Bouwens and Pipeleers 1998; li et al., 2010) and the findings that cells derived from rodent and human islets were multiple potency (Smukler et al., 2011) have further confirmed the possibility of presence of stem cells in adult pancreas. For this reason, human pancreatic ducts have been the target material for insulin-producing cells (Gmyr et al., 2004). Unfortunately the experiment protocol seemed not be optimal enough and generating insulin-producing cells from these duct cells is remaining illusive. Further investigation is required to determine whether there would be possible means to increase beta cells from the stem cells to treat diabetes in newly diagnosed diabetes patients together with immune modulation drugs.

1.2 Immunosuppression approach

When the patient is newly diaganisd as type 1 diabetes, there is often associated with a "honey-noon" phenominon. It is thought that there are new beta cells generated during this transient phase of disease. Earlier clinical trial using immunosuppressive drugs to inhibit the T cells did show the improvement in insulin secretion but at the price of worsening renal functions (Mirouze et al., 1986; Mandrup-Poulsen et al., 1990). These are believed to be the side effects of the immunosuppressive drugs to the kidneys while modulating the autoimmunity to protect beta cells. In 1990s, the most widely used drugs is cyclosporine, which is known to be toxic to beta cells (Hahn et al., 1986), will also damage the beta cells overtime. The trials with less cell toxic drugs such as anti-CD3 or anti-CD4 antibodies also showed some benefits in altering the disease course (Chatenoud et al., 1993; Phillips et al., 2000; Herold et al., 2002) but the hope of increasing new beta cells suficient to cure the disease still meets difficulty (Keymeulen et al., 2005). It is believed that the time to initiate such treatment is crucial as the ability to increase new beta cells is limited. This treatment could be used to prevent type 1 diabetes in risk population when there is still a surficient number of beta cells and with potential renewing beta cells, if such a population is identified.

1.3 Pancreas organ transplantation vs. islet cell transplantation

Human pancreas transplantation has been the main option for replacing the lost beta cells in type 1 diabetes patients since 1960s (Kelly et al., 1967; Hermon-Taylor 1970). Even now it is still the best option to treat diabetes. The insulin independency following pancreas organ transplantation is around 70-90% when the surgical procedures are successful. However, it is a major surgical procedure and is normally reserved for kidney and pancreas

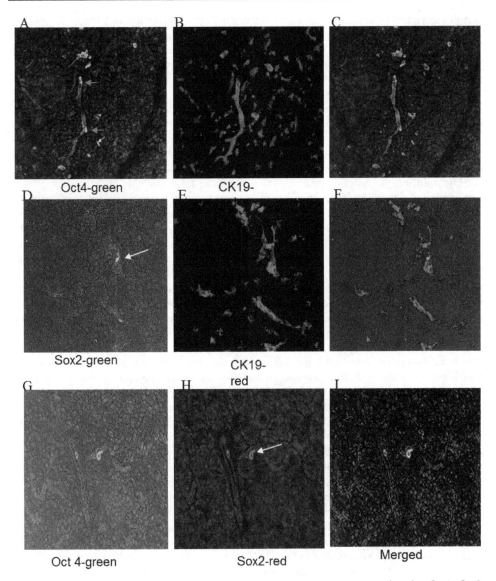

Typical immunohistochemical staining images of human pancreas sections for the Oct4, Sox2 expressing cells and their localization relevant to CK19+ve cells. Panel A and G show Oct4+ve cells (green) within the ductal structures and their surrounding area in a scattering pattern. Majority Oct4+ve cells were shown cytopalsmic staining with only small number cells shown nuclei staining (arrowed). B and E show the CK19+ve duct cells (red) and C is the merged of A and B. Panel D (green) and H (red) show Sox2 positive cells. F is the merge of D and E. Panel I is the merged of G (Oct4+ve, Green) and H (Sox2+ve Cells, Red), showing the colocalization of Oct4 and Sox2 positive cells.

Fig. 1. Immunohistochemical statining of the Oct-4 and Sox2 cells in human adult pancreas sections

simultaneous transplantations just because it is a big operation procedure. Most old patients are not suitable for this approach as they are unable to tolerate the surgical procedures. The operation itself is associated with 10% mortality and mobility; often the patients need a second or third operation to correct the problem of exocrine enzyme leakage.

Human islet transplantation provides an alternative mean to restore the lost beta cells and it become a realistic option for a group of type 1 diabetes patients with bristle diabetes condition, especially for the group of patients with hypoglycaemia unawareness (Shapiro et al. 2000). The advantage for this approach is that it is a minor and less invasive procedure and a more safe approach for the replacement of lost beta cells. The disadvantages are that human pancreas is to be digested with a blend of collagenases and specialized proteases and human islets are purified from the exocrine tissues (Ricordi et al., 1989). Some islets are damaged during the isolation procedures. In addition, approximately 20-50% islets are lost under current density centrifugation purification techniques, which is based on the density differential between endocrine cells and exocrine cells. Therefore, it needs 2-3 pancreases to provide enough islet cell mass (~10,000 Islet IEQ/kg body weight) for one recipient. The human islets are then transplanted into the patient's liver via port vein, where the islets will set down in liver. The islets will function in the higher insulin concentration environment as comparison with those within pancreas. Therefore, this will require islets to work harder and lead to exhaustion of islets themselves. As the islets are digested away from the exocrine tissues, they are also cut away from the vascular system, which provides islets with essential nutrients, oxygen and neuron-regulating molecules and need to be revisualization following transplant. During the period of avascular state, the islets are very vulnerable to any attack, such as inflammatory factors and the cytotoxicity of the immunosuppressive drugs, as the cells take in nutrients and oxygen through passive perfusion, which is very inefficient. Since the body immune system destroys tissues it recognises as "foreign" and the nature of autoimmune disease in the patients, immunosuppressive drugs are given to the patients before, during and after transplant to protect the grafts from allo-rejection and the reoccurrence of autoimmunity. The immune regulation medication has several drawbacks currently. First, the immunosuppressive drugs have significant side effects and some patients cannot tolerate one or another immunosuppressive regimens. The patients have to take the drugs life long in order to protect the islet grafts and to prevent from getting sensitisation against donor tissues. There would be some implications for the risk of tumour generation, as the recipients may not have the full immune capacity to fight tumour cells although there is no such report yet. For the reason of toxicity of the immunosuppressive drugs, this approach is only suitable for a small group of patients. It is not yet suitable for young children simply it is not worthy taking immunosuppressive drugs. Secondly, the drugs also show some degrees of toxicity to beta cells and the drugs will reduce the islet cell mass overtime. The long-term prospect of islet transplantation currently is not yet satisfactory, with only ~13% of transplant patients remaining insulin independence for >5 years, although most patients still have endogenous C-peptide product and benefit from the better control of their blood glucose (Ryan et al., 2005). Thirdly, as to the drawback mentioned above, it requires 2-3 donor organs to generate enough islet cell mass to reach to >10,000 islet IEQ/kg body weight of the recipient. The large islet IEQ is needed because some islets will not survive during the avascular state, which deprive themselves of essential nutrients and oxygen, and the toxicity of immune modulation agents. This will obviously worsen the situation on the already limited supply of donor organs. Fourthly, the reoccurrence autoimmune attack on the grafts developed overtime, which seemed to be able to escape the current immunosuppressive regimens applied. The future work should concentrate on protecting islets during and post-transplantation and development of less toxic immune suppression drugs.

Despite the drawback mentioned above, for patients with bristle diabetic conditions and patients with pancreatectomy (due to prolonged pancreatitis), the beta cell replacement still remains the best option. To make this beta cell replacement as a wider applicable approach for the treatment of diabetes patients, the limitation of glucose responsive insulin-producing cells is the key obstacle and must be addressed. For patients with type 2 diabetes, current islet cell transplantation is insufficient as the demand for insulin-producing cells for these patients is far greater than type 1 diabetes patients. However, this approach could be applied to patients with type 2 diabetes, if the cell source of insulin surrogates is unlimited. For the later, there is only one need, that is, to prevent the allo-graft rejection.

2. Generation of glucose responsive insulin-producing cells

Many type of cells have been used to generate glucose responsive insulin-producing cells with limited success. These include the differentiation of embryonic and adult stem cells and transdifferentiation from other types of cells into insulin producing cells (Fujikawa et al., 2005; Zhao et al., 2005 and 2008; Kroon et al., 2008; Boyd et al., 2009; Tateishi et al., 2008; Zhou et al., 2008; Gabr et al., 2008; Zhang et al., 2009; Cai et al., 2010). However, the success has been limited to small animal models. The focus of this chapter is to briefly discuss the potentiality involved in our laboratories.

2.1 Islet cells replication *in vitro*

Islets of Langerhans are the endocrine mini-organs consisted of 4 major different endocrine cells: α-cells controlling the release of glucagon; β-cells for insulin, δ-cells for somatostatin and the pp cells-polypeptide. These 4 types of endocrine cells work together in a complex interplay in the maintaining of homeostasis of blood glucose level. Islet cells need to stay together as a cluster to function better as indicated by the finding that single Min 6 (mouse beta cell line) cells do not express and secret insulin as well as those when the Min 6 cells are forming as a cluster-called pseudoislets (Hauge-Evans et al., 1999). Human islets cultured in monolayer tend to lose the capacity gradually to express insulin within 5 weeks (Fig.2). Human islet cells cultured in 3-dimension seemed to be able to retain beta cell phenotype. However cells, particularly those at the centre of the clusters, will die due to necrosis if the cells cultured as 3-dimensional manner for too long. This is because that cells located in the centre of the 3-dimension will depend on the perfusion of nutrients and oxygen, which is very insufficient. We therefore developed a method to culture the cells in a rotation manner between monolayer culture (2-dimension) and cluster culture (3-dimension), the cells have acquired the survive signal through the 2-dimensional culture and can also maintain the capacity to express insulin through the 3-dimensional culture. The cells can maintain this capacity to express insulin and respond to glucose challenge for >4 months *in vitro*. When the cells were transplanted into SCID (an immune deficient mouse) mice, rendered diabetes by the injection of straptozotosin (STZ), they were able to correct the hyperglycaemia and maintaining the homeostasis of blood glucose (Fig. 3; Zhao et al., 2002). The beauty of this model is to provide a prototype model to analyse beta cell differentiation. The ability of beta cells to proliferate *in vitro* has been demonstrated in many studies (Beattie et al., 1999; 2000

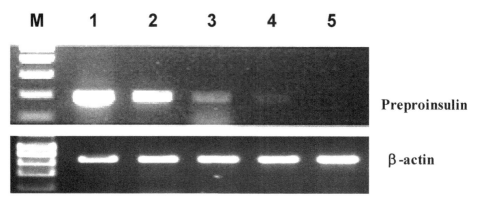

Preproinsulin

β-actin

Semi-quantitative RT- PCR analysis. 5 weeks continuously monolayer cultured human islet cells were induced to express insulin. Total RNA were isolated from each different condition. cDNA derived from 4ng of total RNA were used to amplify preproinsulin and actin. 5 = 5weeks monolayer cultured human islet cells.

Fig. 2. Analyses the expression of insulin in continual monolayer culture

and 2002; Halvorsen et al., 2000; Gershengorn et al., 2004; Lechner et al., 2005; Ouziel-Yahalom et al., 2006;) and was directly confirmed in a study with GFP labelled beta cells using a lentinvirus system (Russ et al., 2008). However, the purpose of *ex vivo* expansion of human islets is to increase the glucose responsive insulin-producing cells for research and eventually for transplantation to treat diabetes. Unfortunately, making the proliferated insulin-producing cells to express insulin again in a glucose responsive manner is still a big challenge to us. Using a lentinvirus labelling system developed by Russ and colleagues, we were able to show that a small percentage of beta cells (GFP expressing cells) were found to be positive for insulin and Ki67--a proliferation marker *in vitro* (Fig. 4; Zhao et al., unpublished). This result illustrated that beta cells have the potential to be expanded *ex vivo*. The question is how to make this more efficient to achieve large number of cells for the treat of diabetes patients.

2.2 Human exocrine cells

From the development point of view, exocrine cells are the excellent candidate materials for insulin-producing cells as they share the same origin with the pancreatic endocrine cells (Slack 1995). Mouse exocrine cells have shown the flexibility to be converted into insulin-producing cells following chemical treatment (Lardon at al., 2004; Baeyens et al., 2005; Zhou et al., 2008). Therefore, there is good reason to believe that it is possible to convert human exocrine cells into endocrine cells. In terms of cell number, exocrine cells consist of 90% pancreatic cells with approximate 40-50 folds of their endocrine cell count apart, which consists of less than ~2% of total pancreatic cells. Secondly, it is already available. Following human islet isolation, the exocrine cells will be the waste material and are discarded at end. Thirdly, following dedifferentiation there is no obvious difference between the two types of cells. Both cells began to express CK19—a ductal cell marker. This is interesting because that both types of cells are derived from ductal cells during pancreas development (Slack 1995). Whether to differentiate into exocrine cells or into endocrine cells is under the complex interplays of complex genes at that stage. Gene Ptf1a may play a big role in the

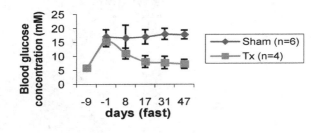

B

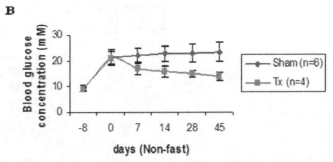

Blood glucose level (mM) of the STZ induced diabetic SCID mice before and after transplantation of long term cultured islets or sham control. Time of transplantation and sham was assigned as 0 day (d) and the time before surgery was indicated as –d. A shows the overnight fasting blood glucose level, solid square = islet cell transplanted (Tx), and the solid diamond shape = sham control. B shows the non-fasting blood glucose levels, solid square = islet cell transplanted (Tx), and solid diamond shape = sham control. The decrease in blood glucose levels was significant in both fasting and non-fasting with student t pair-test at P<0.023 and P<0.002 respectively. The difference in blood glucose levels between transplantation and sham groups was also significant (P<0.02and 0.023 respectively).

Fig. 3. Analyses of the blood glucose levels in mice transplanted with long term cultured human islet cells

determination of cells to exocrine cell fate (Dong et al., 2008). The mechanism of how exocrine cells being converted into endocrine cells is not clear and under our experimental conditions, it requires the gene products from beta cells and the right differentiation environments. Under the Pdx-1 gene influence, exocrine cells express some beta cell phenotype marker following differentiation induction with a cocktail of differentiation inducers (GLP-1, activin A, betacellulin, nicotinamide and glucose, Zhao et al., 2005) and expressed low level of insulin (Fig. 5) *in vitro*. The time to introduce Pdx-1 is seemed to be critical, although we did not have biomarkers to match this window exactly for the gene induction. We speculated that a short window existed during the dedifferentiation of exocrine cells. During which, exocrine cells would be more ready to be induced to express beta cell markers. The cells showed a glucose response *in vitro* when challenged with glucose. But the response was not typical as the background secretion is too high and the challenge secretion is too low in comparison with islet cells, suggesting the insulin-producing cells were immature. As predicted, these cells matured further following transplant in SCID mice, rendered diabetes with the injection of STZ solution. This approach is sufficient to work in small laboratory animals with ~40% mice recovered from the mild

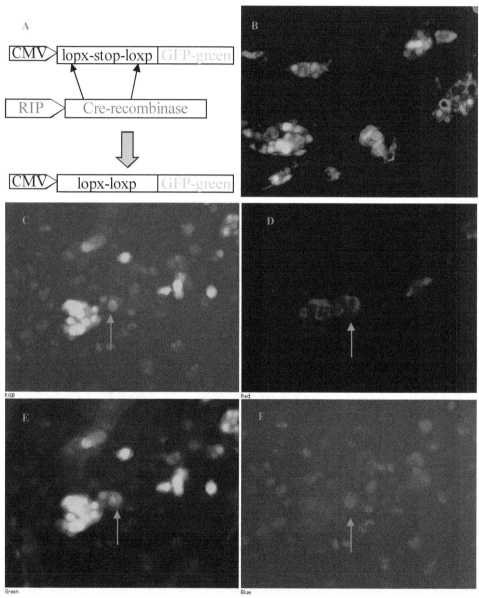

Genomic labelling of human beta cells and differentiation induction assessment. Panel A: the methed used in the labelling of human beta cells (Russ et al., 2008). Panel B: Control experiment of differentiation induction in the labelling beta cells. Beta cells were labelled as green and the cells were staining for insulin (Red). Panel D, E, F were images catched for red (insulin, D), green (beta cells, E) and blue (for Ki67 protein F). Panel C was the merged images of D, E, F. The proliferated beta cell was indicated by the arrow.

Fig. 4. Analyses the potential of proliferated adult human beta cells to reexpress insulin

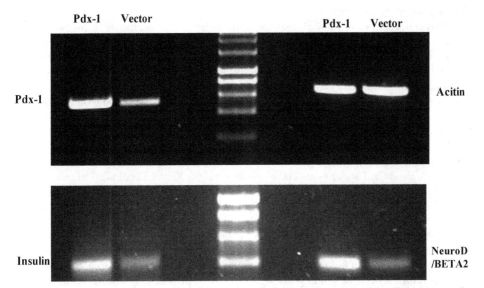

The dedifferentiated human pancreatic exocrine cells expressed insulin and NeuroD1/Beta 2 genes after transfection with Pdx-1 gene and differentiation induction, analysed by semi-quantitative RT-PCR.

Fig. 5. Expression of beta cell phenotype genes in manipulated human non-endocrine pancreatic cells in vitro

diabetes. The grafts showed that glucagon and somatostatin were also expressed in addition to the insulin (Fig.6), indicating that exocrine cells can be converted into whole pancreatic endocrine cells, not just insulin producing cells. Further works are required to explore the full potential of exocrine cells in order to create enough insulin producing materials for the treatment of diabetes.

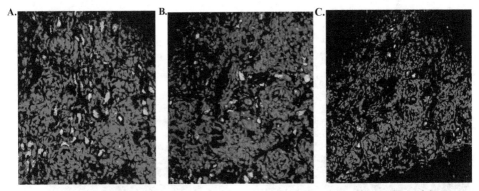

Immunohistochemical staining of the grafts (visulised by confocal microscope) for markers of the pancreatic endocrine cells. Insulin (A, 15±6.7%), Glucagon (B, 8±2.3%) and Somatostatin (C, 3±1.85%) positive cells are shown in green (FITC) and nuclei are stained with propidium iodide (red). Original amplification x40

Fig. 6. The expression of pancreatic endocrine cell hormones in the transdifferentiated cells.

2.3 Mesenchymal stem cell

Mesenchymal stem cells (MSCs) are the nonhematopoietic multipotent progenitor cells found in various adult tissues. Bone marrow derived MSC cells are those cells can adhere to plastic culture flask and proliferate *in vitro* (Kadiyala et al., 1997). The cells have the potential to be expanded *in vitro* in large quantity. MSC under specific differentiation environments can differentiate into cells with phenotypes of many specific tissues, such as bone, adipose and neurons (Pittenger et al., 1999; Deans and Moseley 2000; Deng et al., 2006; Gabr et al., 2008). MSC has the capacity to modulate host immune cells (see review papers in Bunnell et al., 2011) and express molecule help themselves evade the immune attack (El Haddad et al., 2011). The ability of MSC to become insulin-producing cells has been in debates and been controversy (Lechner et al., 2004; Taneera et al., 2006; Butle et al., 2007; Moriscot et al., 2005; Timper et al., 2006; Lee et al., 2006; Karnieli et al., 2007; Lavazais et al., 2007; Hasegawa et al., 2007; Denner et al., 2007). Human bone marrow MSC express low level of Oct4 and Sox2 as well Pdx-1 — an important gene involve in the development of beta cells and the maintaining of beta cell phenotype in adult, indicative that these cells could be differentiated into glucose responsive insulin- producing cells. Under the influence of the gene products of Pdx-1, NeuroD1/BETA2 and Ngn3, the MSC express insulin gene *in vitro* following differentiation induction with a cocktail of differentiation inducers (GLP-1, activin A, betacellulin, nicotinamide and glucose). The cells seemed lacking insulin storage capacity and secreted insulin as it was synthesised. Therefore these cells were not glucose responsive *in vitro*. Following transplantation into SCID diabetes mice, the cells were able to mature further and expressed most beta cell phenotype gene markers, such as Glut-2 and Kir6.2 (Fig. 7A) and insulin processing enzymes, but the cells did not express Sur1 gene and therefore did not have a functional K-ATP channel. Interestingly the cells also expressed glucagon gene, indicating that some cells also differentiated into α-cells (Fig.7B) in addition to insulin producing cells. Nevertheless, the hyperglycaemia in the transplanted mice was corrected despite that the transplanted mice had some impairment in glucose tolerant in comparison with mice transplanted with human islets (Fig. 8 and Zhao et al., 2008). These

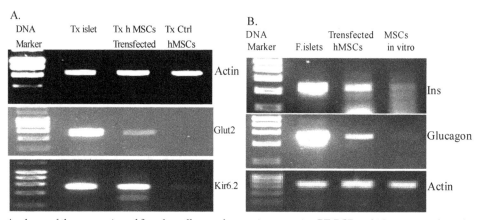

Analyses of the expression of β and α cell genes by semi-quatatative RT-PCR on kidneys transplanted with the cells.

Fig. 7. Gene expression analyses on the transplanted kidneys by semi-quatative RT-PCR

data suggested that the MSC achieve partial glucose responsiveness through non-ATP K channel mechanism. The MSC did not form any teratoma structures *in vivo*; making it an idea candidate to be beta cell surrogates for the treatment of diabetes.

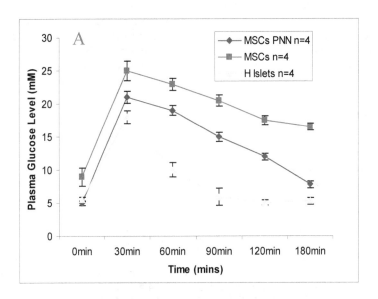

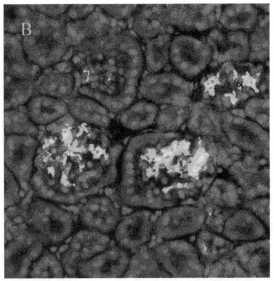

Panel A. Mice transplanted wtih the Pdx-1, Ngn3 and euroD1/Beta2 genes shows response to glucose challenge During a glucose tolerlant test. Panel B shows the manipulated human MSC expressing insulin (green fluorescence) in diabetic mice.

Fig. 8. Functional analyses in mice transplanted with human MSC cells

3. Conclusion and future direction of investigation

There are mounting evidences including our own data described above suggested that insulin-producing cells can be generated from many cells through the differentiation of stem cells (embryonic stem cells to adult stem cells) or via the transdifferentiation mechanisms. However, there are challenges ahead. The most urgent tasks are 1) to optimise the differentiation protocols to make them more efficiency by optimising the differentiation inducers and the extracellular environments; 2) to identify the molecular mechanisms associated with the differentiation to allow the translation of bench discovery to bedside treatments; 3) to enhance the efficacy to increase the cell mass for human usage.

4. References

Baeyens L. De Breuck S.. Lardon J... Mfopou J. K.Rooman I. Bouwens L. (2005) In vitro generation of insulin-producing cells from adult exocrine pancreatic cells. Diabetologia 48: 49–57

Beattie GM, Itkin-Ansari P, Cirulli V, Leibowitz G, Lopez AD, Bossie S, Mally MI, Levine F, Hayek A (1999): Sustained proliferation of PDX-1_ cells derived from human islets. *Diabetes* 48:1013–1019

Beattie GM, Leibowitz G, Lopez AD, Levine F, Hayek A (2000): Protection from cell death in cultured human fetal pancreatic cells. *Cell Transplant*9:431– 438,

Beattie GM, Montgomery AM, Lopez AD, Hao E, Perez B, Just ML, Lakey JR, Hart ME, Hayek A (2002): A novel approach to increase human islet cell mass while preserving _-cell function. *Diabetes* 51:3435–3439

Bonner-Weir S, Baxter LA, Schuppin GT, Smith FE (1993) A second pathway for regeneration of adult exocrine and endocrine pancreas. A possible recapitulation of embryonic development. Diabetes. 42:1715-20

Bouwens, L., and Pipeleers, D.G. (1998) Extra-insular beta-cells associated with ductules are frequent in adult human pancreas. Diabetologia, 41:629–633.

Boyd, A. S. & Wood, K. J (2009): Variation in MHC expression between undifferentiated mouse ES cells and ES cell-derived insulin-producing cell clusters. *Transplantation* 87, 1300–1304

Butler AE, Huang A, Rao PN, Bhushan A, Hogan WJ et al. (2007) Hematopoietic stem cells derived from adult donors are not a source of pancreatic beta-cells in adult nondiabetic humans. Diabetes. 56(7): 1810-6.

Bunnell BA, Betancourt AM, Sullivan DE. New concepts on the immune modulation mediated by mesenchymal stem cells. Stem Cell Res Ther. 2010 Nov 11;1(5):34.

Cai J, Yu C, Liu Y, Chen S, Guo Y, Yong J, Lu W, Ding M, Deng H (2009). Generation of homogeneous PDX1(+) pancreatic progenitors from human ES cell-derived endoderm cells. J Mol Cell Biol. 2010 Feb;2(1):50-60.

Chatenoud L, Thervet E, Primo J, Bach JF (1994): Anti-CD3 antibody induces long-term remission of overt autoimmunity in nonobese diabetic mice. *Proc Natl Acad Sci U S A* 91:123–127

Deans RJ, Moseley AB (2008). Mesenchymal stem cells: biology and potential clinical uses. Exp Hematol;28:875-884.

Deng J, Petersen BE, Steindler DA, Jorgensen ML, Laywell ED (2006). Mesenchymal stem cells spontaneously express neural proteins in culture and are neurogenic after transplantation. Stem Cells.24(4):1054-64.

Denner L, Bodenburg Y, Zhao JG, Howe M, Cappo J, Tilton RG, Copland JA, Forraz N, McGuckin C, Urban R. Stark (2007) Directed engineering of umbilical cord blood stem cells to produce C-peptide and insulin. Cell Prolif. 40(3):367-80.

Dong PD, Provost E, Leach SD, Stainier DY (2008). Graded levels of Ptf1a differentially regulate endocrine and exocrine fates in the developing pancreas. Genes Dev. 22(11):1445-50.

Dor Y, Brown J, Martinez OI, Melton DA (2004) Adult pancreatic beta-cells are formed by self-duplication rather than stem-cell differentiation. Nature. 429:41-6

Dudek, R.W., Lawrence, I.E., Hill, R.S., and Johnson, R.C. (1991) Induction of islet cytodifferentiation by fetal mesenchyme in adult pancreatic ductal epithelium. Diabetes, 40:1041-1048.

El Haddad N, Heathcote D, Moore R, Yang S, Azzi J, Mfarrej B, Atkinson M, Sayegh MH, Lee JS, Ashton-Rickardt PG, Abdi R (2011). Mesenchymal stem cells express serine protease inhibitor to evade the host immune response. Blood.117(4):1176-83.

Finegood DT, Weir GC, Bonner-Weir S (1999). Prior streptozotocin treatment does not inhibit pancreas regeneration after 90% pancreatectomy in rats. Am J Physiol. 276(5 Pt 1):E822-7.

Fujikawa T, Oh SH, Pi L, Hatch HM, Shupe T, Petersen BE (2005) Teratoma formation leads to failure of treatment for type I diabetes using embryonic stem cell-derived insulin-producing cells. Am J Pathol.166(6):1781-91.

Gabr, M. M., Sobh, M. M., Zakaria, M. M., Refaie, A. F. & Ghoneim, M. A (2008). Transplantation of insulin-producing clusters derived from adult bone marrow stem cells to treat diabetes in rats. *Exp. Clin. Transplant.* 6, 236–243

Geddes J, Schopman JE, Zammitt NN, Frier BM. (2008). "Prevalence of impaired awareness of hypoglycaemia in adults with Type 1 diabetes." Diabet.Med. 25(4): 501-504.

Gershengorn MC, Hardikar AA, Wei C, Geras-Raaka E, Marcus-Samuels B, Raaka BM (2004): Epithelial-to-mesenchymal transition generates proliferative human islet precursor cells. *Science* 306:2261–2264

Guz Y, Nasir I, Teitelman G (2001) Regeneration of pancreatic beta cells from intra-islet precursor cells in an experimental model of diabetes. Endocrinology 142: 4956-68

Gmyr V, Belaich S, Muharram G, Lukowiak B, Vandewalle B, Pattou F, Kerr-Conte (2004). Rapid purification of human ductal cells from human pancreatic fractions with surface antibody CA19-9. Biochem Biophys Res Commun. 320(1):27-33.

Hahn HJ, Laube F, Lucke S, Klöting I, Kohnert KD, Warzock R (1986). Toxic effects of cyclosporine on the endocrine pancreas of Wistar rats. Transplantation. 41(1):44-7.

Halvorsen TL, Beattie GM, Lopez AD, Hayek A, Levine F (2000): Accelerated telomere shortening and senescence in human pancreatic islet cells stimulated to divide in vitro. *J Endocrinol* 166:103–109

Hasegawa Y, Ogihara T, Yamada T, Ishigaki Y, Imai J, Uno K, Gao J, Kaneko K, Ishihara H, Sasano H, Nakauchi H, Oka Y, Katagiri H (2007). Bone marrow (BM) transplantation promotes beta-cell regeneration after acute injury through BM cell mobilization. Endocrinology. 148(5):2006-15.

Hauge-Evans AC, Squires PE, Persaud SJ, Jones PM (1999). Pancreatic beta-cell-to-beta-cell interactions are required for integrated responses to nutrient stimuli: enhanced Ca2+ and insulin secretory responses of MIN6 pseudoislets. Diabetes. 48(7):1402-8.

Hermon-Taylor J (1970). [A review of pancreatic transplantation in man, and function of the pancreaticoduodenal graft]. Proc R Soc Med. 63(5):436.

Herold KC, Hagopian W, Auger JA, Poumian-Ruiz E, Taylor L, Donaldson D, Gitelman SE, Harlan DM, Xu D, Zivin RA, Bluestone JA (2002): Anti-CD3 monoclonal antibody in new-onset type 1 diabetes mellitus. N Engl J Med 346:1692–1698

Kadiyala S, Young RG, Thiede MA, Bruder SP (1997). Culture expanded canine mesenchymal stem cells possess osteochondrogenic potential in vivo and in vitro. Cell Transplant. 6(2):125-34.

Karnieli O, Izhar-Prato Y, Bulvik S, Efrat S (2007) Generation of Insulin-producing Cells From Human Bone Marrow Mesenchymal Stem Cells By Genetic Manipulation. Stem Cells. 25:2837-44.

Kelly W D, Lillehei R C, Merkel F K, Idezuki Y & Goetz F C (1967) Surgery 61, 827

Keymeulen B, Vandemeulebroucke E, Ziegler AG, Mathieu C, Kaufman L, Hale G, Gorus F, Goldman M, Walter M, Candon S, Schandene L, Crenier L, De Block C, Seigneurin JM, De Pauw P, Pierard D, Weets I, Rebello P, Bird P, Berrie E, Frewin M, Waldmann H, Bach JF, Pipeleers D, Chatenoud L (2005): Insulin needs after CD3-antibody therapy in new-onset type 1 diabetes. N Engl J Med 352:2598 –2608

Kroon E, Martinson LA, Kadoya K, Bang AG, Kelly OG, Eliazer S, Young H, Richardson M, Smart NG, Cunningham J, Agulnick AD, D'Amour KA, Carpenter MK, Baetge EE (2008). Pancreatic endoderm derived from human embryonic stem cells generates glucose-responsive insulin-secreting cells in vivo. Nat. Biotechnol. 26, 443–452

Lardon J, Huyens N, Rooman I, Bouwens L (2004) Exocrine cell transdifferentiation in dexamethasone-treated rat pancreas. Virchows Arch. 444:61-5

Lavazais E, Pogu S, SaÃ¯ P, Martignat L (2007). Cytokine mobilization of bone marrow cells and pancreatic lesion do not improve streptozotocin-induced diabetes in mice by transdifferentiation of bone marrow cells into insulin-producing cells. Diabetes Metab.33(1):68-78

Lechner A, Yang YG, Blacken RA, Wang L, Nolan AL, Habener JF. (2004) No evidence for significant transdifferentiation of bone marrow into pancreatic beta-cells in vivo. Diabetes. 53: 616-23.

Lechner A, Nolan AL, Blacken RA, Habener JF (2005): Redifferentiation of insulin-secreting cells after in vitro expansion of adult human pancreatic islet tissue. Biochem Biophys Res Commun 327:581–588

Lee RH, Seo MJ, Reger RL, Spees JL, Pulin AA, Olson SD, Prockop DJ. (2006) Multipotent stromal cells from human marrow home to and promote repair of pancreatic islets and renal glomeruli in diabetic NOD/scid mice. Proc. Natl. Acad. Sci. U.S.A. 103: 17438-43.

Li WC, Rukstalis JM, Nishimura W, Tchipashvili V, Habener JF, Sharma A, Bonner-Weir S (2010). Activation of pancreatic-duct-derived progenitor cells during pancreas regeneration in adult rats. J Cell Sci. 2010;123(Pt 16):2792-802.

Mandrup-Poulsen T, Mølvig J, Andersen HU, Helqvist S, Spinas GA, Munck M. Steno Memorial Hospital, Gentofte, Denmark (1990). Lack of predictive value of islet cell antibodies, insulin antibodies, and HLA-DR phenotype for remission in cyclosporin-treated IDDM patients. The Canadian-European Randomized Control Trial Group. Diabetes. 39(2):204-10.

Mirouze J, Rodier M, Richard JL, Lachkar H, Monnier L (1986). Trial of mild immunosuppression by methisoprinol in acute onset diabetes mellitus: effects on rate and duration of remission. Diabetes Res. 3(7):359-62.

Moriscot C, de Fraipont F, Richard MJ, Marchand M, Savatier P, Bosco D, Favrot M, Benhamou PY. (2005) Human bone marrow mesenchymal stem cells can express insulin and key transcription factors of the endocrine pancreas developmental pathway upon genetic and/or microenvironmental manipulation in vitro. Stem Cells. 23: 594-603.

Nano R, Clissi B, Melzi R, Calori G, Maffi P, Antonioli B, Marzorati S, Aldrighetti L, Freschi M, Grochowiecki T, Socci C, Secchi A, Di Carlo V, Bonifacio E, Bertuzzi F. (2005). "Islet isolation for allotransplantation: variables associated with successful islet yield and graft function." Diabetologia 48(5): 906-12.

Ouziel-Yahalom L, Zalzman M, Anker-Kitai L, Knoller S, Bar Y, Glandt M, Herold K, Efrat S (2006): Expansion and redifferentiation of adult human pancreatic islet cells. *Biochem Biophys Res Commun* 341:291–298

Phillips JM, Harach SZ, Parish NM, Fehervari Z, Haskins K, Cooke A (2000): Nondepleting anti-CD4 has an immediate action on diabetogenic effector cells, halting their destruction of pancreatic beta cells. *J Immunol* 165:1949 –1955

Pittenger MF, Mackay AM, Beck SC, Jaiswal RK, Douglas R, Mosca JD, Moorman MA, Simonetti DW, Craig S, Marshak DR. (1999). Multilineage potential of adult human mesenchymal stem cells. Science 284:143-147.

Pour, P.M. (1994) Pancreatic centroacinar cells. The regulator of both exocrine and endocrine function. Int. J. Pancreatol., 15:51–64.

Ricordi C, Lacy PE, Scharp DW (1989). Automated islet isolation from human pancreas. Diabetes. 38 Suppl 1:140-2.

Russ HA, Bar Y, Ravassard P, Efrat S (2008).In vitro proliferation of cells derived from adult human beta-cells revealed by cell-lineage tracing. Diabetes 57(6):1575-83

Ryan EA, Paty BW, Senior PA, Bigam D, Alfadhli E, Kneteman NM, Lakey JR, Shapiro AM. (2005). Five-year follow-up after clinical islet transplantation. *Diabetes* 54: 2060-9.

Shapiro AM, Lakey JR, Ryan EA, Korbutt GS, Toth E, Warnock GL, Kneteman NM, Rajotte RV. (2000). Islet transplantation in seven patients with type 1 diabetes mellitus using a glucocorticoid-free immunosuppressive regimen." N Engl J Med 343(4): 230-8.

Shapiro AM, Ricordi C, Hering BJ, Auchincloss H, Lindblad R, Robertson RP, Secchi A, Brendel MD, Berney T, Brennan DC, Cagliero E, Alejandro R, Ryan EA, DiMercurio B, Morel P, Polonsky KS, Reems JA, Bretzel RG, Bertuzzi F, Froud T, Kandaswamy R, Sutherland DE, Eisenbarth G, Segal M, Preiksaitis J, Korbutt GS, Barton FB, Viviano L, Seyfert-Margolis V, Bluestone J, Lakey JR. (2006). International trial of the Edmonton protocol for islet transplantation. N Engl J Med 355(13): 1318-30.

Slack JM (1995) Developmental biology of the pancreas. Development. 121: 1569-80

Smukler SR, Arntfield ME, Razavi R, Bikopoulos G, Karpowicz P, Seaberg R, Dai F, Lee S, Ahrens R, Fraser PE, Wheeler MB, van der Kooy D (2011). The adult mouse and human pancreas contain rare multipotent stem cells that express insulin. Cell Stem Cell. 8(3):281-93.

Taneera J, Rosengren A, Renstrom E, Nygren JM, Serup P, Rorsman P, Jacobsen SE. (2006) Failure of transplanted bone marrow cells to adopt a pancreatic beta-cell fate. Diabetes. 55: 290-6.

Tateishi K, He J, Taranova O, Liang G, D'Alessio AC, Zhang Y (2008). Generation of insulin secreting islet-like clusters from human skin fibroblasts. *J. Biol. Chem.* 283, 31601–31607

Timper K, Seboek D, Eberhardt M, Linscheid P, Christ-Crain M, Keller U, Müller B, Zulewski H. (2006) Human adipose tissue-derived mesenchymal stem cells differentiate into insulin, somatostatin, and glucagon expressing cells. Biochem. Biophys. Res. Commun. 341: 1135-40.

Wang RN, Kloppel G, Bouwens L (1995). Duct- to islet-cell differentiation and islet growth in the pancreas of duct-ligated adult rats. Diabetologia. 38:1405-11

Zhang D, Jiang W, Liu M, Sui X, Yin X, Chen S, Shi Y, Deng H (2009). Highly efficient differentiation of human ES cells and iPS cells into mature pancreatic insulin-producing cells. *Cell Res.* 19, 429–438

Zhao M, Christie MR, Heaton N, George S, Amiel S, Cai Huang G (2002).Amelioration of streptozotocin-induced diabetes in mice using human islet cells derived from long-term culture in vitro. Transplantation. 73(9):1454-60.

Zhao M, Amiel SA, Christie MR, Rela M, Heaton N, Huang GC (2005). Insulin-producing cells derived from human pancreatic non-endocrine cell cultures reverse streptozotocin-induced hyperglycaemia in mice. Diabetologia. 48(10):2051-61.

Zhao M, Amiel SA, Christie MR, Muiesan P, Srinivasan P, Littlejohn W, Rela M, Arno M, Heaton N, Huang GC (2007). Evidence for the presence of stem cell-like progenitor cells in human adult pancreas. J Endocrinol.195(3):407-14.

Zhao M, Amiel SA, Ajami S, Jiang J, Rela M, Heaton N, Huang GC (2008). Amelioration of streptozotocin-induced diabetes in mice with cells derived from human marrow stromal cells. PLoS One. 3(7):e2666.

Zhou, Q., Brown, J., Kanarek, A., Rajagopal, J. & Melton, D. A (2008). *In vivo* reprogramming of adult pancreatic exocrine cells to beta-cells. *Nature* 455, 627–632

10

Metabolic Control Targets for Patients with Type 1 Diabetes in Clinical Practice

María Gloria Baena-Nieto, Cristina López-Tinoco,
Jose Ortego-Rojo and Manuel Aguilar-Diosdado
Endocrinology & Nutrition Service, Puerta del Mar Hospital, Cadiz,
Spain

1. Introduction

Diabetes and its micro- and macro-vascular complications constitute one of the principal social-health problems world-wide. It has high impact on the quality of life and prognosis of the individuals affected, as well as high direct and indirect economic costs to the Public Health Service. Following the publication of benchmark studies in the 1990s which indicated that the maintenance of glycaemia levels as close as possible to normality is associated with a lower incidence, progression and severity of the complications, the optimisation of metabolic control has been converted to a core therapeutic objective (DCCT, 1993; Herman, 1999; UKPDS, 1998). The tools for the management of diabetes have advanced spectacularly in these past few years, not only for the control of glycaemia but also for its measurement. As such, currently, there is a wide variety of drugs available with different mechanisms of action which, alone or in combination, enable a reasonable metabolic control in the majority of cases. Although insulin has been used for >80 years, the biggest advances in the mode of use have been over the last two decades. This change has been due, in great part, to: 1) development of new sources of insulin (analogues of insulin) together with the development and fine-tuning of different forms of its administration (continuous subcutaneous insulin infusion; CSII) in search of profiles of activity closer to the normal physiologic state; 2) change in philosophy in the therapeutic planning of diabetes, such that the strategies of co-responsibility and flexibility of life-style have become fundamental aspects; 3) introduction of self-control using capillary glycaemia (SCCG) in daily practice (De Witt & Hirsch, 2003); 4) recent incorporation in clinical practice of the use of glucose sensors, continuous glucose monitoring systems (CGMS) that generate the maximum information on modifications of glucose levels in plasma along the course of the whole day.

This review centres on the importance, in clinical practice, of the metabolic control targets for patients with DM type 1. Difficulties in achieving glycaemia goals using multiple insulin injection with new insulin analogues, and modern technologies such as CGMS and CSII are extensively analysed.

2. Importance of glycaemia control in the treatment of diabetes

Traditionally, the conventional therapy has been orientated towards achieving acceptable levels of glycaemia and stable clinical status in the asymptomatic patient. Intensive treatment of diabetes, according to the protocol of the Diabetes Control and Complications Trial (DCCT), consists in a therapeutic design orientated towards achieving almost normal levels of glycaemia. Included are: a rigorous educative plan with frequent actions for a life-style change, an insulin regimen with three or more daily injections (multiple doses of insulin), or CIIS and programme of SCCG four of more per day (DCCT, 1995).

Over the past few years there have been several studies evaluating the effect on the appearance and progression of the micro-vascular complications of diabetes using a strict control of glycaemia with intensive treatment (Herman, 1999). The most significant was the DCCT study published in 1993 (DCCT, 1993). Included were more than 1000 patients with DM type I and the results demonstrated that maintaining the levels of glucose within a range closest to normality, tended to reduce the appearance of retinopathy by 76%, nephropathy by 56% and neuropathy by 60%. The DCCT established the targets of glycaemia control and of glycosylated haemoglobin (HbA1c) in patients with DM type 1, together with the need to perform measurement of capillary glycaemia as part of the intensive treatment regimen.

In DM type 2, the Kumamoto study (Shichiri et al., 2000) with a design similar to the DCCT, demonstrated that intensive treatment (target of HbA1c <7%) reduced the risk of retinopathy by 69% and nephropathy by 70%. The United Kingdom Prospective Diabetes Study (UKPDS) published in 1998, demonstrated that intensive long-term treatment of the hyperglycaemia also reduced the appearance of micro-vascular complication in patients recently diagnosed with DM type 2 (UKPDS, 1998).

These studies demonstrated definitively that the better the control of glycaemia the tighter the association with the decrease in the rates of micro-vascular complications (retinopathy and nephropathy). Follow-up studies of the DCCT (DCCT-EDIC; 2000; Martin et al., 2006) and of the UKPDS (Holman et al., 2008) have highlighted that once the intensive treatment is established in the two groups with evidence of their benefits, those that had been performed earlier retain their benefits as the product of a "metabolic legacy".

Despite that many epidemiologic studies and meta-analyses (Selvin et al., 2004; Stettler et al., 2006) having clearly demonstrated a direct relationship between HbA1c and the incidence of cardiovascular disease (CVD), the potential of intensive control of glycaemia to reduce CVD has not been delineated, as yet. In the DCCT, no differences were observed between the groups with respect to the appearance of CVD events. However, at 8 years of conclusion of the study, the patients who had been assigned to the intensive treatment group had a 42% reduction in CVD and a 57% reduction in the risk of non-fatal myocardial infarction, stroke or death, compared to those who had been assigned to the standard treatment arm of the trial (Nathan et al., 2005). It has been demonstrated recently that, as with DM type 2, the benefit of intensive glycaemia control in patients with DM type 1 persists over decades (DCCT-EDIC, 2009).

In the UKPDS, a reduction was observed of 16% in the risk of CVD in the intensive treatment group, although this difference did not reach statistical significance. However, at 10 years of follow-up, a reduction in non-fatal acute myocardial infarction and in all-cause mortality of 13 and 27%, respectively (Holman et al., 2008) was demonstrated in the participants initially assigned to intensive control of glycaemia, compared to those assigned to conventional control. Nevertheless, the results of three large studies (ACCORD, Ismail-Beigi et al., 2010; ADVANCE, Patel et al., 2008; VADT, Duckworth at al., 2009) that had investigated the effect of glycaemia control in DM type 2, were unable to demonstrate that the intensive control of glycaemia achieved any reduction in the CVD, even though the patients were DM type 2 of long duration and with high risk of CVD.

Maintaining levels of glycaemia that are practically normal carries a series of notable risk. Among these is the increase in episodes of slight as well as of severe hypoglycaemia. The investigators in the EDIC study (Nathan et al., 2005) observed CVD benefits associated with intensive glycaemia control, but not in those with a level of HbA1c <6.5%. In the initial publications of the ACCORD study, the greater rates of mortality were produced in the 2 extreme categories of HbA1c, independently of the regimen of treatment. Also, the decreases in survival in the patients with lower HbA1c levels were related, at least in part, to the appearance of hypoglycaemia. As such, episodes of severe hypoglycaemia in patients with advanced disease need to be prevented, and not with the intention of achieving normal, or near normal, levels of HbA1c (<6.5%) in those in whom achieving normal levels safely do not appear probable.

2.1 Objectives of glycaemia control

The recommendations for glycaemia control targets in adults, in pregnant and in non-pregnant women are shown in Table 1. The recommendations are based on the blood levels of glucose which correlate with levels of HbA1c at 7%. The targets need to be individualised for each patient, and it is necessary to be assured of achieving them. In young and healthy patients that know the symptoms of hypoglycaemia and recover from them relatively easily, the targets need to approximate to the levels of glycaemia observed in persons without diabetes. However, the objectives of control are more strict during gestation, and more permissive for persons who have difficulties noting the symptoms of hypoglycaemia as well as those who present with severe hypoglycaemia or for those whose episodes of hypoglycaemia can be particularly dangerous (for example, patients with heart disease, cerebrovascular pathology or autonomic neuropathy). As such, in adults with limited life expectancy or advanced vascular disease, it would be more appropriate to have less strict targets. Post-prandial hyperglycaemia is defined as values of glycaemia >140 mg/dL at two hours after a meal. It is a frequent phenomenon that is unnoticed in the determination of HbA1c and basal glycaemia since it is already present when the levels of HbA1c are optimum. Several studies have shown that the levels of post-prandial glycaemia are strongly related to the CVD risk (Cavalot et al., 2006; Ceriello, 2005; European Diabetes Epidemiology Group, 1999;). Curiously, the contribution of post-prandial glycaemia appears to be more evident in patients with well-controlled diabetes (contribution of about 70% to the HbA1c when it is <7% and about 40% when it is >7.3%). However, the targets of post-prandial glycaemia using SCCG are controversial. In some epidemiology studies, values of elevated glucose following oral glucose load test have been associated with an increased risk of CVD, independently of the fasting plasma glucose level. Also, the phenomenon appears intimately linked with CVD such as endothelial dysfunction which is aggravated by post-prandial hyperglycaemia (Ceriello et al., 2002). The majority of authors recommend values of HbA1c <7% as the appropriate metabolic control objective (American Diabetes Association, 2011)

Achieving a good metabolic control in DM type 1 is not an easy issue. Results reported in international studies on the degree of metabolic control in 13,612 patients from Sweden (Katarina et al., 2007) and 27,035 from Austria and Germany (Gerstl et al., 2008) showed that only 21.2% and 27%, respectively, of type 1 DM patients have HbA1c <7%. We studied a cohort of patients with type 1 DM (n = 489) followed-up from 2005 to 2007. During the study period, the mean HbA1c decreased from 7.78% to 7.36% and the frequency of patients with HbA1c <7% increased from 24.6% to 27.1% and those with a mean HbA1c of >8% decreased from 42.6% to 38.7% (Baena et al., 2008).

HbA1c	< 7%
Pre-prandial plasma glucose	70-130 mg/dL
Post-prandial plasma glucose	<180 mg/dL
The objectives need to be individualised based on: • Duration of the diabetes • Life expectancy • Associated co-morbidities • Known CVD or advanced micro-vascular complications • Severe hypoglycaemia, or inadvertent To improve objectives of post-prandial glucose if HbA1c was beyond the target despite pre-prandial glucose levels	
In pregnancy: HbA1c Pre-prandial plasma glucose Post-prandial plasma glucose	6% 60-99 mg/dL 100-129 mg/dL

Table 1. Recommended objectives for glycaemia control, in patients with diabetes

3. Glucose monitoring in patients with diabetes

SCCG is an essential component of intensive treatment, and the core of the DCCT publication is the enormous increase in its diffusion and utilisation. As a result of this, the new technologies applied to these systems have evolved rapidly, giving rise to successive new measures on the market.

HbA1c is the reference pattern to assess long-term glycaemia control and, together with the measured glucose, determines the guidelines for adjustments in treatment of diabetes by the attending physician.

As we have stated earlier, in the past few years there has been in increase in the evidence showing the influence of post-prandial hyperglycaemia and glycaemia control, on the development of diabetic complications (Ceriello, 2003).

SCCG consists of determining the capillary blood glucose of the patient, using the glucometer. It carries information complementary to HbA1c levels, such as fasting and post-prandial glucose, detection of hypoglycaemia, information on the daily glucose variability, etc. This enables optimisation of treatment, above all in patients receiving intensive therapy. However, the information provided by the glucometer refers to a specific moment in time. For greater and better information on glycaemic changes there needs to be continuous glucose monitoring systems (CGMS) that perform several measurements per hour and, as such, produce averaged information over the course of the day.

3.1 Indications for self-monitoring of glycaemia in patients with DM type 1

Type 1 diabetes is characterised by frequent fluctuation in glycaemia. SCCG is the method-of-choice and the timing is decided according the needs of the individual patient as well as the targets of the therapeutic regimen. There are no studies that demonstrate the efficacy of SCCG alone in improving the glycaemia control in patients with DM type 1, but they are an integral part of the treatment. The results of the DCCT study demonstrated that intensive treatment is the most appropriate option for the majority of patients with DM type 1. The two modalities of intensive treatment (multiple doses of insulin and continuous subcutaneous infusion of insulin) involved targets of glycaemia control close to normality, with a higher risk of hypoglycaemia (DCCT, 1993). To prevent episodes of asymptomatic hypoglycaemias and hyperglycaemias and, as such, to perform an appropriate adjustment of the insulin dose, it is necessary to frequently supervise the glycaemic levels. In the DCCT study there was a need for at least 4 SCCG measurements per day (pre-prandial and at bedtime) and post-prandial measurements were performed when the levels of HbA1c were not appropriate despite the values of the pre-prandial SCCG values being within the pre-established control targets. Further, a SCCG measurement was indicated at 3:00 a.m. once a week.

It is not clear what would be the optimum frequency of the capillary glucose measurements in patients with DM type 1, although there are various studies that have demonstrated that the increase in the self-control of glycaemia improves the metabolic control in these patients Currently, the majority of patients with DM type 1 and with gestational diabetes treated with insulin need to have at least 3 SCCG per day (ADA, 2011) (grade A evidence), which should be individualised according to the characteristics of the patient and the therapeutic targets. In general, it is recommended that measurements regularly before meals and, on occasions, one or two hours after, and at night-time, provide information that is very useful for therapeutic optimisation (Bergenstal & Gavin, 2005).

The latest clinical practice guide of the American Diabetes Association (ADA) establishes the following recommendations based on the scientific evidence (ADA, 2011):

- Achieving a strict glycaemia control requires SCCG as an integral part of the therapeutic strategy (grade A evidence).
- The patients treated with multiple doses of insulin need to perform SCCG 3 or more times a day (grade A evidence).
- In patients treated with les than 3 doses of insulin, oral agents or single diabetic treatment, the SCCG is useful in achieving glycaemia control targets within the context of a specific educative program (grade E evidence).
- To achieve the targets of post-prandial glycaemia control there needs to post-prandial SCCG performed (grade E evidence).
- There is a need to instruct the patient on the usefulness of the SCCG, and to evaluate the technique and its use regularly so that the data obtained can be used in treatment adjustment (grade E evidence).

3.2 Modalities of self-monitoring of glycaemia
3.2.1 Self-monitoring the level of blood sugar using the glucometer

SCCG requires a capillary blood sample obtained, usually, from finger-prick using a micro-lancet and using a glucose meter. The majority of glucose meters currently available generate plasma values by the device reader, or directly in plasma, or by multiplying the whole blood value by 1.12 so that the value is comparable with that from the laboratory (Valeri et al., 2004).

The measurement of glucose using the modern enzymatic methods (hexokinase or glucose oxidase) generates a rapid, reliable and precise measurement. The strips impregnated with these enzymes collect the blood sample and are read by the device in a short period of time (Goldstein et al., 2004).

The majority of machines have a memory to save the previous results, and some even have the option of downloading to a computer and with printer graphics to enable the analysis of the data and to optimise the metabolic self-monitoring. Some devices enable patients to record data such as the medication dose or the presence of symptoms. The most recent are smaller sized and require less quantity of blood for the analysis. For patients with impaired sight, there are devices that can adapt to voice synthesizer to deliver an audible version of the result. Most results can be obtained within about 5 seconds, depending on the characteristics of the apparatus (Bode et al., 2001).

In some countries such as the USA, there are currently available certain glucometers that use other different sites than that of the finger to obtain the blood sample, in an attempt to reduce the discomfort of the finger-prick. In a study performed on one of these devices that obtained blood from the arm it is noted that reliable results were obtained that were less painful than the finger prick (Fineberg et al., 2001).

3.2.2 Continuous monitoring of glucose - glucose sensors

Over the last decade the SCCG system has been the only measurement available for the monitoring of glycaemia levels. Despite its unquestioned usefulness, it is an invasive technique, tedious for the patient, generates limited information at any specific time, and without additional information to establish trends.

The concentration of glucose in the interstitial tissues is reflected in its concentration in capillary and venous blood, since the glucose diffuses into interstitial tissue to equilibrate both compartments. Based on this, the CGMS measures the glucose concentration in the interstitial liquid of the subcutaneous cellular tissue in a minimally invasive manner, using a sensor subcutaneously located. The CGMS can detect glycaemia oscillations continuously, such that maximum information can be generated on the direction, magnitude, duration, frequency and possible causes of the fluctuations of glycaemia over the long-term course of the day. Hence, it is very useful in optimising the treatment of patients with diabetes (Maran et al., 2005) (Garg, 2009). It precludes the limitations of information of the CGMS system of intensive treatment in the cases of detection in periods of inadvertent hypo- and hyperglycaemia (Klonoff, 2005). However, the sensors currently available do not have the precision of capillary glucometers and, hence, the use is approved as a complement, and not as a substitution, for SCCG.

The invasive intravascular sensors measure plasma glucose directly and has been used to monitor hospitalised patients. However, there have not been any studies published on their functioning and usefulness in extended groups of patients (Klonoff, 2005).

3.2.2.1 Types of glucose sensors

Continuous monitoring of glucose was introduced in the 1970s, with a complex system termed biostator or artificial pancreas. Subsequently, new generation sensors appeared, with mixed results.

Currently, there are 4 types of CGMS approved by the FDA available on the international market: CGMS® (Continuous Glucose Monitoring System) such as the Guardian®, the Guardian Real Time®, the Paradigm Real Time® (Medtronic MiniMed, Northridge, CA, USA); the GlucoDay® system (Menarini Diagnostics, Florence, Italy); the Seven® system (DexCom Inc., San Diego, CA, USA); and the Freestyle Navigator® monitor (Abbott Laboratories, Alameda, CA, USA) (Gross et al., 2000). Table 2 compares the main features of the currently available systems.

CGMS, approved by the FDA in 1999 was the first generation of sensors commercialised and, as such, the most widely used and, for which, there is the most clinical experience available. It is composed of a subcutaneous sensor and an external monitor. It needs to be

	Guardian, Guardian RT, Paradigm RT	Glucoday	Freestyle Navigator	Seven System
Range of glucose values (mg/dL)	40-400	40-400	20-500	40-400
Life-span of sensor (days)	3 in USA/ 6 in Europe	2	5	7
Warm-up period (hours)	2	2	10 (1 for latest system)	2
Calibration frequency	Every 12 h	One point	Post-insertion: -10, 12, 24, 72h -1, 2, 10, 24, 72h (latest system)	Every 72 hours
Sensor device	Amerometric sensor	Microdialysis glucose	Amperometric sensor	Amperometric sensor
Results timing	Retrospective	Retrospective and Real time	Real Time	Real Time
Sensor site	In situ	External	In situ	In situ
Frequency of blood glucose display (min)	5	3	1	5
Rate-of-change arrows	Yes	No	Yes	Yes
Integrate with pump	Yes (Paradigm RT)	No	No	No
Accuracy (error grid) (%)	61.7-76.3	64-88	76.3-81.7	70.4
Limitations	- Life span of 3 days (USA) - Update glycaemia data on the screen every 5 minutes - Calibrations are required every 2- 3 days	- Large system - Life span of 2 days - Skin irritation - No rate- of- change arrows	- Large sensor and transmitter - Warm- up period of 10 hours (first sensor)- - Calibration time programming required - Must use Freestyle strips for calibration - High cost	- Update glycaemia data on the screen every 5 minutes - Does not permit selecting specific points above

Table 2. Main features of the currently available CGMS devices (Torres et al, 2010)

calibrated a minimum of 4 times a day using measured capillary glucose levels, presenting an out-of-phase between the level of glycaemia and the sensor signal of about 4 minutes (Gross et al., 2000).

In the past few years, progressively improved new models have been developed. In 2004, the FDA approved the Guardian Monitor®, with improvements on the previous system that included an alarm not only to signal hyperglycaemia but also for hypoglycaemia. One year later the Guardian MiniMed Real Time® appeared on the market: It was the first continuous glucose monitor that provided the measurements of glucose in real time, every 5 minutes, and with direct connection to a CSII. The Paradigm Real Time® was approved in 2006 as the first sensor integrated with a CSII (Paradigm REAL-time 522/722) enabling it to create a closed circuit. More recently, MiniMed Paradigm Veo® system has been commercialised. It includes CSII with a CGMS with a mechanism that enables the infusion of insulin to be delayed when the levels of glucose are below the specified range. All these systems require at least 2 calibrations per day.

Another type of sensor known as the GlucoDay® system became available on the market in 2002. Its system is based on the technique of micro-dialysis applied to the interstitial fluid that, as has been commented-upon above, provides a reading of the glucose concentration in the subcutaneous cellular tissue that is very similar to the plasma value (Poscia et al.,2003; Varalli et al., 2003). The data collected can be visualised permanently in real time and to be used subsequently for different analyses regarding the behaviour of the glucose concentrations, such as its graphic representation. This system shows high precision and reliability, including at low glucose concentrations (Maran et al., 2002).

The Seven System® was approved by the FDA in 2007. It enables real time readings with measurements performed every 5 minutes and with a latency of 12 hours. It is the only one proven for use over a period of 7 days. The results can be stored for subsequent analyses. The system includes alarms that can be programmed not only for hyperglycaemia but also for hypoglycaemia. It needs to be calibrated every 12 hours with capillary glucose values. A new version is the Seven Plus System® which has improved not only the functionality but also has many additional functions included.

The latest system approved by the FDA in 2008 is the Freestyle Navigator® which has introduced important improvements to the CGM system (McGarraugh, 2009). It enables readings in real time following a latency period of 10 hours (1 hour in the more advanced versions). The concentration of glucose is measured every minute and enables analyses to be made every 10 minutes. The calibration requires capillary glucose measurement (only 4-5 in the first period). It has alarms not only for excessively elevated glucose levels but also for glucose decrease.

3.2.2.2 Clinical indications for continuous glucose monitoring (CGM)

The clinical applications for continuous glucose monitoring (CGM) have not, as yet, been well established. The system can be useful in determining patterns of glycaemia over a 24h period and to detect inadvertent hypoglycaemia. However, its role in improving control of diabetes is, as yet, unclear.

Currently, there are studies and preliminary data on the possible uses; the most extensive studies have focused on the detection of asymptomatic hypoglycaemia. Several studies show an elevated frequency of asymptomatic hypoglycaemia, especially during the nocturnal period and, above all, in patients with DM type 1, detected using CGMS, which have been underestimated with the conventional self-monitoring systems (DeVries et al., 2004). The CGMS also captures values of glucose which can change over a short period of time and, for which, it is not always practical to wait months to evaluate the reductions in the levels of HbA1c. CGM can show the time during which the patients remain in the glucose range that is normal, low or elevated. These values can be more useful than a single point when integrating the data such as the HbA1c levels. Prolonged exposure to intermediate levels of glucose may be preferred in some patients compared to the frequent peaks of hyperglycaemia and hypoglycaemia. This can obviate therapeutically targeting different HbA1c levels in response to oscillating levels of glucose. The CGMS can detect these oscillations as well as measure the mean amplitude and the index of variability of the glycaemia. As such, predictive information on trends during the different times of the day can be obtained (Manuel-y-Keenoy et al., 2004). The CGMS can also be used to evaluate the response of the glycaemia profile to specific treatment or therapeutic modalities such as, for example, the use of multiple doses of insulin vs. the CIIS (Weintrob et al., 2004). There are several studies that show the usefulness of CGMS in modifying treatment and achieving better metabolic control (Edelman et al., 2009; Hirsch et al., 2008; Leinung et al., 2010). Some authors consider this its most important use. In adolescents, apart from being a useful tool to improve glycaemia control, it also promotes communication and motivation of the patient (Schaepelynck-Bélicar et al., 2003) .

According to the data available, beneficial effects in metabolic control can be exercised in pregnant women with diabetes, but more studies are necessary to evaluate the reality of reducing perinatal complications (Festin, 2008).

As such, the possible indications of CGM comprise those situations that require detailed information on the fluctuations of glycaemia: diagnostic confirmation and management of hypoglycaemia (undetected hypoglycaemias or nocturnal hypoglycaemias); therapeutic adjustments in patients who do not achieve the control targets (discrepancy between HbA1c and capillary glycaemia, pregestational diabetes); diabetic educational tool (impact of intake on the glycaemia profile), physical exercise, intercurrent situations; diabetes and hospitalisation (unit for the treatment of the critically-ill patients and/or intensive coronary care), pancreatic tissue transplant and clinical investigation.

According to the recommendations of the American Diabetes Association (ADA, 2011), the CGM can be indicated in selected adult patients with DM type 1 on treatment with intensive insulin therapy to decrease the level of HbA1c (recommendation grade A). As well, CGM can be indicated in children, adolescents, and young adults in whom the adherence to treatment would be high (recommendation grade C). In patients with inadvertent hypoglycaemias, the CGM would be indicated as a complement to the SCCG.

3.2.2.3 Inconveniences

Currently, the CGMS is approved for the use in supplementing SCCG due to the inherent problems: limited level of precision for the isolated measurement of glucose, above all, at decreased levels (Klonoff, 2004); the need to calibrate the sensor several times a day using capillary measurements; short period of use (2-7 days) (Kovatchev et al., 2008).

Minimally invasive CGMS can present secondary effects related to the continuous measure of interstitial fluid. It can cause slight local distress at the site of catheter insertion which can occur on rare occasions. Further, because of its complicated technique, these systems require help from the health-care professional team (Tanenberg et al., 2004).

The major limitation of CGMS is, however, the current absence of scientific evidence of its usefulness. Methodologically appropriate studies are necessary to evaluate precisely the impact of these systems on improving the metabolic control in patients with diabetes, and their effect on hypoglycaemia decrease. The use can be extended in the future but CGMS needs to be improved with respect to the accuracy of glucose measurement, convenience for the patient, integration with other technologies such as CIIS.

4. Treatment of diabetes

As commented-upon earlier, intensive therapy of DM type 1 has been consolidated as the therapeutic strategy of choice since it has been demonstrated to delay the appearance and progression of the chronic complications (DCCT, 1993; Nathan et al., 2005). This strategy consists of multiple daily subcutaneous injections, or the use of CIIS with adjustment of insulin according to the intake of carbohydrates and the level of glycaemia (ADA, 2011).

4.1 Treatment with multiple doses of insulin

The objective of intensive insulin therapy is to arrive at levels of glycaemia close to that of normal, using a regimen of insulin similar to physiological conditions. To achieve this, basal insulin treatment (1 or 2 doses per day with intermediate or low insulin) is accompanied by pre-prandial bolus of quick-acting insulin which is adjusted according to the pre-prandial glycaemia and the intake of carbohydrates. To correctly fulfil this type of therapy, collaboration on the part of the patient is necessary and can be achieved with motivation and information using an appropriate program of diabetes education. As has been highlighted earlier, this type of treatment needs to be accompanied with frequent monitoring with capillary measurements.

Intensive therapy is associated with more frequent hypoglycaemias. Since the DCCT publication, analogues of fast- and slow-acting insulins have been developed which, currently, form the basis of intensive treatment with multiple doses of insulin. These insulin analogues have been associated with a lower risk of hypoglycaemias, and a comparable decrease in HbA1c. Among the analogues of slow-acting insulin are glargine and detemir. Glargine insulin is almost identical to human insulin, except for certain modifications in the molecular structure that enables delaying the absorption in subcutaneous tissue resulting in prolonged duration without peaks of activity. It can be administered at any time of the day without impairing its effectiveness. Detemir insulin is another slow-acting analogue that has a fatty acid in its structure that enables it to bind to albumin in the subcutaneous tissue and its slow release prolongs its action in the blood stream. Both insulins, glargine and detemir, have similar efficacy, similar to the NPH, and are especially indicated in patients with recurring hypoglycaemias (Sing et al., 2009).

The fast-acting insulin analogues have modifications in the molecular structure which facilitate more rapid absorption into the bloodstream. Currently, there are three fast-acting analogues (lispro, aspart and glulisine) whose duration of action and effects are similar. They commence action within 5-15 minutes of subcutaneous administration, with a maximum peak at 30-90 minutes and a duration of 2-4 hours. Compared to standard insulin that begins its effects at 30-45 minutes from injection and has a duration of 4-6 hours, the new fast-acting analogues decrease the post-prandial glucose peak more quickly, can be injected immediately before meals, and decrease hypoglycaemias (Plank et al., 2005; Porcellati et al., 2008). The election of one or other insulin for multiple dose therapy would depend on the characteristics of the patient. No one type of insulin has been elected as treatment-of-choice because a clear benefit on metabolic control has not as yet been demonstrated in a generic manner.

4.2 Continuous Insulin Infusion Systems (CIIS)

Pumps for CIIS are electro-mechanical, portable and small, with the administration of insulin from a reservoir at a programmable rate via a flexible catheter through a cannular inserted subcutaneously. This system delivers insulin continuously at a rhythm that is termed "basal rate" and which can be increased or decreased according to the requirements of the patient. In basal rate, the control of hepatic production of pre-prandial and overnight glucose is an objective. Further, the pump can provide specific amounts of extra "bolus" insulin which can administered before the intake allows the post-prandial glycaemia to become elevated. It can, as well, correct specific increases in glycaemia caused by other circumstances. Insulins used in the CIIS are exclusively fast-acting. Standard human, and preferably, the analogues lispro, aspart and glulisine, are used since these offer less variability in absorption, and show a pharmacokinetic profile closer to that of the physiologic state (Hirsch, 2005; Radermecker & Scheen, 2004).

Using CIIS in patients with DM type 1 began in the decade of the 1970s but, despite being effective in metabolic control, the initial devices had high risk of sepsis and thrombosis. At the start of the decade of the 1980s, evidence was communicated of an increase in mortality in patients having the CIIS; data that were not subsequently confirmed (Teutsch et al., 1984). The use of CIIS does not perform very well against the possibility of severe hypoglycaemia (Lock & Rigg, 1981) and frank ketoacidosis which was highlighted in some articles (Home & Marshall, 1984). The impact of the results of the DCCT became decisive for the widespread use of insulin pumps. The study highlighted a significant reduction in the levels of HbA1c in patients treated with CIIS compared with those who received multiple daily doses of insulin (DCCT, 1995). Since then, the use of CIIS has accelerated exponentially, and what was a research tool has become an established type of treatment for selected patients with DM type 1 (Cummins et al., 2010). On the other hand, the important technological development over the past few years has been to reduce the size of the pump considerably, to increase the benefits and to improve their safety. In the past decade, several studies have confirmed that therapy with CIIS has advantages in metabolic control while achieving greater decreases in the levels of HbA1c (Cummins et al., 2010; Pańkowska et al., 2009; Pickup & Sutton, 2008; Torres et al., 2009). Further, this improvement in glycaemia control is achieved with a lower quantity of insulin (Jeitler et al., 2008; Torres et al., 2009). Hence, CIIS has become established as the preferred modality of treatment, and an alternative to the multiple doses of insulin for those selected patients who do not achieve the target of glycaemia control with multiple injections of insulin (Bruttomesso et al., 2009).

The patients with DM type 1 treated with multiple injections of insulin frequently present with the "dawn phenomenon" which consists of a sharp increase in glucose in the small hours of the morning; increase due to the increase in the counter-regulatory hormones that occur during this period and which are not sufficiently counteracted by long-acting insulin administered at bedtime. The therapy with CIIS, enables basal infusion to be anticipated and programmed, which can be useful in controlling this phenomenon by increasing the basal rhythm to that suitable for the individual's needs (Bruttomesso et al., 2009; Cummins et al., 2010).

When CIIS therapy was used initially, there were cases of severe hypoglycaemia reported which brought the safety of the system into question (Lock & Rigg, 1981). In the subsequent years, the devices available were safer and used fast-acting analogues of insulin which resulted in reduction in the frequency of the severe hypoglycaemias. This form of treatment can achieve and maintain a grade of better metabolic control than can be achieved with multiple doses of insulin; the incidence of hypoglycaemia being significantly less, including at night (Pickup & Sutton, 2008; Torres et al., 2009). Brittle diabetes, with frequent and unannounced glycaemia oscillations, is improved with CIIS therapy.

Oscillations in glycaemia are reduced due to the use of fast-acting insulin analogues whose absorption variability is much lower than other insulins, and with which there is the possibility of programming different rhythms of infusion (Bruttomesso et al., 2008; Pickup et al., 2006).

The accumulated experience of CIIS use in children and adolescents is very promising. This modality of treatment reduces the incidence of acute complications, not only hypoglycaemias but also ketoacidosis, together with improved metabolic control, increased adherence to the treatment and promotion of family involvement. Treatment with CIIS in the paediatric population is safe and efficacious and represents a valid option in selected patients of whatever age provided that there is always appropriate family and health-care professional support (Boland et al., 1999; Danne et al., 2008; DiMeglio et al., 2004). The results of the use of CIIS in pregestational diabetes have not been quite conclusive. Although some trials had observed benefits in metabolic control (Lapolla et al., 2003), more studies are needed to confirm their advantages in achieving maternal and foetal objectives, and regards their safety during the gestation (Cummins et al., 2010; Mukhopadhyay et al., 2007; Volpe et al., 2010).

There are several studies that have found that the CIIS improves the quality-of-life of the patients because it allows better flexibility in relation to food intake and towards the conduct of various planned or unplanned activities. The considerable acceptance of this modality among users is due to the individual not being obliged to link food intake and social activities to insulin administration since several hours can elapse between the activities; as occurs when multiple dose insulin is used. The intake can be delayed or omitted and the content varied. Also, the intensity of the exercise can be modified as can the timing of the activity without compromising the glycaemia control target (EQuality1 Study Group, 2008; Radermecker & Scheen, 2004; Torres et al., 2009). The advantages of CIIS are summarised in Table 3.

Improvement in metabolic control
Correction of the dawn phenomenon
Decrease in hypoglycaemias
Improvement in brittle diabetes
Effective in adults, adolescents and children
Flexibility and improvement in quality-of-life

Table 3. Advantages of CIIS

Interruption of insulin delivery by mechanical failure in the system of infusion leads quickly to hypoglycaemia and ketoacidosis due to the absence of a subcutaneous deposit of insulin (Krzentowski et al., 1983). This and other similar circumstances are preventable by training the individual to identify a potential episode, to warn and to treat the elevated levels of glycaemia (Guilhem et al., 2006). At the site of insertion of the cannular there may appear atrophy, hypertrophy, pruritus, erythema and infection. In the majority of cases the clinical picture is slight and related to inadequate hygiene in the techniques used. Systematic rotation and changing the catheter a maximum of every 3 days would decrease, or pre-empt, these complications (Guilhem et al., 2006). The better strategy to prevent these complications is to instruct the patients using specific educative programs that highlight frequent monitoring of the glycaemia, objectives of glycaemia control, calculation of dietary carbohydrates and the adaptation of daily fluctuations in glycaemia induced by intake, physical exercise and situations of stress or illness. Further, family help and social environment are important for outcomes (Jeandidier et al., 2008; Tamborlane et al., 2003). The indications for CSII treatment are not universally established. Appropriate patient selection is fundamental in minimising the risks that these devices can involve. The best results are obtained in psychologically stable patients, with sufficient intellectual capacity, highly motivated and supervised by a multi-disciplinary team. CIIS therapy requires a specifically formed team of healthcare professionals with sufficient time dedication to their patients not only for the training but also for clinical follow-up. The circumstances for CIIS treatment apply to any age in achieving good metabolic outcomes (Bruttomesso et al., 2009; Cummins et al., 2010). The indications more widely accepted are collected in Table 4

HbA1c >7% despite good adherence to therapy with multi-injection systems
Severe hypoglycaemias, recurrent, nocturnal or inadvertent
Significant dawn phenomenon
Brittle diabetes. Wide glycaemia variation, independent of HbA1c
Planned pregnancy if no good control with multi-injection
Need for flexible life-style
Low insulin requirements (<20 UI/day)

Table 4. Indications for CIIS

4.3 CIIS monitoring

Frequent monitoring of glycaemia is a highly positive factor in obtaining good results with CIIS therapy (Shalitin et al., 2010). The information provided by CGMS enables better adaptation not only to the rhythm of basal infusion but also to the bolus. If it is accepted that if the patients treated with CIIS are more motivated, the outcomes resulting from the application of CGMS in this group could be greater (Leinung et al., 2010; Raccah et al., 2009). Currently, better practical advantages are to be gained in the *in situ* subcutaneous sensors with continuous reading in real time which integrate the CGMS in a continuous infusion of insulin using wireless communication; the technique termed continuous interactive monitoring. In this mode, the users of CIIS can adapt the insulin infusion and diet to the real metabolic status. This is possible because the information generated by CGMS allows for the detection of inadvertent hypoglycaemias, information on trends and speed-of-change of glucose, and provides help in planning the bolus to reduce the duration of the hyperglycaemic episode (Hirsch, 2009). A recent innovation has consisted of semi-automatic models that, apart from integrating the insulin infusion and the CGMS, automatically incorporates the delay in infusion over 2 hours in case of having produced an alarm for hypoglycaemia but had not obtained a response from the user (Hirsch et al., 2008a).

Real time information is an important advance in self-care by the patients but, as well, implies a challenge in applying this technology with safety and rigor. In the past 10 years the precision of these systems has improved and the durability of the sensor has increased up to 6-7 days. However, one important limitation is that none of the sensors currently available have the precision of the standard glucometers. This is because they do not measure the blood sugar directly but, rather, evaluate glucose in the subcutaneous interstitial fluid. The defects in precision are related to the low concentration of glucose in the interstitial fluid, the specific dynamics of the glucose in the capillary and interstitial fluids and the delays inherent in the measurement (Torres et al., 2010).

The patients with CIIS who are candidates for CGMS systems need to be very motivated and to have received verbal and written information in a program of therapeutic education. The effect is to avoid false expectations and to recognise the limitations of these systems. The educative program would be orientated towards training, management of the devices, and in the interpretation of the measurements of glucose in real time; all orientated towards achieving the euglycaemia state (Gilliam & Hirsch, 2009; Hirsch et al., 2008a; Juvenile Diabetes Research Foundation Continuous Glucose Monitoring Study Group, 2009a). In principle, the ideal candidate would be a patient with DM type 1, with excellent motivation and optimum therapeutic education, who has not been able to achieve HbA1c levels <7%.

Several studies have demonstrated that the use of CGMS in patients with CIIS has advantages in metabolic control, with significant decreases in the levels of HbA1c (Bergenstal et al., 2010; Deiss et al., 2006; Hirsch et al., 2008b; Juvenile Diabetes Research Foundation Continuous Glucose Monitoring Study Group, 2008) and less glycaemia variability (Garg et al., 2006; Kordonouri et al., 2010). Some studies have, as well, demonstrated improvement in the frequency of hypoglycaemia (Garg et al., 2006; Juvenile Diabetes Research Foundation Continuous Glucose Monitoring Study Group, 2009b; Leinung et al., 2010). The best results have been obtained in relation of adherence to the CGMS systems; continuous use being more efficient than intermittent use (Hirsch et al., 2008b; Juvenile Diabetes Research Foundation Continuous Glucose Monitoring Study Group, 2008, 2009a; Raccah et al., 2009) but, in practice, can be more difficult to fulfil (O'Connell et al., 2009).

A list of possible indication for the use of CGMS is summarised in Table 5 (American Diabetes Association, 2011; Fabiato et al., 2009).

Patients with DM type 1, excellent motivation and optimum therapeutic education, but who have not been able to achieve HbA1c <7%
Severe hypoglycaemias, inadvertent hypoglycaemias or fear of hypoglycaemias that impede achieving the targets of glycaemia control
Brittle diabetes
Planned pregnancy with difficulties achieving appropriate glycaemia control
Children and adolescents with significant glucose variability or frequent hypoglycaemias, severe or inadvertent despite adjustments of the therapies. It is indispensable that they and/or the family are motivated and have appropriate training.

Table 5. Indications for interactive CGMS

5. Future research

The challenge to achieve an optimum metabolic control in type 1 DM is being progressively better addressed. New insulins and technological devices have been designed to mimic beta cell function. However, to translate these findings into the clinical practice new research and clinical trials are needed. Technological advances have enabled the development of new CIIS devices with better performance in programming and for calculating optimal dose of insulin required. Systems security alerts are getting better, and the availability of sensors that promote CIIS devices has been a promising development. A closed-loop system should include an implantable continuous glucose sensor, an insulin pump and an algorithm control leading to insulin infusion adjusted to the glucose concentrations (Kumareswaran et al., 2009). In the future, combined use of insulin pumps and glucose sensors could become an effective and safe strategy, with minimal constraints in optimising metabolic control in diabetic patients to achieve glycaemia very close to normal (Hirsch, 2009; Keenan et al., 2010; Kowalski, 2009). Finally, we note that both CIIS therapy and the use of CGMS are expensive. The implementation of these technologies requires public health systems that have sufficient resources to initiate treatment and to ensure appropriate monitoring by the users. Further studies are needed on cost and effectiveness of these systems (Cummins et al., 2010; Fabiato et al., 2009; Huang et al., 2010).

6. Conclusions

Several prospective studies in Type 1 DM have demonstrated the tight association existing between glycaemia and the development of micro- and macro-angiopathy complications. The most significant study (the DCCT study) demonstrated that intensive treatment was accompanied by a reduction in the appearance and progression of the micro-vascular complications. Subsequent analyses of the DCCT study population demonstrated that the beneficial effects persisted even after the intervention and that they are extended to adverse cardiovascular events, as well. To achieve this objective, treatment of DM continues to be enriched by several novel therapeutic approaches. These have increased with the incorporation of insulin analogues and the introduction and optimisation of devices for the administration of insulin (continuous infusion system, CIIS) which achieves profiles of activity closer to the physiological equivalent. Several studies have demonstrated that the treatment with CIIS improves glycaemia variation with greater decrease in the HbA1c, less hypoglycaemias, and no increase in the frequency of ketoacidosis. Methods for evaluating response to treatment have been progressively improved. Recent clinical evidence has demonstrated that the glycaemia profile of the patients with DM, especially type 1 DM, is characterised by wide fluctuations related to physical activity, diet, and the specific treatment administered. The impact and the consequences of these variations are only partially known. Hence, the possibility of having continuous information available on glucose levels is an attractive option. Glucose sensors or CGMS provide maximum information on the changes in plasma glucose levels along the course of the day, and can be used in optimising treatment in patients with DM. However, the clinical applications of the CGMS have not, as yet, been well established.

7. Acknowledgments

This study was financed, in part, by grants from the Andalusia Department of Health (CTS-368). The authors declare that there is no conflict of interest that would prejudice the impartiality of this scientific work. Editorial assistance was by Peter R. Turner.

8. References

ADVANCE Collaborative Group; Patel, A., MacMahon, S., Chalmers, J., Neal, B., Billot, L., Woodward M., & Marre M. (2008). Intensive blood glucose control and vascular outcomes in patients with type 2 diabetes. *N Engl J Med*, Vol. 358, No. 24, (Jun. 2008), pp. 2560-2572, ISSN 0028-4793.

Alemzadeh, R., Lopnow, C., Parton, E., Kirby, & M. (2003). Glucose sensor evaluation of glycemic inestability in pediatric type 1 diabetes mellitus. *Diabetes Technol Ther*, Vol. 5, No. 2, (Jul. 2003), pp. 167-73. ISSN 1520-9156.

American Diabetes Association (2011). Standards of medical care in diabetes-2011. Diabetes Care, Vol. 34, Suppl. 1, (Jan. 2011), pp. S11-S61, ISSN 0149-5992.

Avignon, A., Radauceanu, A., & Monnier, L. (1997) Nonfasting plasma glucose is a better marker of diabetic control than fasting plasma glucose in type 2 diabetes. *Diabetes Care*, Vol. 20, (Dec. 1997) pp. 1822-1826, ISSN 0149-5992.

Baena, G., Carral, F., Roca, M., Cayón, M., Ortego, J., Escobar-Jiménez, L., Torres, I., Gavilán, I., Doménech, I., García, A., Coserria, C., López-Tinoco, C., & Aguilar-Diosdado, M. (2008). Can the metabolic control targets established for patients with type 1 diabetes be achieved in clinical practice? *Endocrino Nutr*, Vol. 55, No. 10, pp. 442-447, ISSN 1575-0922.

Bergenstal, R.M., & Gavin, J.R. (2005). The role of self-monitoring of blood glucose in the care of people with diabetes: report of a global consensus conference. *Am J Med*, Vol. 118, (Oct. 2005) pp. 1-6, ISSN 0002-9343.

Bergenstal, R.M., Tamborlane, W.V., Ahmann, A., Buse, J.B., Dailey, G., Davis, S.N., Joyce, C., Peoples, T., Perkins, B.A., Welsh, J.B., Willi, S.M., Wood, M.A. & STAR 3 Study Group (2010). Effectiveness of sensor-augmented insulin-pump therapy in type 1 diabetes. N Engl J Med, Vol. 363, No. 4, (Jul. 2010), pp. 311-320, ISSN 0028-4793.

Bode, B.W., Sabbad, H., & Davidson, P.C. (2001). What`s ahead in glucose monitoring? New techniques hold promise for improved ease and accuracy. *Postgrad Med*, Vol. 109, No. 4, (April 2001), pp. 41-9, ISSN 0032-5481.

Boland, E.A., Grey, M., Oesterle, A., Fredrickson, L. & Tamborlane, W.V. (1999). Continuous subcutaneous insulin infusion. A new way to lower risk of severe hypoglycaemia, improve metabolic control, and enhance coping in adolescents with type 1 diabetes. *Diabetes Care*, Vol. 22, No. 11, (Nov. 1999), pp. 1779-1784, ISSN 0149-5992.

Bruttomesso, D., Crazzolara, D., Maran, A., Costa, S., Dal Pos, M., Girelli, A., Lepore, G., Aragona, M., Iori, E., Valentini, U., Del Prato, S., Tiengo, A., Buhr, A., Trevisan, R., & Baritussio, A. (2008). In type 1 diabetic patients with good glycaemic control, blood glucose variability is lower during continuous subcutaneous insulin infusion than during multiple daily injections with insulin glargine. Diabet Med, Vol. 25, No. 3, (Mar. 2008), pp. 326-332, ISSN 0742-3071.

Bruttomesso, D., Costa, S. & Baritussio, A. (2009). Continuous subcutaneous insulin infusion (CSII) 30 years later: still the best option for insulin therapy. *Diabetes Metab Res Rev*, Vol. 25, No. 2, (Feb. 2009), pp. 99-111, ISSN 1520-7552.

Cavalot, F., Petrelli, A., Traversa, M., Bonomo, K., Fiora, E., Conti, M., Anfossi, G., Costa, G., & Trovati, M. (2006) Post-prandial blood glucose is a stronger predictor of cardiovascular events than fasting blood glucose in type 2 diabetes mellitus, particularly in women: lessons from the San Luigi Gonzaga Diabetes Study. *J Clin Endocrinol Metab*, Vol. 91, No. 3, (Dec. 2005) pp. 813-9, ISSN 0021-972X.

Ceriello, A., Taboga, C., Tonutti, L., Quagliaro, L., Piconi, L., Bais, B., Da Ros, R., & Motz, E. (2002). Evidence for an independent and cumulative effect of post-prandial hypertriglyceridemia and hyperglycemia on endothelial dysfunction and oxidative stress generation: effects of short- and long-term simvastatin treatment. *Circulation*, Vol. 106, No. 2, (Sept. 2002), pp. 1211- 1218, ISSN 0009-7322.

Ceriello, A. (2003). New insights on oxidative stress and diabetic complications may lead to a «causal» antioxidant therapy. *Diabetes Care*, Vol. 26, No. 5, pp. 1589-96, ISSN 0149-5992.

Ceriello, A. (2005). Post-prandial hyperglycemia and diabetes complications. Is it time to treat?. *Diabetes*, Vol. 54, No. 1, (Dec. 2004) pp. 1-7, ISSN 0012-1797.

Cooper, M., Glasziou, P., Grobbee, D., Hamet, P., Harrap, S., Heller, S., Liu, L., Mancia, G., Mogensen, CE., Pan, C., Poulter, N., Rodgers, A., Williams, B., Bompoint, S., de Galan, B.E., Joshi, R., & Travert, F. (2008). *Intensive Blood*, pp. 2560–2572, ISSN 1533-4406.

Cummins, E., Royle, P., Snaith, A., Greene, A., Robertson, L., McIntyre, L., & Waugh N. Clinical effectiveness and cost-effectiveness of continuous subcutaneous insulin infusion for diabetes: systematic review and economic evaluation. *Health Technol Assess*, Vol. 14, No. 11, (Feb. 2010), pp. 1-181, ISSN 1366-5278.

Danne, T., Battelino, T., Jarosz-Chobot, P., Kordonouri, O., Pánkowska, E., Ludvigsson, J., Schober, E., Kaprio, E., Saukkonen, T., Nicolino, M., Tubiana-Rufi, N., Klinkert, C., Haberland, H., Vazeou, A., Madacsy, L., Zangen, D., Cherubini, V., Rabbone, I., Toni, S., de Beaufort, C., Bakker-van Waarde, W., van den Berg, N., Volkov, I., Barrio, R., Hanas, R., Zumsteg, U., Kuhlmann, B., Aebi, C., Schumacher, U., Gschwend, S., Hindmarsh, P., Torres, M., Shehadeh, N., Phillip, M., & PedPump Study Group. (2008). Establishing glycaemic control with continuous subcutaneous insulin infusion in children and adolescents with type 1 diabetes: experience of the PedPump Study in 17 countries. *Diabetologia*, Vol. 51, No. 9, (Sept. 2008), pp. 1594-1601, ISSN 0012-186X

DCCT-EDIC. (2000). Retinopathy and nephropathy in patients with type 1 diabetes four years after a trial of intensive therapy. The Diabetes Control and Complications Trial/Epidemiology of Diabetes Interventions and Complications Research Group. *N Engl J Med*, Vol. 342, No. 6, (Feb. 2000), pp. 381–389, ISSN 0028-4793.

De Witt, D.E., & Hirsch, I.B. (2003). Outpatient insulin therapy in type 1 and type 2 diabetes mellitus: scientific review. *JAMA*, Vol. 289, No. 17, (May 2003), pp. 2254-2264, ISSN 0098-7484.

Deiss, D., Bolinder, J., Riveline, J.P., Battelino, T., Bosi, E., Tubiana-Rufi, N., Kerr, D. & Phillip, M. (2006). Improved glycemic control in poorly controlled patients with type 1 diabetes using real-time continuous glucose monitoring. Diabetes Care, Vol. 29, No. 12, (Dec. 2006), pp. 2730-2732, ISSN 0149-5992.

DeVries, J.H., Wentholt, I.M., Masurel, N., Mantel, I., Poscia, A., Maran, A., & Heine, R.J. (2004). Nocturnal hypoglycaemia in type 1 diabetes: consequences and assessment. *Diabetes Metab Res Rev*, Vol. 20, (Nov. 2004) pp. 43-6, ISSN 1520-7552.

Diabetes Control and Complications Trial Research Group. (1993). The effect of intensive treatment of diabetes on the development and progression of long-term complications in insulin-dependent diabetes mellitus. *N Engl J Med*, Vol. 329, No. 14 , (Sept. 1993), pp.977-986, ISSN 0028-4793.

Diabetes Control and Complications Trial Research Group. (1995). Implementation of treatment protocols in the Diabetes Control and Complications Trial. *Diabetes Care*, Vol. 18, No. 3, (Mar. 1995), pp. 361–376 ISSN 0149-5992

Diabetes Control and Complications Trial/Epidemiology of Diabetes Interventions and Complications (DCCT/EDIC) Research Group, Nathan, D.M., Zinman, B., Cleary, P.A., Backlund, J.Y., Genuth, S., Miller, R., & Orchard, T.J. (2009). Modern day clinical course of type 1 diabetes mellitus after 30 years' duration: the diabetes control and complications trial/epidemiology of diabetes interventions and complications and Pittsburgh epidemiology of diabetes complications experience (1983–2005). *Arch Intern Med*, Vol. 169, No. 14, (Jul. 2009), pp. 1307–1316, ISSN 0003-9926.

DiMeglio, L.A., Pottorff, T.M., Boyd, S.R., France, L., Fineberg, N., & Eugster E.A. (2004). A randomized, controlled study of insulin pump therapy in diabetic preschoolers. *J Pediatr*, Vol. 145, No. 3, (Sept. 2004), pp. 380-384, ISSN 0022-7476.

Duckworth, W., Abraira, C., Moritz, T., Reda, D., Emanuele, N., Reaven, P.D., Zieve, F.J., Marks, J., Davis, S.N., Hayward, R., Warren, S.R., Goldman, S., McCarren, M., Vitek, M.E., Henderson, W.G., Huang, G.D., & VADT Investigators. (2009). Glucose control and vascular complications in veterans with type 2 diabetes. *N Engl J Med*. Vol. 360, No. 2, (Jan. 2009), pp. 129–139, ISSN 0028-4793.

Edelman, S.V., & Bailey, T.S. (2009) Continuous glucose monitoring health outcomes. *Diabetes Technol Them*, Vol. 11, No. 1, (Jul. 2009), pp. 68-74, ISSN 1520-9156.

EQuality1 Study Group-Evaluation of quality of life and costs in diabetes type 1, Nicolucci, A., Maione, A., Franciosi, M., Amoretti, R., Busetto, E., Capani, F., Bruttomesso, D., Di Bartolo, P., Girelli, A., Leonetti, F., Morviducci, L., Ponzi, P., & Vitacolonna E. (2008). Quality of life and treatment satisfaction in adults with type 1 diabetes: a comparison between continuous subcutaneous insulin infusion and multiple daily injections. Diabet Med, Vol. 25, No. 2, (Feb. 2008), pp. 213-220, ISSN 0742-3071.

Ellison, J.M., Stegmann, J.M., Colner, S.L., Michael, R.H., Sharma, M.K., Ervin, K.R., & Horwithz, D.L. (2001). Rapid changes in post-prandial blood glucose produce concentration differences at finger, forearm, and thigh sampling sites. *Diabetes Care*, Vol. 25, No. 6, (May 2005) pp. 961-964, ISSN 0149-5992.

Esmatjes, E., Flores, L., Vidal, M., Rodriguez, L., Cortes, A., Almirall, L., Ricart, M.J., & Gomis, R. (2003). Hypoglycaemia after pancreas transplantation: usefulness of a continuous glucose monitoring system. *Clin Transplant*, Vol. 17, No. 6, (Feb. 2002) pp. 534-538, ISSN 0902-0063.

Fabiato, K., Buse, J., Duclos, M., Largay, J., Izlar, C., O'Connell, T., Stallings, J., & Dungan, K. (2009). Clinical experience with continuous glucose monitoring in adults. Diabetes Technol Ther, Vol. 11, Suppl. 1, (Jun. 2009), pp. S93-S103, ISSN 1520-9156.

Farmer, A., Wade, A., Goyder, E., Yudkin, P., French, D., Craven, A., Holman, R., Kinmonth, A.L., & Neil, A. (2007). Impact of self monitoring of blood glucose in the management of patients with non-insulin treated diabetes: open parallel group randomised trial. *BMJ*, Vol. 335, No. 7611, (Jun. 2007) pp. 1-8, ISSN 0959-535X.

Festin, M. (2008). Continuous glucose monitoring in women with diabetes during pregnancy. *BMJ*, Vol. 337, No. 1472, (Sept. 2008), pp. 1472, ISSN 0959-535X.

Fineberg, S.E., Bernstein, R.M., Laffel, L.M., & Schwartz, S.L. (2001). Use of an automated device for alternative site blood glucose monitoring. *Diabetes Care*, Vol. 24, No. 7, (Jul. 2001), pp. 1217-1220, ISSN 0149-5992.

Garg, S., Zisser, H., Schwartz, S., Bailey, T., Kaplan, R., Ellis, S., & Jovanovic, L. (2006). Improvement in glycemic excursions with a transcutaneous, real-time continuous glucose sensor: a randomized controlled trial. Diabetes Care, Vol. 29, No. 1, (Jan. 2006), pp. 44-50, ISSN 0149-5992

Garg, S.K. (2009). Role of continuous glucose monitoring in patients with diabetes using multiple daily insulin injections. *Infusystems International*. Vol. 8, No. 3, pp. 17-21.

Gerstl, E., Rabl, W., Rosenbauer, J., Grobe, H., Hofer, S., Krause, U., & Holl, R.W. (2008). Metabolic control as reflected by HbA1c in children, adolescents and young adults with type-1 diabetes mellitus: combined longitudinal analysis including 27035 patients from 207 centers in Germany and Austria during the last decade. *Eur J Pediatr*, Vol. 167, No. 4, (April 2008), pp. 447-453, ISSN 0340-6199.

Gilliam, L.K. & Hirsch, I.B. (2009). Practical aspects of real-time continuous glucose monitoring. Diabetes Technol Ther, Vol. 11, Suppl. 1, (Jun. 2009), pp. S75-S82, ISSN 1520-9156.

Goldstein, D.E., Lorenz, R.A., Malone, J.I., Nathan, D., & Peterson, C.M. (2004). Test of glycemia in diabetes. *Diabetes Care*, Vol. 27, Suppl. 1, (Jan. 2004), pp. 1761-1773, ISSN 0149-5992.

Gross, T.M., Einhorn, D., Kayne, D.M., Reed, J.H., White, N.H., & Mastrototaro, J.J. (2000). Performance evaluation of the MiniMed continuous glucose monitoring system during patient home use. *Diabetes Technol Ther*, Vol. 2, No. 1, (April 2001), pp. 49-56, ISSN 1520-9156.

Guerci, B., Tubiana-Rufi, N., Bauduceau, B., Bresson, R., Cuperlier, A., Delcroix,. C., Durain, D., Fermon, C., Le Floch, J.P., Le Devehat, C., Melki, V., Monnier, L., Mosnier-Pudar, H., Taboulet, P., & Hanaire-Broutin, H. (2005). Advantages to using capillary blood beta-hydroxybutyrate determination for the detection and treatment of diabetic ketosis. *Diabetes Metab*, Vol. 31, No. 4, Pt. 1, (Sept. 2005), pp. 401-406, ISSN 0742-3071.

Guilhem, I., Leguerrier, A.M., Lecordier, F., Poirier, J.Y., & Maugendre, D. (2006). Technical risks with subcutaneous insulin infusion. *Diabetes Metab*, Vol. 32, No. 3, (Jun. 2006), pp. 279-284, ISSN 0742-3071.

Diabetes Control and Complications Trial Research Group. (1999). Glucose tolerance and mortality: comparison of WHO and American DiabetesmAssociation diagnostic criteria. The DECODE study group. Collaborative analysis Of Diagnostic criteria in Europe. *Lancet*, Vol. 354, No. 9179, (Aug. 1999), pp. 617-21, ISSN 0140-6736.

Hanas, R. (2002). Selection for and initiation of continuous subcutaneous insulin infusion. Proceedings from a workshop. *Horm Res*, Vol. 57, Suppl. 1, (2002), pp. 101-104, ISSN 0301-0163.

Herman, W.H. (1999). Glycemic control in diabetes. *BMJ*, Vol. 319, No. 7202, (Jul. 1999), pp. 104-106, ISSN 0959-535X.

Hirsch, I.B. (2005). Insulin Analogues. *N Engl J Med*, Vol. 352, No. 2, (Jan. 2005), pp. 174-183, ISSN 0028-4793

Hirsch, I.B., Amstrong, D., Bergenstal, R.M., Buckingham, B., Childs, B.P., Clarke, W.L., Peters, A., & Wolpert H. (2008a). Clinical application of emerging sensor technologies in diabetes management: consensus guidelines for continuous glucose monitoring (CGM). *Diabetes Technol Ther*, Vol. 10, No. 4, (Aug. 2008), pp. 232-244, ISSN 1520-9156.

Hirsch, I.B., Abelseth, J., Bode, B.W., Fischer, J.S., Kaufman, F.R., Mastrototaro, J., Parkin, C.G., Wolpert, H.A., & Buckingham, B.A. (2008b). Sensor-augmented insulin pump therapy: results of the first randomized treat-to-target study. *Diabetes Technol Ther*, Vol. 10, No. 5, (Oct. 2008), pp. 377-383, ISSN 1520-9156.

Hirsch, I.B. (2009). Realistic expectations and practical use of continuous glucose monitoring for the endocrinologist. *J Clin Endocrinol Metab*, Vol. 94, No. 7, (Jul. 2009), pp. 2232-2238, ISSN 0021-972X.

Holman, R.R., Paul, S.K., Bethel, M.A., Matthews, D.R., & Neil, H.A. (2008). 10-year follow-up of intensive glucose control in type 2 diabetes. *N Engl J Med*, Vol. 359, No. 15, (Oct. 2008), pp. 1577– 1589, ISSN 0028-4793.

Home, P.D., & Marshall, S.M. (1984). Problems and safety of continuous subcutaneous insulin infusion. *Diabet Med*, Vol. 1, No. 1, (May 1984), pp. 41-44, ISSN 0742-3071.

Huang, E.S., O'Grady, M., Basu, A., Winn, A., John, P., Lee, J., Meltzer, D., Kollman, C., Laffel, L., Tamborlane, W., Weinzimer, S., Wysocki T., & Juvenile Diabetes Research Foundation Continuous Glucose Monitoring Study Group. (2010). The cost-effectiveness of continuous glucose monitoring in type 1 diabetes. Diabetes Care, Vol. 33, No. 6, (Jun. 2010), pp. 1269-1274, ISSN 0149-5992.

Ismail-Beigi, F., Craven, T., Banerji, M.A., Basile, J., Calles, J., Cohen, R.M., Cuddihy, R., Cushman, W.C., Genuth, S., Grimm, R.H. Jr., Hamilton, B.P., Hoogwerf, B., Karl, D., Katz, L., Krikorian, A., O'Connor, P., Pop-Busui, R., Schubart, U., Simmons, D., Taylor, H., Thomas, A., Weiss, D., Hramiak, I., & ACCORD trial group. (2010). Effect of intensive treatment of hyperglycaemia on micro-vascular outcomes in type 2 diabetes: an analysis of the ACCORD randomized trial. *Lancet*. Vol. 376, No. 9739, (Aug. 2010), pp. 419–430, ISSN 0140-6736.

Jeandidier, N., Riveline, J.P., Tubiana-Rufi, N., Vambergue, A., Catargi, B., Melki, V., Charpentier, G., & Guerci B. (2008). Treatment of diabetes mellitus using an external insulin pump in clinical practice. *Diabetes Metab*, Vol. 34, No. 4 ,Pt. 2, (Sept. 2008), pp. 425-438, ISSN 0742-3071.

Jeitler, K., Horvath, K., Berghold, A., Gratzer, T.W., Neeser, K., Pieber, T.R., & Siebenhofer, A. (2008). Continuous subcutaneous insulin infusion versus multiple daily insulin injections in patients with diabetes mellitus: systematic review and meta-analysis. *Diabetologia*, Vol. 51, No. 6, (Jun. 2008), pp. 941-951, ISSN 0012-186X

Juvenile Diabetes Research Foundation Continuous Glucose Monitoring Study Group, Tamborlane, W.V., Beck, R.W., Bode, B.W., Buckingham, B., Chase, H.P., Clemons, R., Fiallo-Scharer, R., Fox, L.A., Gilliam, L.K., Hirsch, I.B., Huang, E.S., Kollman, C., Kowalski, A.J., Laffel, L., Lawrence, J.M., Lee, J., Mauras, N., O'Grady, M., Ruedy, K.J., Tansey, M., Tsalikian, E., Weinzimer, S., Wilson, D.M., Wolpert, H., Wysocki, T., & Xing, D. (2008). Continuous glucose monitoring and intensive treatment of type 1 diabetes. *N Engl J Med*, Vol. 359, No. 14, (Oct. 2008), pp. 1464-1476, ISSN 0028-4793.

Juvenile Diabetes Research Foundation Continuous Glucose Monitoring Study Group, Beck, R.W., Buckingham, B., Miller, K., Wolpert, H., Xing, D., Block, J.M., Chase, H.P., Hirsch, I., Kollman, C., Laffel, L., Lawrence, J.M., Milaszewski, K., Ruedy, K.J., & Tamborlane, W.V. (2009a). Factors predictive of use and of benefit from continuous glucose monitoring in type 1 diabetes. *Diabetes Care*, Vol. 32, No. 11, (Nov. 2009), pp. 1947-1953, ISSN 0149-5992.

Juvenile Diabetes Research Foundation Continuous Glucose Monitoring Study Group, Bode, B., Beck, R.W., Xing, D., Gilliam, L., Hirsch, I., Kollman, C., Laffel, L., Ruedy, K.J., Tamborlane, W.V., Weinzimer, S., & Wolpert, H. (2009b). Sustained benefit of continuous glucose monitoring on A1C, glucose profiles, and hypoglycemia in adults with type 1 diabetes. Diabetes Care, Vol. 32, No. 11, (Nov. 2009), pp. 2047-2049, ISSN 0149-5992.

Katarina, E., Cederholm, J., Nilson, P., Gudbjornsdottir, S., & Eliasson, B. (2007). Glycemic and risk factor control in type 1 diabetes. Result from 13612 patients in a national diabetes register. *Diabetes Care*, Vol. 30, No. 3, (Mar. 2007), pp. 496-502, ISSN 0149-5992.

Keenan, D.B., Cartaya, R., & Mastrototaro, J.J. (2010). The pathway to the closed-loop artificial pancreas: research and commercial perspectives. *Pediatr Endocrinol Rev*, Vol. 7, Suppl. 3, (Aug. 2010), pp. 445-451, ISSN 1565-4753.

Klonoff, D.C. (2004). The need for separate performance goals for glucose sensors in the hypoglycemic, normomglycemic, and hyperglycaemic ranges. *Diabetes Care*, Vol. 27, No. 3, (Mar. 2004), pp. 834-836, ISSN 0149-5992.

Klonoff, D.C. (2005). Continuous glucose monitoring. Roadmap for 21st century diabetes therapy. *Diabetes Care*, Vol. 28, No. 5, (May 2008), pp. 1231-9, ISSN 0149-5992.

Kordonouri, O., Pankowska, E., Rami, B., Kapellen, T., Coutant, R., Hartmann, R., Lange, K., Knip, M., & Danne, T. (2010). Sensor-augmented pump therapy from the diagnosis of childhood type 1 diabetes: results of the Paediatric Onset Study (ONSET) after 12 months of treatment. Diabetologia, Vol. 53, No. 12, (Dec. 2010), pp. 2487-2495, ISSN 0012-186X.

Kowalski, A.J. (2009). Can we really close the loop and how soon? Accelerating the availability of an artificial pancreas: a roadmap to better diabetes outcomes. *Diabetes Technol Ther*, Vol. 11, Suppl. 1, (Jun. 2009), pp. S113-S119, ISSN 1520-9156.

Kovatchev, B., Anderson, S., Heinemann, L., & Clarke, W. (2008). Comparison of the numerical and clinical accuracy of four continuous glucose monitors. *Diabetes Care*, Vol. 31, No. 6, (Jun. 2008), pp. 1160-1164, ISSN 0149-5992.

Krzentowski, G., Scheen, A., Castillo, M., Luyckx, A.S., & Lefebvre, P.J. (1983). A 6-hour nocturnal interruption of a continuous subcutaneous insulin infusion. Metabolic and hormonal consequences and scheme for a prompt return to adequate control. *Diabetologia*, Vol. 24, No. 5, (May 1983), pp. 314-318, ISSN 0012-186X.

Kumareswaran, K., Evans, M.L., & Hovorka, R. (2009). Artificial pancreas: an emerging approach to treat type 1 diabetes. *Expert Rev Med Devices*, Vol. 6, No. 4, (Jul. 2009), pp. 401-410, ISSN 1743-4440.

Lapolla, A., Dalfrà, M.G., Masin, M., Bruttomesso, D., Piva, I., Crepaldi, C., Tortul, C., Dalla Barba, B., & Fedele, D. (2003). Analysis of outcome of pregnancy in type 1 diabetics treated with insulin pump or conventional insulin therapy. *Acta Diabetol*, Vol. 40, No. 3, (Sept. 2003), pp. 143-149, ISSN 0940-5429.

Leinung, M., Thompson, S., & Nardacci, E. (2010). Benefits of continuous glucose monitor use in clinical practice. *Endocr Pract*, Vol. 16, No. 3, (May-Jun. 2010), pp. 371-375, ISSN 1530-891X.

Lock, D.R., & Rigg, L.A. (1981). Hypoglycemic coma associated with subcutaneous insulin infusion by portable pump. *Diabetes Care*, Vol. 4, No. 3, (May-Jun. 1981), pp. 389-391, ISSN 0149-5992.

Malmberg, K., Ryden, L., Efendic, S., Herlitz, J., Nicol, P., Waldenstrom, A., Wedel, H., & Welin, L. (1995). Randomized trial of insulin-glucose infusion followed by subcutaneous insulin treatment in diabetic patients with acute myocardial infarction (DIGAMI study): effects of mortality at 1 year. *J Am Coll Cardiol*, Vol. 26, No. 1 (Jul. 1995), pp. 57-65, ISSN 0735-1097.

Manuel-y-Keenoy, B., Vertommen, J., Abrams, P., Van Gaal, L., De Leeuw, I., Messeri, D., & Poscia, A. (2004). Post-prandial glucose monitoring in type 1 diabetes mellitus: use of a continuous subcutaneous monitoring device. *Diabetes Metab Res Rev*, Vol. 20, Suppl. 2, (Dec. 2004), pp. S24-31, ISSN 1520-7552.

Maran, A., Crepaldi, C., Tiengo, A., Grassi, G., Vitali, E., Pagano, G., Bistoni, S., Calabrese, G., Santeusanio, F., Leonetti, F., Ribaudo, M., Di Mario, U., Annuzzi, G., Genovese, S., Riccardi, G., Previti, M., Cucinotta, D., Giorgino, F., Bellomo, A., Giorgino, R., Poscia, A., & Varalli, M. (2002). Continuous subcutaneous glucose monitoring in diabetic patients: a multicenter analysis. *Diabetes Care*, Vol. 25, No. 2, (Feb. 2002), pp. 347-52, ISSN 0149-5992.

Martin, C.L., Albers, J., Herman, W.H., Cleary, P., Waberski, B., Greene, D.A., Stevens, M.J., Feldman, E.L., & DCCT/EDIC Research Group. (2006). Neuropathy among the diabetes control and complications trial cohort 8 years after trial completion. *Diabetes Care*, Vol. 29, No. 2, (Feb. 2006), pp. 340–344, ISSN 0149-5992.

McGarraugh, G. (2009). The chemistry of commercial continuous glucose monitors. *Diabetes Technol Ther*, Vol. 11. Suppl. 1, (Jun. 2009), pp. 17-24, ISSN 1520-9156.

Mukhopadhyay, A., Farrell, T., Fraser, R.B., & Ola, B. (2007). Continuous subcutaneous insulin infusion vs intensive conventional insulin therapy in pregnant diabetic women: a systematic review and metaanalysis of randomized, controlled trials. *Am J Obstet Gynecol*, Vol. 197, No. 5, (Nov. 2007), pp. 447-456, ISSN 0002-9378.

Nathan, D.M., Cleary, P.A., Backlund, J.Y., Genuth, S.M., Lachin, J.M., Orchard, T.J., Raskin, P., Zinman, B., & Diabetes Control and Complications Trial/Epidemiology of Diabetes Interventions and Complications (DCCT/EDIC) Study Research Group. (2005). Intensive diabetes treatment and cardiovascular disease in patients with type 1 diabetes. N Engl J Med, Vol. 353, No. 25, (Dec. 2005), pp. 2643-2653, ISSN 0028-4793

O'Connell, M.A., Donath, S., O'Neal, D.N., Colman, P.G., Ambler, G.R., Jones, T.W., Davis, E.A., & Cameron, F.J. (2009). Glycaemic impact of patient-led use of sensor-guided pump therapy in type 1 diabetes: a randomised controlled trial. *Diabetologia*, Vol. 52, No. 7, (Jul. 2009), pp. 1250-1257, ISSN 0012-186X

Ohkubo, Y., Kishikawa, H., Araki, E., Miyata, T., Isami, S., Motoyoshi, S., Kojima, Y., Furuyoshi, N., & Shichiri, M. (1995). Intensive insulin therapy prevents the progression of diabetic micro-vascular complications in Japanese patients with non-insulin dependent diabetes mellitus: a randomized prospective 6-year study. *Diabetes Res Clin Pract*, Vol. 28, No. 2, (May 1995), pp. 103-17, ISSN 0168-8227.

Pańkowska, E., Błazik, M., Dziechciarz, P., Szypowska, A., & Szajewska, H. (2009). Continuous subcutaneous insulin infusion vs. multiple daily injections in children with type 1 diabetes: a systematic review and meta-analysis of randomized control trials. Pediatr Diabetes, Vol. 10, No. 1, (Feb. 2009), pp. 52-58, ISSN 1399-543X.

Pickup, J.C., Kidd, J., Burmiston, S., & Yemane, N. (2006). Determinants of glycaemic control in type 1 diabetes during intensified therapy with multiple daily insulin injections or continuous subcutaneous insulin infusion: importance of blood glucose variability. *Diabetes Metab Res Rev*, Vol. 22, No. 3, (May-Jun. 2006), pp. 232-237, ISSN 1520-7552.

Pickup, J.C., & Sutton, A.J. (2008). Severe hypoglycaemia and glycaemic control in type 1 diabetes: meta-analysis of multiple daily insulin injections compared with continuous subcutaneous insulin infusion. *Diabet Med*, Vol. 25, No. 7, (Jul. 2008), pp. 765-774, ISSN 0742-3071.

Plank, J., Siebenhofer, A., Berghold, A., Jeitler, K., Horvath, K., Mrak, P., & Pieber, T.R. (2005). Systematic review and meta-analysis of short-acting insulin analogues in patients with diabetes mellitus. *Arch Intern Med*, Vol. 165, No.12. (Jun. 2005), pp. 1337-1344, ISSN 0003-9926.

Porcellati, F., Rossetti, P., Busciantella, N.R., Marzotti, S., Lucidi, P., Luzio, S., Owens, D,R., Bolli, G.B., & Fanelli, C.G. (2007). Comparison of pharmacokinetics and dynamics of the long-acting insulin analogs glargine and detemir at steady state in type 1 diabetes: a double-blind, randomized, crossover study. *Diabetes Care*, Vol. 30, No.10 (Oct. 2007) pp. 2447-52. ISSN 0149-5992

Poscia, A., Mascini, M., Moscone, D., Luzzana, M., Caramenti, G., Cremonesi, P., Valgimigli, F., Bongiovanni, C., & Varalli, M. (2003). A microdialysis technique for continuous subcutaneous glucose monitoring in diabetic patients (part 1). *Biosens Bioelectron*, Vol. 18, No. 7, (Jul. 2003), pp. 891-898, ISSN 0956-5663.

Raccah, D., Sulmont, V., Reznik, Y., Guerci, B., Renard, E., Hanaire, H., Jeandidier, N., & Nicolino, M. (2009). Incremental value of continuous glucose monitoring when starting pump therapy in patients with poorly controlled type 1 diabetes: the RealTrend study. *Diabetes Care*, Vol. 32, No. 12, (Dec. 2009), pp. 2245-2250, ISSN 0149-5992.

Radermecker, R.P., & Scheen, A.J. (2004). Continuous subcutaneous insulin infusion with short-acting insulin analogues or human regular insulin: efficacy, safety, quality of life, and cost-effectiveness. *Diabetes Metab Res Rev*, Vol. 20, No. 3 , (May-Jun. 2004), pp. 178-188, ISSN 1520-7552.

Schaepelynck-Bélicar, P., Simonin, G., & Lassmann-Vague, V. (2003). Improved metabolic control in diabetic adolescents using the continuous glucose monitoring system. *Diabetes Metab*, Vol. 29, No. 6, (Dec. 2003), pp. 608-612, ISSN 0742-3071.

Selvin, E., Marinopoulos, S., Berkenblit, G., Rami, T., Brancati, F.L., Powe, N.R., & Golden, S.H. (2004). Meta-analysis: glycosylated hemoglobin and cardiovascular disease in diabetes mellitus. *Ann Intern Med*, Vol. 141, No. 6, (Sept. 2004), pp. 421–431, ISSN 0003-4819.

Shalitin, S., Gil, M., Nimri, R., de Vries, L., Gavan, M.Y., & Phillip, M. (2010). Predictors of glycaemic control in patients with Type 1 diabetes commencing continuous subcutaneous insulin infusion therapy. *Diabet Med*, Vol. 27, No. 3, (Mar. 2010), pp. 339-347, ISSN 0742-3071.

Shichiri, M., Kishikawa, H., Ohkubo, Y., & Wake, N. (2000). Long-terms results of de Kumamoto Study on Optimal Diabetes Control in Type 2 Diabetic Patients. *Diabetes Care*, Vol. 23, Suppl. 2, (April 2000), pp. B21-B29, ISSN 0149-5992

Simon, J., Gray, A., Clarke, P., Wade, A., Neil, A., Farmer, A., & Diabetes Glycaemic Education and Monitoring Trial Group. (2008). Cost effectiveness of self monitoring of blood glucose in patients with non-insulin treated type 2 diabetes: economic evaluation of data from the DiGEM trial. *BMJ*, Vol. 336, No. 7654, (May 2008), pp. 1177-1180, ISSN 0959-535X.

Singh, S.R., Ahmad, F., LaI, A., Yu, C., Bai, Z., & Bennett, H.C. (2009). Efficacy and safety of insulin analogues for the management of diabetes mellitus: a meta-analysis. CMAJ Vol. 17, No. 4, (Feb. 2009), pp. 385-97, ISSN 1488-2329.

Skyler, J.S. (2009). Continuous glucose monitoring: An overview of its development. *Diabetes Technol Ther*, Vol. 11, Suppl. 1, (Jun. 2009), pp. 5-10, ISSN 1557-8593.

Stettler, C., Allemann, S., Jüni, P., Cull, C.A., Holman, R.R., Egger, M., Krähenbühl. S., & Diem, P. (2006). Glycemic control and macrovascular disease in types 1 and 2 diabetes mellitus: Meta-analysis of randomized trials. *Am Heart J*, Vol. 152, No. 1, (Jul. 2006), pp. 27–38, ISSN 0002-8703.

Tamborlane, W.V., Fredrickson, L.P., & Ahern, J.H. (2003). Insulin pump therapy in childhood diabetes mellitus: guidelines for use. *Treat Endocrinol*, Vol. 2, No. 1, (Jan. 2003), pp. 11-21, ISSN 1175-6349.

Tanenberg, R., Bode, B., Lane, W., Levetan, C., Mestman, J., Harmel, A.P., Tobian, J., Gross, T., & Mastrototaro, J. (2004). Use of the continuous glucose monitoring system to guide therapy in patients with insulin-treated diabetes: a randomized controlled trial. *Mayo Clin Proc*, Vol. 79, No. 12, (Dec. 2004), pp. 1521-6, ISSN 0025-6196.

Teutsch, S.M., Herman, W.H., Dwyer, D.M., & Lane, J.M. (1984). Mortality among diabetic patients using continuous insulin-infusion pumps. *N Eng J Med*, Vol. 310, No. 6, (Feb. 1984), pp. 361-368, ISSN 0028-4793.

Torres, I., Ortego, J., Valencia, I., García-Palacios, M.V., & Aguilar-Diosdado, M. (2009). Benefits of continuous subcutaneous insulin infusion in type 1 diabetes previously treated with multiple daily injections with once-daily glargine and pre-meal analogues. *Exp Clin Endocrinol Diabetes*, Vol. 117, No. 8, (Sept. 2009), pp. 378-385, ISSN 0947-7349.

Torres, I., Baena, M.G., Cayon, M., Ortego-Rojo, J., & Aguilar-Diosdado, M. (2010). Use of sensors in the treatment and follow-up of patients with diabetes mellitus. *Sensors*, Vol. 10, No. 8, (Aug. 2010), pp. 7404-7420, ISSN 1424-8220.

U.K. Prospective Diabetes Study (UKPDS) Group. (1998). Intensive blood glucose control with sulphonylureas or insulin compared with conventional treatment and risk of complications in patients with type 2 diabetes. *Lancet*, Vol. 352, No. 9131, (Sept. 1998), pp. 837-853, ISSN 0140-6736.

Varalli, M., Marelli, G., Maran, A., Bistoni, S., Luzzana, M., Cremonesi, P., Caramenti, G., Valgimigli, F., & Poscia, A. (2003). A microdialysis technique for continuous subcutaneous glucose monitoring in diabetic patients (part 2). *Biosens Bioelectron*, Vol. 18, No. 7, (Jul. 2003), pp. 899-905, ISSN 0956-5663.

Valeri, C., Pozsilli, P., & Leslie, D. (2004). Glucose control in diabetes. *Diabetes Metab Res Rev*, Vol. 20, Suppl. 2 (Nov-Dec. 2004), pp. S1-8, ISSN 1520-7552.

Volpe, L., Pancani, F., Aragona, M., Lencioni, C., Battini, L., Ghio, A., Resi, V., Bertolotto, A., Del Prato, S., & Di Cianni, G. (2010). Continuous subcutaneous insulin infusion and multiple dose insulin injections in Type 1 diabetic pregnant women: a case-control study. *Gynecol Endocrinol*, Vol. 26, No. 3, (Mar. 2010), pp. 193-196, ISSN 0951-3590.

Weintrob, N., Schechter, A., Benzaquen, H., Shalitin, S., Lilos, P., Galatzer, A., & Phillip, M. (2004). Glycemic patterns detected by continuous subcutaneous glucose sensing in children and adolescents with type 1 diabetes mellitus treated by multiple daily injections vs continuous subcutaneous insulin infusion. *Arch Pediatr Adolesc Med*, Vol. 158, No. 7, (Jul. 2004), pp. 677-84, ISSN 1072-4710.

Welschen, L.M., Nijpels, G., Dekker, J.M., Heine, R.J., Stalman, W.A., & Bouter, L.M. (2005). Self-monitoring of blood glucose in patients with type 2 diabetes who are not using insulin: a systematic review. *Diabetes Care*, Vol. 28, No. 6, (Jun. 2005), pp. 1510-1517, ISSN 0149-5992.

Permissions

The contributors of this book come from diverse backgrounds, making this book a truly international effort. This book will bring forth new frontiers with its revolutionizing research information and detailed analysis of the nascent developments around the world.

We would like to thank Gianluca Aimaretti, Paolo Marzullo and Flavia Prodam, for lending their expertise to make the book truly unique. They have played a crucial role in the development of this book. Without their invaluable contribution this book wouldn't have been possible. They have made vital efforts to compile up to date information on the varied aspects of this subject to make this book a valuable addition to the collection of many professionals and students.

This book was conceptualized with the vision of imparting up-to-date information and advanced data in this field. To ensure the same, a matchless editorial board was set up. Every individual on the board went through rigorous rounds of assessment to prove their worth. After which they invested a large part of their time researching and compiling the most relevant data for our readers. Conferences and sessions were held from time to time between the editorial board and the contributing authors to present the data in the most comprehensible form. The editorial team has worked tirelessly to provide valuable and valid information to help people across the globe.

Every chapter published in this book has been scrutinized by our experts. Their significance has been extensively debated. The topics covered herein carry significant findings which will fuel the growth of the discipline. They may even be implemented as practical applications or may be referred to as a beginning point for another development. Chapters in this book were first published by InTech; hereby published with permission under the Creative Commons Attribution License or equivalent.

The editorial board has been involved in producing this book since its inception. They have spent rigorous hours researching and exploring the diverse topics which have resulted in the successful publishing of this book. They have passed on their knowledge of decades through this book. To expedite this challenging task, the publisher supported the team at every step. A small team of assistant editors was also appointed to further simplify the editing procedure and attain best results for the readers.

Our editorial team has been hand-picked from every corner of the world. Their multi-ethnicity adds dynamic inputs to the discussions which result in innovative outcomes. These outcomes are then further discussed with the researchers and contributors who give their valuable feedback and opinion regarding the same. The feedback is then collaborated with the researches and they are edited in a comprehensive manner to aid the understanding of the subject.

Apart from the editorial board, the designing team has also invested a significant amount of their time in understanding the subject and creating the most relevant covers. They scrutinized every image to scout for the most suitable representation of the subject and create an appropriate cover for the book.

The publishing team has been involved in this book since its early stages. They were actively engaged in every process, be it collecting the data, connecting with the contributors or procuring relevant information. The team has been an ardent support to the editorial, designing and production team. Their endless efforts to recruit the best for this project, has resulted in the accomplishment of this book. They are a veteran in the field of academics and their pool of knowledge is as vast as their experience in printing. Their expertise and guidance has proved useful at every step. Their uncompromising quality standards have made this book an exceptional effort. Their encouragement from time to time has been an inspiration for everyone.

The publisher and the editorial board hope that this book will prove to be a valuable piece of knowledge for researchers, students, practitioners and scholars across the globe.

List of Contributors

Ichiro Sakata and Takafumi Sakai
Saitama University, Japan

Francisca Lago
SERGAS Santiago University Clinical Hospital, Research Laboratory 7 (Molecular and Cellular Cardiology), Santiago de Compostela, Spain

Rodolfo Gómez, Javier Conde, Morena Scotece and Oreste Gualillo
SERGAS Santiago University Clinical Hospital, Research Laboratory 9 (NEIRID LAB, Laboratory of Neuro Endocrine Interactions in Rheumatology and Inflammatory Diseases), Santiago de Compostela, Spain

Carlos Dieguez
University of Santiago de Compostela, Department of Physiology, Santiago de Compostela, Spain

Malin Hedengran Faulds and Karin Dahlman-Wright
Karolinska Institutet, Sweden

Carmen Sanz, Isabel Roncero, Elvira Alvarez, Verónica Hurtado and Enrique Blázquez
University Complutense of Madrid, Medical School and CIBERDEM, Department of Cellular Biology and Department of Biochemistry and Molecular Biology, Spain

Guangzhong Wang, Caiyun Sun, Haoran Lin and Wensheng Li
State Key Laboratory of Biocontrol, Institute of Aquatic Economic Animals and Guangdong Provincial Key Laboratory for Aquatic Economic Animals, School of Life Sciences, Sun Yat-Sen University, Guangzhou,
P. R. China

Takahiro Yoshikawa
Department of Sports Medicine, Osaka City University Graduate School of Medicine, Osaka, Japan

Ana Gordon, José C. Garrido-Gracia, Rafaela Aguilar, Carmina Bellido, Juana Martín de las Mulas and José E. Sánchez-Criado
University of Córdoba, Spain

Colin G. Scanes
University of Wisconsin Milwaukee, USA

Guo Cai Huang and Min Zhao
Department of Diabetes and Endocrinology, King's College London School of Medicine, London, Great Britain

María Gloria Baena-Nieto, Cristina López-Tinoco, Jose Ortego-Rojo and Manuel Aguilar-Diosdado
Endocrinology & Nutrition Service, Puerta del Mar Hospital, Cadiz, Spain

Printed in the USA
CPSIA information can be obtained
at www.ICGtesting.com
JSHW011401221024
72173JS00003B/370